D0767826

DEATH AND DYING
END-OF-LIFE CONTROVERSIES

ISSN 1532-2726

DEATH AND DYING
END-OF-LIFE CONTROVERSIES

Sandra M. Alters

INFORMATION PLUS® REFERENCE SERIES
Formerly Published by Information Plus, Wylie, Texas

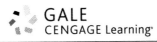
GALE
CENGAGE Learning·

Detroit • New York • San Francisco • New Haven, Conn • Waterville, Maine • London

Death and Dying: End-of-Life Controversies

Sandra M. Alters

Kepos Media, Inc.: Paula Kepos and Janice Jorgensen, Series Editors

Project Editors: Kimberley McGrath, Kathleen J. Edgar, Elizabeth Manar

Rights Acquisition and Management: Margaret Chamberlain-Gaston, Kimberly Potvin

Composition: Evi Abou-El-Seoud, Mary Beth Trimper

Manufacturing: Cynde Lentz

For product information and technology assistance, contact us at **Gale Customer Support, 1-800-877-4253.**
For permission to use material from this text or product, submit all requests online at **www.cengage.com/permissions.**
Further permissions questions can be e-mailed to **permissionrequest@cengage.com**

Cover photograph: © Natalia Bratslavsky/Shutterstock.com.

Gale
27500 Drake Rd.
Farmington Hills, MI 48331-3535

ISBN-13: 978-0-7876-5103-9 (set)
ISBN-13: 978-1-4144-8135-7

ISBN-10: 0-7876-5103-6 (set)
ISBN-10: 1-4144-8135-7

ISSN 1532-2726

This title is also available as an e-book.
ISBN-13: 978-1-4144-9726-6 (set)
ISBN-10: 1-4144-9726-1 (set)
Contact your Gale sales representative for ordering information.

Printed in the United States of America
1 2 3 4 5   16 15 14 13 12

FD289

TABLE OF CONTENTS

PREFACE

Death and Dying: End-of-Life Controversies is part of the *Information Plus Reference Series*. The purpose of each volume of the series is to present the latest facts on a topic of pressing concern in modern American life. These topics include the most controversial and studied social issues of the 21st century: abortion, capital punishment, care for the elderly, crime, health care, the environment, immigration, minorities, social welfare, women, youth, and many more. Even though this series is written especially for high school and undergraduate students, it is an excellent resource for anyone in need of factual information on current affairs.

By presenting the facts, it is the intention of Gale, Cengage Learning to provide its readers with everything they need to reach an informed opinion on current issues. To that end, there is a particular emphasis in this series on the presentation of scientific studies, surveys, and statistics. These data are generally presented in the form of tables, charts, and other graphics placed within the text of each book. Every graphic is directly referred to and carefully explained in the text. The source of each graphic is presented within the graphic itself. The data used in these graphics are drawn from the most reputable and reliable sources, such as from the various branches of the U.S. government and from private organizations and associations. Every effort has been made to secure the most recent information available. Readers should bear in mind that many major studies take years to conduct and that additional years often pass before the data from these studies are made available to the public. Therefore, in many cases the most recent information available in 2012 is dated from 2009 or 2010. Older statistics are sometimes presented as well, if they are landmark studies or of particular interest and no more-recent information exists.

Even though statistics are a major focus of the *Information Plus Reference Series*, they are by no means its only content. Each book also presents the widely held positions and important ideas that shape how the book's subject is discussed in the United States. These positions are explained in detail and, where possible, in the words of their proponents. Some of the other material to be found in these books includes historical background, descriptions of major events related to the subject, relevant laws and court cases, and examples of how these issues play out in American life. Some books also feature primary documents or have pro and con debate sections that provide the words and opinions of prominent Americans on both sides of a controversial topic. All material is presented in an evenhanded and unbiased manner; readers will never be encouraged to accept one view of an issue over another.

HOW TO USE THIS BOOK

Death is one of the universal human experiences. This and its ultimately unknowable nature combine to make it a topic of great interest to most Americans. How we die and how we deal with the deaths of others evokes profound religious or ethical issues, or both, about which many people hold strong beliefs. When these beliefs are in conflict with those of others, this can result in some of the most serious and divisive controversies in the United States. This book examines how Americans deal with death, with a particular focus on the highly charged political and moral issues of living wills, life-sustaining treatments, end-of-life care funding, and physician-assisted suicide.

Death and Dying: End-of-Life Controversies consists of 11 chapters and three appendixes. Each chapter is devoted to a particular aspect of death and dying in the United States. For a summary of the information that is covered in each chapter, please see the synopses that are provided in the Table of Contents. Chapters generally begin with an overview of the basic facts and background information on the chapter's topic, then proceed to examine subtopics of particular interest. For example, Chapter 4: The End of Life: Medical Considerations first addresses trends in the causes of death. The chapter then focuses on life-sustaining treatments, including cardio-pulmonary resuscitation, mechanical ventilation, artificial nutrition and hydration, and kidney dialysis. Disorders of consciousness—persistent vegetative state/unresponsive wakefulness syndrome, the minimally conscious state, and locked-in syndrome—are then investigated along with ways to manage these conditions. The chapter ends with a discussion of organ donation and transplantation. Readers can find their way through a chapter by looking for the section and subsection headings, which are clearly set off from the text. They can also refer to the book's extensive Index if they already know what they are looking for.

Statistical Information

The tables and figures featured throughout *Death and Dying: End-of-Life Controversies* will be of particular use to readers in learning about this issue. These tables and figures represent an extensive collection of the most recent and important statistics on death, as well as related issues—for example, graphics cover the death rates for the 15 leading causes of death, the percentage of high school students who attempted suicide and whose suicide attempt required medical attention, Medicare enrollees and expenditures by Medicare program and type of serv-ice, the advance health care directive, and public opinion on the moral acceptability of doctor-assisted suicide. Gale, Cengage Learning believes that making this infor-mation available to readers is the most important way to fulfill the goal of this book: to help readers understand the issues and controversies surrounding death and dying in the United States and reach their own conclusions.

Each table or figure has a unique identifier appearing above it, for ease of identification and reference. Titles for the tables and figures explain their purpose. At the end of each table or figure, the original source of the data is provided.

To help readers understand these often complicated statistics, all tables and figures are explained in the text. References in the text direct readers to the relevant sta-tistics. Furthermore, the contents of all tables and figures are fully indexed. Please see the opening section of the Index at the back of this volume for a description of how to find tables and figures within it.

Appendixes

Besides the main body text and images, *Death and Dying: End-of-Life Controversies* has three appendixes.

The first is the Important Names and Addresses directory. Here, readers will find contact information for a number of government and private organizations that can provide further information on aspects of death and dying. The second appendix is the Resources section, which can also assist readers in conducting their own research. In this section, the author and editors of *Death and Dying: End-of-Life Controversies* describe some of the sources that were most useful during the compilation of this book. The final appendix is the detailed Index. It has been greatly expanded from previous editions and should make it even easier to find specific topics in this book.

ADVISORY BOARD CONTRIBUTIONS

The staff of Information Plus would like to extend its heartfelt appreciation to the Information Plus Advisory Board. This dedicated group of media professionals pro-vides feedback on the series on an ongoing basis. Their comments allow the editorial staff who work on the project to continually make the series better and more user-friendly. The staff's top priority is to produce the highest-quality and most useful books possible, and the Information Plus Advisory Board's contributions to this process are invaluable.

The members of the Information Plus Advisory Board are:

- Kathleen R. Bonn, Librarian, Newbury Park High School, Newbury Park, California
- Madelyn Garner, Librarian, San Jacinto College, North Campus, Houston, Texas
- Anne Oxenrider, Media Specialist, Dundee High School, Dundee, Michigan
- Charles R. Rodgers, Director of Libraries, Pasco-Hernando Community College, Dade City, Florida
- James N. Zitzelsberger, Library Media Department Chairman, Oshkosh West High School, Oshkosh, Wisconsin

COMMENTS AND SUGGESTIONS

The editors of the *Information Plus Reference Series* welcome your feedback on *Death and Dying: End-of-Life Controversies*. Please direct all correspondence to:

Editors
Information Plus Reference Series
27500 Drake Rd.
Farmington Hills, MI 48331-3535

CHAPTER 1
DEATH THROUGH THE AGES: A BRIEF OVERVIEW

Strange, is it not? That of the myriads who Before us pass'd the door of Darkness through, Not one returns to tell us of the Road, Which to discover we must travel too.

—Omar Khayyám, *Rubáiyát of Omar Khayyám*

Death is the inevitable conclusion of life, a universal destiny that all living creatures share. Even though all societies throughout history have realized that death is the certain fate of human beings, different cultures have responded to it in different ways. Through the ages, attitudes toward death and dying have changed and continue to change, shaped by religious, intellectual, and philosophical beliefs and conceptions. In the 21st century advances in medical science and technology continue to influence ideas about death and dying.

ANCIENT TIMES

Archaeologists have found that as early as the Paleolithic period, about 2.5 million to 3 million years ago, humans held metaphysical beliefs about death and dying—those beyond what humans can know with their senses. Tools and ornaments excavated at burial sites suggest that the earliest ancestors believed that some element of a person survived the dying experience.

The ancient Hebrews (c. 1020–586 BC), while acknowledging the existence of the soul, were not preoccupied with the afterlife. They lived according to the commandments of their God, to whom they entrusted their eternal destiny. By contrast, the early Egyptians (c. 2900–950 BC) thought that the preservation of the dead body (mummification) guaranteed a happy afterlife. They believed a person had a dual soul: the *ka* and the *ba*. The *ka* was the spirit that dwelled near the body, whereas the *ba* was the vitalizing soul that lived on in the netherworld (the world of the dead). Similarly, the ancient Chinese (c. 2500–1000 BC) also believed in a dual soul, one part of which continued to exist after the death of the body. It was this spirit that the living venerated during ancestor worship.

Among the ancient Greeks (c. 2600–1200 BC), death was greatly feared. Greek mythology—which was full of tales of gods and goddesses who exacted punishment on disobedient humans—caused the living to follow rituals meticulously when burying their dead so as not to displease the gods. Even though reincarnation is usually associated with Asian religions, some Greeks were followers of Orphism, a religion that taught that the soul underwent many reincarnations until purification was achieved.

THE CLASSICAL AGE

Mythological beliefs among the ancient Greeks persisted into the classical age. The Greeks believed that after death the psyche (a person's vital essence) lived on in the underworld. The Greek writer Homer (c. eighth century–c. seventh century BC) greatly influenced classical Greek attitudes about death through his epic poems the *Iliad* and the *Odyssey*. Greek mythology was freely interpreted by writers after Homer, and belief in eternal judgment and retribution continued to evolve throughout this period.

Certain Greek philosophers also influenced conceptions of death. For example, Pythagoras of Samos (c. 570–c. 490 BC) opposed euthanasia ("good death" or mercy killing) because it might disturb the soul's journey toward final purification as planned by the gods. On the contrary, Socrates (469–399 BC) and Plato (428–347 BC) believed people could choose to end their life if they were no longer useful to themselves or the state.

Like Socrates and Plato, the classical Romans (c. 509–264 BC) believed a person suffering from intolerable pain or an incurable illness should have the right to choose a "good death." They considered euthanasia a "mode of dying" that allowed a person to take control of an intolerable situation and distinguished it from suicide, an act considered to be a shirking of responsibilities to one's family and to humankind.

THE MIDDLE AGES

During the European Middle Ages (500–1485) death—with its accompanying agonies—was accepted as a destiny everyone shared, but it was still feared. As a defense against this phenomenon that could not be explained, medieval people confronted death together, as a community. Because medical practices during this era were crude and imprecise, the ill and dying person often endured prolonged suffering. However, a long period of dying gave the dying individual an opportunity to feel forewarned about impending death, to put his or her affairs in order, and to confess his or her sins. The medieval Roman Catholic Church, with its emphasis on the eternal life of the soul in heaven or hell, held great power over people's notions of death.

By the late Middle Ages the fear of death had intensified due to the Black Death—the great plague of 1347 to 1351. The Black Death killed more than 25 million people in Europe alone. Commoners not only watched their neighbors stricken but also saw church officials and royalty struck down: Queen Eleanor of Aragon and King Alfonso XI (1311–1350) of Castile met with untimely deaths, as did many at the papal court in Avignon, France. With their perceived "proper order" of existence shaken, the common people became increasingly preoccupied with their own death and with the Last Judgment, God's final and certain determination of the character of each individual. Because the Last Judgment was closely linked to an individual's disposition to heaven or hell, the event of the plague and such widespread death was frightening.

THE RENAISSANCE

From the 14th through the 16th centuries Europe experienced new directions in economics, the arts, and social, scientific, and political thought. Nonetheless, the obsession with death did not diminish with this "rebirth" of Western culture. A new self-awareness and emphasis on humans as the center of the universe further fueled the fear of dying.

By the 16th century many European Christians were rebelling against religion and stopped relying on church, family, and friends to help ease their passage to the next life. The religious upheaval of the Protestant Reformation of 1520, which emphasized the individual nature of salvation, caused further uncertainties about death and dying.

The 17th century marked a shift from a religious to a more scientific exploration of death and dying. Lay people drifted away from the now disunited Christian church toward the medical profession, seeking answers in particular to the question of "apparent death," a condition in which people appeared to be dead but were not. In many cases unconscious patients mistakenly believed to be dead were hurriedly prepared for burial by the clergy, only to "come back to life" during burial or while being transported to the cemetery.

An understanding of death and its aftermath was clearly still elusive, even to physicians who disagreed about what happened after death. Some physicians believed the body retained some kind of "sensibility" after death. Thus, many people preserved cadavers so that the bodies could "live on." Alternatively, some physicians applied the teachings of the Catholic Church to their medical practice and believed that once the body was dead, the soul proceeded to its eternal fate and the body could no longer survive. These physicians did not preserve cadavers and pronounced them permanently dead.

THE 18TH CENTURY

The fear of apparent death that took root during the 17th century resurfaced with great intensity during the 18th century. Coffins were built with contraptions that enabled any prematurely buried person to survive and communicate from the grave. (See Figure 1.1.)

For the first time, the Christian church was blamed for hastily burying its "living dead," particularly because

FIGURE 1.1

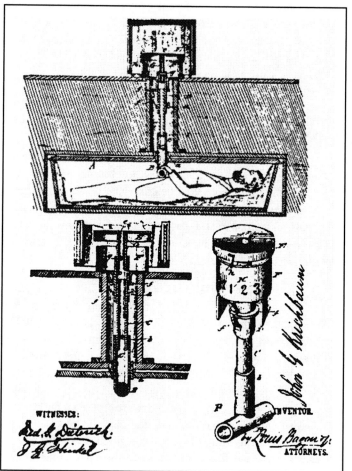

Device for indicating life in buried persons, 1882.

it had encouraged the abandonment of pagan burial traditions such as protracted mourning rituals. In the wake of apparent death incidents, more long burial traditions were revived.

THE 19TH CENTURY

Premature and lingering deaths remained commonplace during the 19th century. Death typically took place in the home following a long deathbed watch. Family members prepared the corpse for viewing in the home, not in a funeral parlor. However, this practice changed during the late 19th century, when professional undertakers took over the job of preparing and burying the dead. They provided services such as readying the corpse for viewing and burial, building the coffin, digging the grave, and directing the funeral procession. Professional embalming and cosmetic restoration of bodies became widely available, all carried out in a funeral parlor where bodies were then viewed instead of in the home.

Cemeteries changed as well. Before the early 19th century, American cemeteries were unsanitary, overcrowded, and weed-filled places that bore an odor of decay. That began to change in 1831, when the Massachusetts Horticultural Society purchased 72 acres (29 ha) of fields, ponds, trees, and gardens in Cambridge and built Mount Auburn Cemetery. This cemetery became a model for the landscaped garden cemetery in the United States. These cemeteries were tranquil places where those grieving could visit the graves of loved ones and find comfort in the beautiful surroundings.

Literature of the time often focused on and romanticized death. Death poetry, consoling essays, and mourning manuals became available after 1830, which comforted the grieving with the concept that the deceased were released from worldly cares in heaven and that they would be reunited there with other deceased loved ones. The deadly lung disease tuberculosis—called consumption at the time—was pervasive during the 19th century in Europe and the United States. The disease caused sufferers to develop a certain appearance—an extreme pallor and thinness, with a look often described as haunted—that actually became a kind of fashion statement. The fixation on the subject by writers such as Edgar Allan Poe (1809–1849) and the English Romantic poets helped fuel the public's fascination with death and dying. In the late 20th and early 21st centuries the popularization of the Goth look is sometimes associated with the tubercular appearance.

Spiritualism

By the mid-19th century the romanticizing of death took on a new twist in the United States. Spiritualism, in which the living communicate directly with the dead, began in 1848 in the United States with the Fox sisters: Margaret Fox (1833–1893) and Kate Fox (1839–1892) of Hydesville, New York. The sisters claimed to have communicated with the spirit of a man who had been murdered by a former tenant in their house. The practice of conducting "sittings" to contact the dead gained instant popularity. Mediums, such as the Fox sisters, were supposedly sensitive to "vibrations" from the disembodied souls that temporarily lived in that part of the spirit world just outside Earth's limits.

This was not the first time people tried to communicate with the dead. Spiritualism has been practiced in cultures all over the world. For example, many Native Americans believe shamans (priests or medicine men) have the power to communicate with the spirits of the dead. The first book of Samuel recounts the visit of King Saul to a medium at Endor, who summoned the spirit of the prophet Samuel, which predicted the death of Saul and his sons.

The mood in the United States during the 1860s and 1870s was ripe for Spiritualist séances. Virtually everyone had lost a son, husband, or other loved one during the Civil War (1861–1865). Some survivors wanted assurances that their loved ones were all right; others were simply curious about life after death. Those who had drifted away from traditional Christianity embraced this new Spiritualism, which claimed scientific evidence of survival after physical death. This so-called evidence included table rapping, levitation, and materialization that occurred during the séances. In May 1875 a 12-member commission organized by the Russian chemist and inventor Dmitri Ivanovich Mendeleyev (1834–1907) concluded that Spiritualism had no scientific basis and that the séance phenomena resulted from fraud—from mediums consciously deceiving those in attendance by using tricks to create illusions.

THE MODERN AGE

In the last decades of the 20th century, attitudes about death and dying slowly began to change. Aging baby boomers (people born between 1946 and 1964), facing the deaths of their parents, began to confront their own mortality. Even though medical advances continue to increase life expectancy, they have raised an entirely new set of issues that are associated with death and dying. For example, how long should advanced medical technology be used to keep comatose people alive? How should the elderly or incapacitated be cared for? Is it reasonable for people to stop medical treatment, or even actively end their life, if that is what they wish?

Modern medicine plays a vital role in the way people die and, consequently, the manner in which the dying process of a loved one affects relatives and friends. With advancements in medical technology, the dying process can become depersonalized, moving away from the familiar surroundings of home and family to the sterile world of hospitals and strangers. However, the development of the modern hospice movement and the works of the American psychiatrist Elisabeth Kübler-Ross (1926–2004), including the pioneering book *On Death and Dying* (1969), have helped individuals from all walks of life confront the reality of death and restore dignity to those who are dying. Considered to be a highly respected authority on death, grief, and bereavement, Kübler-Ross influenced the medical practices that are undertaken at the end of life, as well as the attitudes of physicians, nurses, clergy, and others who care for the dying.

Hospice Care

The modern hospice movement developed in response to the need to provide humane care to terminally ill patients, while at the same time lending support to their families. The British physician Cicely Saunders (1918–2005) is considered to be the founder of the modern hospice movement—first in England in 1967 and later in Canada and the United States. The soothing, calming care provided by hospice workers is called palliative care, and it aims to relieve patients' pain and the accompanying symptoms of terminal illness, while providing comfort to patients and their families.

Hospice may refer to a place—a freestanding facility or designated floor in a hospital or nursing home—or to a program such as hospice home care, in which a team of health care professionals helps the dying patient and family at home. Hospice teams may involve physicians, nurses, social workers, pastoral counselors, and trained volunteers.

WHY PEOPLE CHOOSE HOSPICE CARE. Hospice workers consider the patient and family to be the "unit of care" and focus their efforts on attending to emotional, psychological, and spiritual needs as well as to physical comfort and well-being. With hospice care, as a patient nears death, medical details move to the background as personal details move to the foreground to avoid providing care that is not wanted by the patient, even if some clinical benefit might be expected.

THE POPULATION SERVED. Hospice facilities served over 1 million people of all ages in 2007, shown as "hospice care discharges" in Figure 1.2 and Table 1.1. Hospice care discharges are people who were in hospice care during the year but left hospice, either because they died or because they no longer needed hospice care. Eighty-three percent (868,100) of hospice care discharges (hospice patients) were 65 years and older in 2007. The category "current hospice care patients" in Table 1.1 refers to the number of patients in hospice at one particular time of the year—a snapshot in time. The annualized figure is the total number served during that year. Approximately 14,400 agencies served both the hospice and the home health care population in 2007. Home health care is medically oriented care in which a patient—

FIGURE 1.2

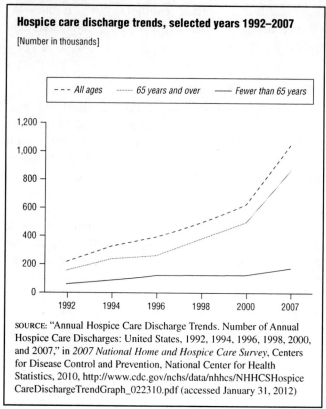

Hospice care discharge trends, selected years 1992–2007

[Number in thousands]

--- All ages   .... 65 years and over   —— Fewer than 65 years

SOURCE: "Annual Hospice Care Discharge Trends. Number of Annual Hospice Care Discharges: United States, 1992, 1994, 1996, 1998, 2000, and 2007," in *2007 National Home and Hospice Care Survey*, Centers for Disease Control and Prevention, National Center for Health Statistics, 2010, http://www.cdc.gov/nchs/data/nhhcs/NHHCSHospice CareDischargeTrendGraph_022310.pdf (accessed January 31, 2012)

often a senior—is helped to recover from an illness or injury at home instead of in a hospital or in a long-term health care facility. Both home health care and hospice care are growing as the population ages.

According to the National Hospice and Palliative Care Organization, in *NHPCO Facts and Figures: Hospice Care in America 2011 Edition* (2012, http://www.nhpco.org/ files/public/Statistics_Research/2011_Facts_Figures.pdf), terminal cancer patients (35.6%) were the largest single group of people served by hospice in 2010. People with heart disease (14.3%) and dementia (13%) were the two next largest groups. Other types of dying patients served by hospice include those with lung disease, strokes, end-stage renal (kidney) disease, liver disease, and human immunodeficiency syndrome/acquired immunodeficiency syndrome (HIV/AIDS).

The National Hospice and Palliative Care Organization notes that a majority of hospice patients die in their place of residence; 66.7% died in their place of residence in 2010. Most often, the patient's place of residence was his or her home (41.1%). Some lived in nursing homes (18%) and died there under hospice care. About one out of five (21.9%) hospice patients died in a hospice inpatient facility, and about one out of 10 (11.4%) died in an acute care hospital in 2010.

TABLE 1.1

Number of home health and hospice care agencies, patients, and discharges, selected years 1992–2007

Type of estimate	1992	1994	1996	1998	2000	2007
Agencies	8,000	10,900	13,500	13,300	11,400	14,400
Current home health-care patients	1,232,200	1,889,400	2,427,500	1,881,800	1,355,300	1,459,900
Fewer than 65 years	298,200	509,500	665,200	589,200	400,100	456,600
65 years and over	933,900	1,367,900	1,753,300	1,292,500	955,200	1,003,400
Current hospice-care patients	52,100	61,000	59,400	79,800	105,500	n/a
Fewer than 65 years	10,400	18,900	13,100	17,300	19,600	n/a
65 years and over	41,600	42,100	46,100	62,600	85,900	n/a
Home health-care discharges (annualized)	3,054,000	5,272,200	7,775,700	7,621,800	7,179,000	n/a
Fewer than 65 years	775,700	1,445,700	2,633,000	2,320,400	2,216,900	n/a
65 years and over	2,278,300	3,778,300	5,137,500	5,301,400	4,962,100	n/a
Hospice-care discharges (annualized)	219,300	328,000	393,200	496,000	621,100	1,045,100
Fewer than 65 years	61,400	88,400	121,100	118,300	126,900	177,000
65 years and over	157,900	239,100	265,200	377,600	494,300	868,100

Notes: 2007 data are based on a redesign of the National Home and Hospice Care Survey (NHHCS). The 2007 NHHCS collected data on only current home health-care patients and hospice care discharges. Numbers may not add to totals because of rounding.
n/a = not available.

SOURCE: "Table 1. Number of Home Health and Hospice Care Agencies, Patients, and Discharges: United States, 1992, 1994, 1996, 1998, 2000, and 2007," in *2007 National Home and Hospice Care Survey*, Centers for Disease Control and Prevention, National Center for Health Statistics, 2010, http://www.cdc.gov/nchs/data/nhhcs/NHHCSTrendTable_022310.pdf (accessed January 31, 2012)

CHAPTER 2
REDEFINING DEATH

TRADITIONAL DEFINITION OF DEATH

The processes of human life are sustained by many factors, but oxygen is a key to life. Respiration and blood circulation provide the body's cells with the oxygen that is needed to perform their life functions. When an injury or a disease compromises respiration or circulation, a breakdown in the oxygen supply can occur. As a result, the cells, deprived of essential life-sustaining oxygen, deteriorate. Using the criteria of a working heart and lungs, defining death was once quite simple: a person was considered dead once he or she stopped breathing or was without a detectable heartbeat.

A NEW CRITERION FOR DEATH

Advances in medical science have complicated the definition of death. Life-saving measures such as cardiopulmonary resuscitation or defibrillation (electrical shock) can restart cardiac activity. The development of the mechanical respirator during the 1950s also prompted a change in the concept of death. An unconscious patient, unable to breathe without assistance, could be kept alive with a respirator and, based on the heart and lung criteria, could not be declared dead.

Further complicating the issue was the transplantation of the first human heart. Experimental organ transplantation has been performed since the early 1900s. During the 1960s transplantation of organs such as kidneys became routine practice. Kidneys could be harvested from a patient whose heart had stopped and who therefore could be declared legally dead. By contrast, a successful heart transplant required a beating heart from a "dead" donor. On December 3, 1967, the South African surgeon Christiaan Barnard (1922–2001) transplanted a heart from a fatally injured accident victim into the South African businessman Louis Washkansky (1913–1967). Washkansky's health declined within a week after the surgery, and he died 18 days later from pneumonia.

Physicians who had been debating how best to handle patients whose life functions were supported mechanically now faced a new dilemma. With the first successful heart transplant, such patients now became potential heart donors, and it became necessary to ensure that a patient was truly dead before the heart was actually removed. Thus, physicians proposed a new criterion for death: irreversible cessation of brain activity, or what many called brain death.

The Harvard Criteria

In 1968 the Ad Hoc Committee of the Harvard Medical School to Examine the Definition of Brain Death was organized. The goal of the Harvard Brain Death Committee, as it was also known, was to redefine death. In August 1968 the committee published the report "A Definition of Irreversible Coma" (*Journal of the American Medical Association*, vol. 205, no. 6). This landmark report, known as the Harvard Criteria, listed the following guidelines for identifying irreversible coma:

- Unreceptivity and unresponsivity—the patient is completely unaware of externally applied stimuli and inner need. He or she does not respond even to intensely painful stimuli.

- No movements or breathing—the patient shows no sign of spontaneous movements and spontaneous respiration and does not respond to pain, touch, sound, or light.

- No reflexes—the pupils of the eyes are fixed and dilated. The patient shows no eye movement even when the ear is flushed with ice water or the head is turned. He or she does not react to harmful stimuli and exhibits no tendon reflexes.

- Flat electroencephalogram (EEG)—this shows lack of electrical activity in the cerebral cortex.

The Harvard Criteria could not be used unless reversible causes of brain dysfunction, such as drug intoxication and hypothermia (abnormally low body temperature—below 90 degrees Fahrenheit [32.2 degrees Celsius] core temperature), had been ruled out. The committee further recommended that the four tests be repeated 24 hours after the initial test.

The Harvard committee stated, "Our primary purpose is to define irreversible coma as a new criterion for death." Despite this, the committee in effect reinforced brain death (a lack of all neurological activity in the brain and brain stem) as the legal criterion for the death of a patient. A patient who met all four guidelines could be declared dead, and his or her respirator could be withdrawn. The committee added, however, "We are concerned here only with those comatose individuals who have no discernible central nervous system activity." Brain death differs somewhat from irreversible coma; patients in deep coma may show brain activity on an EEG, even though they may not be able to breathe on their own. People in a persistent vegetative state are also in an irreversible coma; however, they show more brain activity on an EEG than patients in deep coma and are able to breathe without the help of a respirator. Such patients were not considered dead by the committee's definition because they still had brain activity.

Criticisms of the Harvard Criteria

In 1978 Public Law 95-622 established the ethical advisory body called the President's Commission for the Study of Ethical Problems in Medicine and Biomedical and Behavioral Research. President Ronald Reagan (1911–2004) assigned the commission the task of defining death. In *Defining Death: A Report on the Medical, Legal and Ethical Issues in the Determination of Death* (July 1981, http://bioethics.georgetown.edu/pcbe/reports/past_commissions/defining_death.pdf), the commission reported that "the 'Harvard criteria' have been found to be quite reliable. Indeed, no case has yet been found that met these criteria and regained any brain functions despite continuation of respirator support."

However, the commission noted the following deficiencies in the Harvard Criteria:

- The phrase "irreversible coma" is misleading. Coma is a condition of a living person. A person lacking in brain function is dead and, therefore, beyond the condition called coma.

- The Harvard Brain Death Committee failed to note that spinal cord reflexes can continue or resume activity even after the brain stops functioning.

- "Unreceptivity" cannot be tested in an unresponsive person who has lost consciousness.

- The committee had not been "sufficiently explicit and precise" in expressing the need for adequate testing of brain stem reflexes, especially apnea (absence of the impulse to breathe, leading to an inability to breathe

spontaneously). Adequate testing to eliminate drug and metabolic intoxication as possible causes of the coma had also not been spelled out explicitly. Metabolic intoxication refers to the accumulation of toxins (poisons) in the blood resulting from kidney or liver failure. These toxins can severely impair brain functioning and cause coma, but the condition is potentially reversible.

- Even though all people who satisfy the Harvard Criteria are dead (with irreversible cessation of whole-brain functions), many dead individuals cannot maintain circulation long enough for retesting after a 24-hour interval.

THE GOVERNMENT REDEFINES DEATH

The president's commission proposed in *Defining Death* a model statute, the Uniform Determination of Death Act, the guidelines of which would be used to define death:

- [Determination of Death.] An individual who has sustained either (1) irreversible cessation of circulatory and respiratory functions, or (2) irreversible cessation of all functions of the entire brain, including the brain stem, is dead. A determination of death must be made in accordance with accepted medical standards.

- [Uniformity of Construction and Application.] This act shall be applied and construed to effectuate its general purpose to make uniform the law with respect to the subject of this Act among states enacting it.

Brain Death

In *Defining Death*, the president's commission incorporated two formulations or concepts of the "whole-brain definition" of death. It stated that these two concepts were "actually mirror images of each other. The Commission has found them to be complementary; together they enrich one's understanding of the 'definition' [of death]."

The first whole-brain formulation states that death occurs when the three major organs (heart, lungs, and brain) suffer an irreversible functional breakdown. These organs are closely interrelated, so that if one stops functioning permanently, the other two will also stop working. Even though traditionally the absence of the "vital signs" of respiration and circulation have signified death, this is simply a sign that the brain, the core organ, has permanently ceased to function. Individual cells or organs may continue to live for many hours, but the body as a whole cannot survive for long. Therefore, death can be declared even before the whole system shuts down.

The second whole-brain formulation "identifies the functioning of the whole brain as the hallmark of life because the brain is the regulator of the body's integration." Because the brain is the seat of consciousness and the director of all bodily functions, when the brain dies, the person is considered dead.

Reason for Two Definitions of Death

The president's commission claimed in *Defining Death* that its aim was to "supplement rather than supplant the existing legal concept." The brain-death criteria were not being introduced to define death in a new way. In most cases the cardiopulmonary definition of death would be sufficient. Only comatose patients on respirators would be diagnosed using the brain-death criteria.

Criteria for Determination of Death

The president's commission did not include in the proposed Uniform Determination of Death Act any specific medical criteria for diagnosing brain death. Instead, it had a group of medical consultants develop a summary of currently accepted medical practices. The commission stated in *Defining Death* that "such criteria—particularly as they relate to diagnosing death on neurological grounds—will be continually revised by the biomedical community in light of clinical experience and new scientific knowledge." These Criteria for Determination of Death read as follows (with medical details omitted here):

1. An individual with irreversible cessation of circulatory and respiratory functions is dead. A) Cessation is recognized by an appropriate clinical examination. B) Irreversibility is recognized by persistent cessation of functions during an appropriate period of observation and/or trial of therapy.

2. An individual with irreversible cessation of all functions of the entire brain, including the brainstem, is dead. A) Cessation is recognized when evaluation discloses findings that cerebral functions are absent and brainstem functions are absent. B) Irreversibility is recognized when evaluation discloses findings that the cause of coma is established and is sufficient to account for the loss of brain functions; the possibility of recovery of any brain functions is excluded; and the cessation of all brain functions persists for an appropriate period of observation and/or trial of therapy.

The Criteria for Determination of Death further warn that conditions such as drug intoxication, metabolic intoxication, and hypothermia may be confused with brain death. Physicians should practice caution when dealing with young children and people in shock. Infants and young children, who have more resistance to neurological damage, have been known to recover brain function. Shock victims might not test well due to a reduction in blood circulation to the brain.

Since the development of brain-death criteria in the United States, most countries have adopted the brain-death concept. Nevertheless, determining brain death varies worldwide. One reason has to do with cultural or religious beliefs. For example, in Japan it is believed that the soul lingers in the body for some time after death. Such a belief may influence the length of time the patient is observed before making the determination of death.

There is no federally mandated definition for brain death or method for certifying brain death. Thus, states have adopted the previously described Uniform Determination of Death Act. However, within each hospital, clinical practice is determined by the medical staff and administrative committees. A simplified list of criteria for brain death, which was still current as of April 2012, is listed in Table 2.1.

Even though the practice parameter has been published, several questions arose regarding the American Academy of Neurology's (AAN) guidelines, which were established in 1995. These questions are based on historical criteria. In "Evidence-Based Guideline Update: Determining Brain Death in Adults" (*Neurology*, vol. 74, no. 23, June 8, 2010), Eelco F. M. Wijdicks et al. articulate the questions and seek to answer them. The questions are:

1. Are there patients who fulfill the clinical criteria of brain death who recover neurologic [nervous system] function?

2. What is an adequate observation period to ensure that cessation of neurologic function is permanent?

3. Are complex motor movements that falsely suggest retained brain function sometimes observed in brain death?

4. What is the comparative safety of techniques for determining apnea?

5. Are there new ancillary [secondary] tests that accurately identify patients with brain death?

TABLE 2.1

Criteria for brain death

Coma
Absence of motor responses
Absence of pupillary responses to light and pupils at midposition with respect to dilatation (4–6 mm)
Absence of corneal reflexes
Absence of caloric responses
Absence of gag reflex
Absence of coughing in response to tracheal suctioning
Absence of respiratory drive at $PaCO_2$ that is 60 mm Hg or 20 mm Hg above normal baseline values

SOURCE: Eelco F. M. Wijdicks and Ronald E. Cranford, "Table 3. Clinical Criteria for Brain Death," in "Clinical Diagnosis of Prolonged States of Impaired Consciousness in Adults," *Mayo Clinic Proceedings*, vol. 80, no. 8, August 2005, http://download.journals.elsevierhealth.com/pdfs/journals/0025-6196/PIIS0025619611615863.pdf (accessed January 31, 2012). Data from E. F. M. Wijdicks, "The Diagnosis of the Brain," *New England Journal of Medicine*, no. 344, 2001: 1215-21.

The researchers reviewed studies between January 1996 and May 2009, and they limited their focus to adults aged 18 years and older. The answers that Wijdicks et al. find, which are endorsed by the Neurocritical Care Society, the Child Neurology Society, the Radiological Society of North America, and the American College of Radiology, are:

1. The criteria for the determination of brain death given in the 1995 AAN practice parameter have not been invalidated by published reports of neurologic recovery in patients who fulfill these criteria.

2. There is insufficient evidence to determine the minimally acceptable observation period to ensure that neurologic functions have ceased irreversibly.

3. Complex-spontaneous motor movements and false-positive triggering of the ventilator may occur in patients who are brain dead.

4. There is insufficient evidence to determine the comparative safety of techniques used for apnea testing.

5. There is insufficient evidence to determine if newer ancillary tests accurately confirm the cessation of function of the entire brain.

Wijdicks et al.'s results confirm that Table 2.1 still shows accurate criteria for brain death. In addition, Wijdicks's editorial "The Clinical Criteria of Brain Death throughout the World: Why Has It Come to This?" (*Canadian Journal of Anesthesia*, vol. 53, no. 6, June 2006) maintains his premise that "what is required is standardization of policy, appropriate education of staff, introduction of checklists in intensive care units, and brain death examination by designated, experienced physicians who have documented proficiency in brain death examination." For the care of children, Thomas A. Nakagawa et al. recommend in "Clinical Report—Guidelines for the Determination of Brain Death in Infants and Children: An Update of the 1987 Task Force Recommendations" (*Pediatrics*, vol. 128, no. 3, September 2011) that their care closely follows that given to adults as outlined by Wijdicks et al. More specifically, Nakagawa et al. explain that the care of children should use the Grading of Recommendations Assessment, Development, and Evaluation (GRADE), a standardized methods-and-consensus-based approach that committees use to make death determinations for children.

Brain Death and Persistent Vegetative State

In the past people who suffered severe head injuries usually died from apnea. In the 21st century rapid emergency medical intervention allows them to be placed on respirators before breathing stops. In some cases the primary brain damage may be reversible and unassisted breathing eventually resumes. In many cases, however, brain damage is irreversible, and, if the respirator is not disconnected, it will continue to pump blood to the dead brain.

FIGURE 2.1

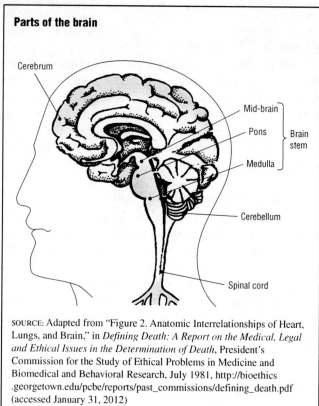

Parts of the brain

SOURCE: Adapted from "Figure 2. Anatomic Interrelationships of Heart, Lungs, and Brain," in *Defining Death: A Report on the Medical, Legal and Ethical Issues in the Determination of Death*, President's Commission for the Study of Ethical Problems in Medicine and Biomedical and Behavioral Research, July 1981, http://bioethics.georgetown.edu/pcbe/reports/past_commissions/defining_death.pdf (accessed January 31, 2012)

The brain stem, traditionally called the lower brain, is usually more resistant to damage from anoxia (oxygen deprivation). Thus, oxygen deprivation may cause irreversible damage to the cerebrum, or higher brain, but may spare the brain stem. (See Figure 2.1.) When the cerebrum is irreversibly damaged yet the brain stem still functions, the patient goes into a persistent vegetative state. Persistent vegetative state patients, lacking in the higher-brain function, are awake but unaware. They swallow, grimace when in pain, yawn, open their eyes, and may even breathe without a respirator.

Table 2.2 lists the criteria for the diagnosis of the persistent vegetative state, which is also called the unresponsive wakefulness syndrome. Steven Laureys et al. explain in "Unresponsive Wakefulness Syndrome: A New Name for the Vegetative State or Apallic Syndrome" (*BMC Medicine*, vol. 8, no. 68, November 1, 2010) that the use of the term *unresponsive wakefulness syndrome* is more appropriate, neutral, and descriptive. According to the researchers:

Our proposal offers the medical community the possibility to adopt a neutral and descriptive name, unresponsive wakefulness syndrome, as an alternative to vegetative state (orapallic syndrome) which we view as outdated. We feel this is a real necessity, given that the term [persistent vegetative state] continues to have strong negative connotations after over 35 years of use, while inadvertently risking comparisons between patients and vegetables and implying persistency from

TABLE 2.2

Criteria for persistent vegetative state (PVS)

- Unaware of surroundings or self
- Exhibits eye-opening and eye-closing cycles
- Has enough autonomic nervous system and hypothalamus function to allow long-term survival with medical care
- Unable to interact with others
- Does not respond in a sustained, reproducible, or purposeful way to sights, sounds, touches, or smells
- Does not provide evidence of understanding language nor an ability to communicate with language
- Cannot control bladder and bowel functions
- May exhibit certain cranial nerve reflexes, such as dilation and constriction of pupils and the gag reflex

SOURCE: Created by Sandra Alters for Gale, 2012

the moment of diagnosis. It should be stressed that [unresponsive wakefulness syndrome] is a clinical syndrome describing patients who fail to show voluntary motor responsiveness in the presence of eyes-open wakefulness which can be either transitory on the way to recovery from (minimal) consciousness or irreversible.

Patients in a persistent vegetative state are not dead, so the brain-death criteria do not apply to them. They can survive for years with artificial feeding and antibiotics for possible infections. In *Defining Death*, the president's commission reported on a patient who remained in a persistent vegetative state for 37 years: Elaine Esposito (1934–1978) lapsed into a coma after surgery in 1941 and died in 1978.

The case of Karen Ann Quinlan (1954–1985) called attention to the ramifications of the persistent vegetative state. In 1975 Quinlan suffered a cardiopulmonary arrest after ingesting a combination of alcohol and drugs. In 1976 Joseph Quinlan was granted court permission to discontinue artificial respiration for his comatose daughter. Even after life support was removed, Karen remained in a persistent vegetative state until she died of multiple infections in 1985.

A more recent case that refocused national attention on the persistent vegetative state was that of Terri Schiavo (1963–2005), who entered a persistent vegetative state in 1990, when her brain was deprived of oxygen during a heart attack that was brought on by an eating disorder. Michael Schiavo, her husband, argued that she would never recover and that she would not want to be kept alive by artificial means. He petitioned a Florida court to remove her feeding tube. In October 2003 a Florida judge ruled that the tube should be removed. However, Schiavo's parents believed their daughter would recover and requested that Jeb Bush (1953–), the governor of Florida, intervene. The Florida legislature subsequently gave Governor Bush the authority to override the courts, and the feeding tube was reinserted six days after its removal. In May 2004 the law that allowed Governor Bush to intervene in the case was

ruled unconstitutional by a Florida appeals court. The case was then appealed to the U.S. Supreme Court, which in January 2005 refused to hear the appeal and reinstate the Florida law. In March 2005 doctors removed Terri's feeding tube. She died 13 days later. An autopsy showed extensive damage throughout the cerebrum.

A similar case followed four years later, in 2009, when Eluana Englaro (1970–2009) died in Italy. She had been in a vegetative state for 17 years after a car accident resulted in her irreversible brain damage. Eluana's father, Beppino, tried for a decade to have his daughter's feeding tube removed, because she did not want to be kept alive by artificial means. He finally succeeded in spite of protests by the Catholic Church. Eluana died four days into the process of having her food and water diminished.

That same year the case of Rom Houben (1963–) was publicized worldwide. When Houben was 20, he was injured in an automobile accident, and his doctors eventually determined that he fell into a persistent vegetative state. Twenty-three years later he was suddenly able to communicate. Houben's doctors were convinced that he had been misdiagnosed and that he had not really been in a persistent vegetative state for all those years. However, experts questioned the man's method of communication, which is called facilitated communication. Maria Cheng explains in "Belgian Coma Patient Can't Talk after All" (Associated Press, February 19, 2010) that facilitated communication is a method by which a speech therapist helps the patient type out his or her thoughts by having the patient guide the therapist's hand. In response to questions raised about the technique, one of Houben's doctors performed tests on the method and determined that it did not work. Further tests have revealed that facilitated communication does not work with patients such as Houben. Claims that Houben could communicate were proven to be false.

Martin M. Monti et al. reveal in "Willful Modulation of Brain Activity in Disorders of Consciousness" (*New England Journal of Medicine*, vol. 362, no. 7, February 18, 2010) that they used functional magnetic resonance imaging technology to determine whether patients in a persistent vegetative state or a minimally conscious state (patients with partial preservation of conscious awareness) had brain activity that reflected "some awareness and cognition." The researchers scanned the brains of 54 previously unresponsive patients. Five of the patients showed brain activity (responsiveness) when researchers asked the patients to imagine themselves playing tennis. One of those five patients was also able to respond to questions with brain activity that is consistent with yes or no answers. Monti et al. expect that using such techniques with patients in a persistent vegetative or minimally conscious state may help to better refine the diagnosis of their condition, provide more appropriate treatment to those who show responsiveness, and establish basic communication with patients who otherwise appear to be unresponsive. See Chapter 4 for more information on disorders of consciousness and the minimally conscious state.

THE NEAR-DEATH EXPERIENCE

The term *near-death experience* was first used by Raymond A. Moody Jr. in *Life after Life: The Investigation of a Phenomenon—Survival of Bodily Death* (1976), a compilation of interviews with people who claimed to have come back from the dead. A decade earlier, the American psychiatrist Elisabeth Kübler-Ross (1926–2004) investigated out-of-body episodes that were recounted by her patients.

The near-death experience is not a phenomenon limited to modern times. It has been recounted in various forms of mysticism and by well-known historical figures such as the Greek philosopher Plato (428–347 BC) and the Benedictine historian and theologian St. Bede the Venerable (c. 673–c. 735). It appears, however, that the development and administration of emergency resuscitation has contributed to widespread reports of near-death experiences.

Some people who were revived after having been declared clinically dead have recounted remarkably similar patterns of experiences. They report leaving their body and watching, in a detached manner, while others tried to save their life. They felt no pain and experienced complete serenity. After traveling through a tunnel, they encountered a radiant light. Some claim they met friends and relatives who have died; many attest to seeing their whole life replayed and of ultimately being given either a choice or a command to return to their body.

Many people who have had a near-death experience believe they have undergone a spiritual event of great importance. For example, they may believe that they saw, or even entered, the afterlife. Studies conducted during the 1990s indicated that the near-death experience might be related to one or more physical changes in the brain. These changes include the gradual onset of anoxia in the brain, residual electrical activity in the brain, the release of endorphins in response to stress, or drug-induced hallucinations produced by drug therapies that are used during resuscitation attempts or resulting from previous drug abuse.

Not everyone who has been close to death has had a near-death experience. These experiences are atypical reactions to trauma, and the involvement of the temporal lobes of the brain in these experiences has been explored by researchers for decades. In "Near-Death Experiences and the Temporal Lobe" (*Psychological Science*, vol. 15, no. 4, April 2004), Willoughby B. Britton and Richard R. Bootzin of the University of Arizona discuss the results of their study of temporal lobe functioning in 43 individuals who had experienced life-threatening events. Of the 43 participants, 23 reported having had near-death experiences during these events. The researchers find that people who reported near-death experiences had more of certain types of temporal lobe activity than those who did not have such experiences. Britton and Bootzin conclude that "altered temporal lobe functioning may be involved in the near-death experience and that individuals who have had such experiences are physiologically distinct from the general population."

In "Heaven Can Wait—or Down to Earth in Real Time: Near-Death Experience Revisited" (*Netherlands Heart Journal*, vol. 16, no. 10, October 2008), C. van Tellingen describes a neurophysiological explanation for near-death experiences. Van Tellingen suggests that as the body's nerve cells and their connections break down, "reminiscences, memories and building stones of the personal identity are 'released' and strengthen a feeling of time travel and life review. Perhaps this situation is more or less comparable with the situation in old age when literally loss of neurons and their connections bring back 'buried' memories and reminiscences." Dean Mobbs and Caroline Watt agree and conclude in "There Is Nothing Paranormal about Near-Death Experiences: How Neuroscience Can Explain Seeing Bright Lights, Meeting the Dead, or Being Convinced You Are One of Them" (*Trends in Cognitive Sciences*, vol. 15, no. 10, August 18, 2011) that "near-death experiences are the manifestation of normal brain function gone awry, during a traumatic, and sometimes harmless, event."

CHAPTER 3
THE END OF LIFE: ETHICAL CONSIDERATIONS

Defining death has become a complex matter. Innovative medical technology, while saving many lives, has also blurred the lines between life and death. The controversy about the definition of death is but one of the ethical issues, or principles of moral conduct, related to end-of-life care and decision making. For example, should a son or daughter request the withdrawal of nutrition and hydration from a parent who is in a persistent vegetative state, especially when he or she knows about the parent's respect for the sanctity of life? Does a physician honor a patient's do-not-resuscitate order when it goes against the physician's ethical convictions? Who should determine when medical care is futile and no longer benefits the dying patient?

The answers to questions about care at the end of life, as well as decisions made by people who are dying and by their loved ones, vary in response to cultural influences, family issues, and spiritual beliefs. Historical, social, cultural, political, and religious convictions shape ethical beliefs about death and guide the actions of health care professionals and people who are terminally ill. For people of faith, religious convictions are vitally important when making end-of-life decisions.

RELIGIOUS TEACHINGS

All major religions consider life sacred. When it comes to death and dying, they take seriously the fate of the soul, be it eternal salvation (as in Christian belief) or reincarnation (as in Buddhist philosophy).

Roman Catholicism

According to Catholic teachings, death is contrary to God's plan for humankind. In the Old Testament of the Bible, the book of Genesis indicates that when God created human beings, he did not intend for them to die. However, when Adam and Eve (the first humans) disobeyed God in the Garden of Eden, physical death was the consequence of their sin. The New Testament of the Bible explains that Jesus was the son of God who, out of love for humankind, was born into the world and died as a man. God raised Jesus from the dead after his crucifixion to live eternally with him in heaven, and Jesus promised humankind the same opportunity. The Vatican notes in *Catechism of the Catholic Church* (August 23, 2002, http://www.vatican.va/archive/ccc_css/archive/catechism/ccc_toc.htm) that according to Christian doctrine, Jesus "transformed the curse of death into a blessing."

HISTORY. Early Christians believed that God was the giver of life, and therefore he alone could take life away. They viewed euthanasia (hastening the death of a dying, suffering patient who requests death) as usurping that divine right. The early Christian philosopher St. Augustine of Hippo (354–430) taught that people must accept suffering because it comes from God. According to Augustine, suffering not only helps Christians grow spiritually but also prepares them for the eternal joy that God has in store for them. Moreover, the healthy were exhorted to minister to the sick not for the purpose of helping to permanently end their suffering, but to ease their pain.

St. Thomas Aquinas (c. 1225–1274), who is considered to be one of the greatest Catholic theologians, taught that ending one's suffering by ending one's life was sinful. To help another take his or her life was just as sinful. However, in 1516 Sir Thomas More (1478–1535), an English statesman, humanist, and loyal defender of the Catholic Church, published *Utopia*, which described an ideal country that was governed by reason. More argued that if a disease is not only incurable but also causes pain that is hard to control, it is permissible to free the sufferer from his or her painful existence. This was a major departure from the medieval acceptance of suffering and death as the earthly price to be paid for eternal life.

RULE OF DOUBLE EFFECT. Catholic moral theologians were said to have developed the ethical principle "Rule of Double Effect." According to this principle, "Effects that would be morally wrong if caused intentionally are permissible if foreseen but unintended." For example, a physician prescribes an increased dosage of the painkiller morphine to ease a patient's pain, not to bring about his or her death. However, it is foreseen that a potent dosage may depress the patient's respiration and hasten death. In *Catechism of the Catholic Church*, the Vatican states that "the use of painkillers to alleviate the sufferings of the dying, even at the risk of shortening their days, can be morally in conformity with human dignity if death is not willed as either an end or a means, but only foreseen and tolerated as inevitable."

ON EUTHANASIA. For several decades, Catholic theologians have debated balancing the preservation of God-given life with the moral issue of continuing medical treatments that are of no apparent value to patients. In "The Prolongation of Life" (1957), Pope Pius XII (1876–1958) states that if a patient is hopelessly ill, physicians may discontinue heroic measures "to permit the patient, already virtually dead, to pass on in peace." He adds that if the patient is unconscious, relatives may request withdrawal of life support under certain conditions.

In 1980 the Vatican published the *Declaration on Euthanasia* (http://www.vatican.va/roman_curia/congregations/cfaith/documents/rc_con_cfaith_doc_19800505_euthanasia_en.html), which is considered to be the official Catholic Church stance against euthanasia. It defines the term: "By euthanasia is understood an action or an omission which of itself or by intention causes death, in order that all suffering may in this way be eliminated." The declaration notes that a person cannot ask for euthanasia no matter what the situation, because it is a "violation of the divine law" and it is almost always an "anguished plea for help and love." The declaration indicates, however, that a dying patient may be administered painkilling medications at the end of life to help him or her be more comfortable.

The Committee for Pro-life Activities of the National Conference of Catholic Bishops states in *Nutrition and Hydration: Moral and Pastoral Reflections* (April 1992, http://www.priestsforlife.org/magisterium/bishops/92-04nutritionandhydrationnccbprolifecommittee.htm) that "in the final stage of dying one is not obliged to prolong the life of a patient by every possible means: 'When inevitable death is imminent in spite of the means used, it is permitted in conscience to take the decision to refuse forms of treatment that would only secure a precarious and burdensome prolongation of life, so long as the normal care due to the sick person in similar cases is not interrupted.'" However, the article "Pope Rules Patients in Permanent Vegetative State May Not be Denied Artificial Nutrition and Hydration" (LifeSiteNews.com, September 14, 2007) notes that the Vatican's Congregation for the Doctrine of the Faith ruled in 2007 that a person in a persistent vegetative state must receive nutrition and hydration. Pope Benedict XVI

(1927–) approved the ruling. Moreover, the Vatican explains in *Catechism of the Catholic Church* that "direct euthanasia" is "morally unacceptable" in any situation under the Fifth Commandment.

The Eastern Orthodox Church

The Eastern Orthodox Church resulted from the division between eastern and western Christianity during the 11th century. Differences in doctrines and politics, among other things, caused the separation. The Eastern Orthodox Church does not have a single worldwide leader such as the Roman Catholic pope. Instead, national jurisdictions called sees are each governed by a bishop.

Eastern Orthodoxy relies on the Scriptures, traditions, and decrees of the first seven ecumenical councils to regulate its daily conduct. Concerning matters of morality in the 21st century, such as the debates on end-of-life issues, contemporary Orthodox ethicists explore possible courses of action that are in line with the "sense of the church." The sense of the church is deduced from church laws and dissertations of the church fathers, as well as from previous council decisions. Their recommendations are subject to further review.

In "The Stand of the Orthodox Church on Controversial Issues" (2012, http://www.goarch.org/ourfaith/ourfaith7101), the Reverend Stanley S. Harakas states, "The Orthodox Church has a very strong pro-life stand which in part expresses itself in opposition to doctrinaire advocacy of euthanasia." However, Harakas notes that "as current Orthodox theology expresses it: 'The Church distinguishes between euthanasia and the withholding of extraordinary means to prolong life. It affirms the sanctity of human life and man's God-given responsibility to preserve life. But it rejects an attitude which disregards the inevitability of physical death.'"

Protestantism

The different denominations of Protestantism have varying positions on euthanasia. Many hold that euthanasia is morally wrong, but they also believe that prolonging life by extraordinary measures is not necessary. In other words, even though few would condone euthanasia, many accept withdrawing life support from a dying patient. Among the Protestant denominations that support this latter view are the Jehovah's Witnesses, the Church of Jesus Christ of Latter-day Saints (Mormons), the Lutheran Church, the Reformed Presbyterians, the Presbyterian Church in America, the Christian Life Commission of the Southern Baptist Convention, and the General Association of the General Baptists.

Some denominations have no official policy on euthanasia. However, many individual ethicists and representatives within these churches agree with other denominations that euthanasia is morally wrong but that futile life support serves no purpose. Among these churches are the Seventh-Day Adventists, the Episcopal Church, and the United Methodist Church.

Christian Scientists believe that prayer heals all diseases. They claim that illnesses are mental in origin and therefore cannot be cured by outside intervention, such as medical help. Some also believe that seeking medical help while praying diminishes or even cancels the effectiveness of the prayers. Because God can heal even those diseases that others see as incurable, euthanasia has no practical significance among Christian Scientists.

The Unitarian Universalist Association, a union of the Unitarian and Universalist Churches, is perhaps the most liberal when it comes to the right to die. The association states in "The Right to Die with Dignity: 1988 General Resolution" (August 24, 2011, http://www.uua.org/social justice/socialjustice/statements/14486.shtml) that "human life has inherent dignity, which may be compromised when life is extended beyond the will or ability of a person to sustain that dignity." Furthermore, "Unitarian Universalists advocate the right to self-determination in dying, and the release from civil or criminal penalties of those who, under proper safeguards, act to honor the right of terminally ill patients to select the time of their own deaths."

Judaism

There are three main branches of Judaism in the United States. The Orthodox tradition adheres strictly to Jewish laws. Conservative Judaism advocates adapting Jewish precepts to a changing world, but all changes must be consistent with Jewish laws and tradition. Reform Judaism, while accepting the ethical laws as coming from God, generally considers the other laws of Judaism as "instructional but not binding."

Like the Roman Catholics, Jews believe that life is precious because it is a gift from God. No one has the right to extinguish life, because one's life is not his or hers in the first place. Generally, rabbis from all branches of Judaism agree that euthanasia is not morally justified. It is tantamount to murder, which is forbidden by the Torah. Moreover, Jewish teaching holds that men and women are stewards entrusted with the preservation of God's gift of life and therefore are obliged to hold on to that life as long as possible.

PROLONGING LIFE VERSUS HASTENING DEATH. Even though Jewish tradition maintains that a devout believer must do everything possible to prolong life, this admonition is subject to interpretation even among Orthodox Jews.

The Torah and the Talmud (the definitive rabbinical compilation of Jewish laws, lore, and commentary) provide the principles and laws that guide Jews. The Talmud offers continuity to Jewish culture by interpreting the Torah and adapting it to the constantly changing situations of Jewish people.

On the subject of prolonging life versus hastening death, the Talmud narrates a number of situations that involve people who are considered "goses" (literally, "the death rattle is in the patient's throat" or "one whose death is imminent"). Scholars often refer to the story of Rabbi Hanina ben Teradyon, who, during the second century, was condemned to be burned to death by the Romans. To prolong his agonizing death, the Romans wrapped him in some wet material. At first, the rabbi refused to hasten his own death; however, he later agreed to have the wet material removed, thus bringing about a quicker death.

Some Jews interpret this Talmudic narration to mean that in the final stage of a person's life, it is permissible to remove any hindrance to the dying process. In this modern age of medicine, this may mean implementing a patient's wish, such as a do-not-resuscitate order or the withdrawal of artificial life support.

Islam

Islam was founded by the prophet Muhammad (c. 570–632) during the seventh century. The Koran, which is composed of Allah's (God's) revelations to Muhammad, and the sunna, Muhammad's teachings and deeds, are the sources of Islamic beliefs and practice. Even though there are many sects and cultural diversities within the religion, all Muslims (followers of Islam) are bound by a total submission to the will of Allah. The basic doctrines of Allah's revelations were systematized into definitive rules and regulations that now make up the sharia (the religious law that governs the life of Muslims).

Muslims look to the sharia for ethical guidance in all aspects of life, including medicine. Sickness and pain are part of life and must be accepted as Allah's will. They should be viewed as a means to atone for one's sins. By contrast, death is simply a passage to another existence in the afterlife. Those who die after leading a righteous life will merit the true life on Judgment Day. The Koran states, "How do you disbelieve in God seeing you were dead and He gave you life and then He shall cause you to die, then He shall give you life, then unto Him you shall be returned?"

Islam teaches that life is a gift from Allah; therefore, no one can end it except Allah. Muhammad said, "Whosoever takes poison and thus kills himself, his poison will be in his hand; he will be tasting it in Hell, always abiding therein, and being accommodated therein forever" (compiled in *Sahih Bukhari*). While an ailing person does not have the right to choose death, even if he or she is suffering, Muslims heed the following admonition from the *Islamic Code of Medical Ethics* (1981): "[The] doctor is well advised to realize his limit and not transgress it. If it is scientifically certain that life cannot be restored, then it is futile to diligently [maintain] the vegetative state of the patient by heroic means.... It is the process of life that the doctor aims to maintain and not the process of dying. In any case, the doctor shall not take a positive measure to terminate the patient's life."

Hinduism

The Eastern religious tradition of Hinduism is based on the principle of reincarnation (the cycle of life, death, and physical rebirth). Hindus believe that death and dying are intricately interwoven with life and that the individual soul undergoes a series of physical life cycles before uniting with Brahman (God). Karma refers to the ethical consequences of a person's actions during a previous life, which determine the quality of his or her present life. A person can neither change nor escape his or her karma. By conforming to dharma (religious and moral law), an individual is able to fulfill obligations from the past life. Life is sacred because it offers one the chance to perform good acts toward the goal of ending the cycle of rebirths.

Therefore, a believer in Hinduism views pain and suffering as personal karma, and serious illness as a consequence of past misdeeds. Death is simply a passage to another rebirth, which brings one closer to Brahman. Artificial medical treatments to sustain life are not recommended, and medical intervention to end life is discouraged. Euthanasia simply interrupts one's karma and the soul's evolution toward final liberation from reincarnation.

Buddhism

Buddhism, like Hinduism, is based on a cycle of reincarnation. To Buddhists, the goals of every life are the emancipation from samsara (the compulsory cycle of rebirths) and the attainment of nirvana (enlightenment or bliss). Like the Hindus, Buddhists believe that sickness, death, and karma are interrelated. The followers of Buddha (563–480 BC), the founder of Buddhism, claim that Buddha advised against taking too strict a position when it comes to issues such as the right to die.

Tenzin Gyatso (1935–), the 14th Dalai Lama, the spiritual leader of Tibetan Buddhism, has commented on the use of mechanical life support when the patient has no chance of recovery. Sogyal Rinpoche explains in *The Tibetan Book of Living and Dying* (1992) that the Dalai Lama advises that each case be considered individually: "If there is no such chance for positive thoughts [Buddhists believe that a dying person's final thoughts determine the circumstances of his or her next life], and in addition a lot of money is being spent by relatives simply to keep someone alive, then there seems to be no point. But each case must be dealt with individually; it is very difficult to generalize."

BIOETHICS AND MEDICAL PRACTICE

Since ancient times, medical practice has been concerned with ethical issues. However, only since the last half of the 20th century have rapid advances in medicine given rise to so many ethical dilemmas. In matters of death and dying the debate continues on issues such as physicians' honoring a patient's do-not-resuscitate order, withholding food and fluids, and withdrawing artificial respiration.

There are four basic tenets of bioethics: autonomy, beneficence, nonmaleficence, and justice. Autonomy refers to self-rule and self-determination. Beneficence is action that is in the best interest of the patient. Nonmaleficence means to do no harm. Justice is the practice of treating patients in comparable circumstances the same way and refers to equitable distribution of resources, risks, and costs. Even though bioethics is subject to change and reinterpretation, medical practice continues to rely on these principles to guide the actions of physicians and other health care providers.

The Hippocratic Oath

The earliest written document to deal with medical ethics is generally attributed to Hippocrates (460–377 BC), who is considered to be the father of medicine. For more than 2,000 years the Hippocratic Oath has been adopted by Western physicians as a code of ethics, defining their conduct in the discharge of their duties. In part, the oath states: "I will follow that method of treatment, which, according to my ability and judgment, I consider for the benefit of my patients, and abstain from whatever is deleterious [harmful] and mischievous. I will give no deadly medicine to anyone if asked, nor suggest any such counsel."

Nonetheless, some scholars claim that the giving of "deadly medicine" does not refer to euthanasia. During the time of Hippocrates, helping a suffering person end his or her life was common practice. Therefore, the oath might have been more an admonition to the medical profession to avoid acting as an accomplice to murder, rather than to refrain from the practice of euthanasia.

Some physicians believe that a literal interpretation of the oath is not necessary. It simply offers guidelines that allow for adaptation to 21st-century situations. In fact, in 1948 the World Medical Association modified the Hippocratic Oath to call attention to the atrocities that were committed by Nazi physicians. Known as the Declaration of Geneva (June 6, 2002, http://www.cirp .org/library/ethics/geneva/), the document reads in part: "I will practice my profession with conscience and dignity; the health of my patient will be my first consideration.... I will not permit considerations of religion, nationality, race, party politics or social standing to intervene between my duty and my patient. I will maintain the utmost respect for human life from the time of conception, even under threat, I will not use my medical knowledge contrary to the laws of humanity."

The Changing Patient-Physician Relationship

Even in ancient times, as can be gleaned from the Hippocratic Oath, physicians believed they knew what was best for their patients. Patients relied on their doctors' ability and judgment and usually did not question the treatments that were prescribed. Doctors were not even required to tell their patients the details of their illness, even if they were terminally ill.

Beginning in the 1960s many patients assumed a more active role in their medical care. The emphasis on preventive medicine encouraged people to take responsibility for their own health. Physicians were treating patients who wanted to be active participants in their health care. Patients also wanted to know more about modern technologies and procedures that were evolving in medicine. With this new health consciousness, physicians and hospitals assumed the responsibility for informing and educating patients, and increasingly were legally liable for failing to inform patients of the consequences of medical treatments and procedures.

To compound the complexity of the changing patient-physician relationship, modern technology, which could sometimes prolong life, was also prolonging death. Historically, physicians had been trained to prevent and combat death, rather than to deal with dying patients, communicate with the patient and the family about a terminal illness, prepare them for an imminent death, or respond to a patient requesting assisted suicide. By the 1980s physicians were facing another issue with which they had not be trained for: administering lethal injections to death-row inmates.

The Death Penalty and the Physician's Role

In 1982 the first lethal injections were used to kill death-row inmates, and these events led to a controversy about whether medical professionals should participate. The drug or drugs are administered intravenously by either a prison employee or a medical professional, but most of the country's leading medical organizations oppose their members' involvement. Nonetheless, many physicians believe that their presence, according to the laws in some states, helps the executions occur in a pain-free manner. They hold that these executions will proceed regardless of their personal convictions. After a cardiac monitor indicates that the inmate's heart has definitively stopped, the inmate is declared dead. A death certificate is filled out, which shows the cause of death. (See Figure 3.1.) The document is filled out by the funeral director and the medical certifier, as it is with all deaths.

Even though there are disagreements over which drugs should be used to carry out executions and which drugs are available for use, states determine their protocols and many states require the presence of a physician at an execution. In the perspective article "When Law and Ethics Collide—Why Physicians Participate in Executions" (*New England Journal of Medicine*, vol. 354, no. 12, March 23, 2006), Atul Gawande of the Brigham and Women's Hospital in Boston, Massachusetts, describes his discussions with a few physicians who became involved in executions. All of them began by wanting to help after being asked. In many instances, they started out by simply monitoring the executions. However, when prison staff had difficulties finding a vein for the needle, these physicians began suggesting where to insert the needle. A few even inserted the needles themselves. As complications arose, some even had to ask that more of a certain drug be administered to guarantee that the inmate's heart had stopped beating. In effect, their role shifted from being innocuous to being nocuous (harmful). When people within the physicians' community learned that they assisted in executions, some of the physicians continued helping the prisons, whereas others decided to stop. Gawande determines that physicians who were employed by the correctional system felt more clearly that their involvement was needed, than physicians who worked in local community clinics and hospitals.

Gawande ends his perspective article by stating:

> The easy thing for any doctor . . . is simply to follow the written rules. But each of us has a duty not to follow rules and laws blindly. In medicine, we face conflicts about what the right and best actions are in all kinds of areas: relief of suffering for the terminally ill, provision of narcotics for patients with chronic pain, withdrawal of care for the critically ill, abortion, and executions, to name just a few. All have been the subject of professional rules and government regulation, and at times those rules and regulations will be wrong. We will then be called on to make a choice. We must do our best to choose intelligently and wisely.

Medical Education in Death and Dying

Prior to and during the 1960s, medical education was seriously deficient in areas related to death and dying. D. Black, D. Hardoff, and J. Nelki provide some evidence for this conclusion in "Educating Medical Students about Death and Dying" (*Archives of Disease in Childhood*, vol. 64, no. 5, May 1989). The researchers note that their review of the medical literature between 1960 and 1971 reveals no articles about the teaching of death and dying to medical students.

However, other medical researchers surveyed medical schools themselves to determine curricular offerings in death, dying, and palliative care (care that relieves symptoms and suffering, rather than treats or cures disease) and found that medical education became less deficient in

FIGURE 3.1

Death certificate

LOCAL FILE NO.   STATE FILE NO.

NAME OF DECEDENT — For use by physician or institution

To Be Completed/Verified By: FUNERAL DIRECTOR:

1. DECEDENT'S LEGAL NAME (Include AKA's if any) (First, Middle, Last)

2. SEX

3. SOCIAL SECURITY NUMBER

4a. AGE-Last Birthday (Years) | 4b. UNDER 1 YEAR — Months / Days | 4c. UNDER 1 DAY — Hours / Minutes | 5. DATE OF BIRTH (Mo/Day/Yr) | 6. BIRTHPLACE (City and State or Foreign Country)

7a. RESIDENCE-STATE | 7b. COUNTY | 7c. CITY OR TOWN

7d. STREET AND NUMBER | 7e. APT. NO. | 7f. ZIP CODE | 7g. INSIDE CITY LIMITS? ☐ Yes ☐ No

8. EVER IN US ARMED FORCES? ☐ Yes ☐ No | 9. MARITAL STATUS AT TIME OF DEATH ☐ Married ☐ Married, but separated ☐ Widowed ☐ Divorced ☐ Never Married ☐ Unknown | 10. SURVIVING SPOUSE'S NAME (If wife, give name prior to first marriage)

11. FATHER'S NAME (First, Middle, Last)

12. MOTHER'S NAME PRIOR TO FIRST MARRIAGE (First, Middle, Last)

13a. INFORMANT'S NAME | 13b. RELATIONSHIP TO DECEDENT | 13c. MAILING ADDRESS (Street and Number, City, State, Zip Code)

14. PLACE OF DEATH (Check only one: see instructions)

IF DEATH OCCURRED IN A HOSPITAL: ☐ Inpatient ☐ Emergency Room/Outpatient ☐ Dead on Arrival

IF DEATH OCCURRED SOMEWHERE OTHER THAN A HOSPITAL: ☐ Hospice facility ☐ Nursing home/Long term care facility ☐ Decedent's home ☐ Other (Specify):

15. FACILITY NAME (If not institution, give street & number) | 16. CITY OR TOWN , STATE, AND ZIP CODE | 17. COUNTY OF DEATH

18. METHOD OF DISPOSITION: ☐ Burial ☐ Cremation ☐ Donation ☐ Entombment ☐ Removal from State ☐ Other (Specify): | 19. PLACE OF DISPOSITION (Name of cemetery, crematory, other place)

20. LOCATION-CITY, TOWN, AND STATE | 21. NAME AND COMPLETE ADDRESS OF FUNERAL FACILITY

22. SIGNATURE OF FUNERAL SERVICE LICENSEE OR OTHER AGENT | 23. LICENSE NUMBER (Of Licensee)

ITEMS 24–28 MUST BE COMPLETED BY PERSON WHO PRONOUNCES OR CERTIFIES DEATH | 24. DATE PRONOUNCED DEAD (Mo/Day/Yr) | 25. TIME PRONOUNCED DEAD

26. SIGNATURE OF PERSON PRONOUNCING DEATH (Only when applicable) | 27. LICENSE NUMBER | 28. DATE SIGNED (Mo/Day/Yr)

29. ACTUAL OR PRESUMED DATE OF DEATH (Mo/Day/Yr) (Spell Month) | 30. ACTUAL OR PRESUMED TIME OF DEATH | 31. WAS MEDICAL EXAMINER OR CORONER CONTACTED? ☐ Yes ☐ No

To Be Completed By: MEDICAL CERTIFIER

CAUSE OF DEATH (See instructions and examples)

32. **PART I.** Enter the chain of events—diseases, injuries, or complications—that directly caused the death. DO NOT enter terminal events such as cardiac arrest, respiratory arrest, or ventricular fibrillation without showing the etiology. DO NOT ABBREVIATE. Enter only one cause on a line. Add additional lines if necessary.

Approximate interval: Onset to death

IMMEDIATE CAUSE (Final disease or condition resulting in death) ------→ a. _____
Due to (or as a consequence of):

Sequentially list conditions, if any, leading to the cause listed on line a. Enter the UNDERLYING CAUSE (disease or injury that initiated the events resulting in death) LAST

b. _____
Due to (or as a consequence of):

c. _____
Due to (or as a consequence of):

d. _____

PART II. Enter other significant conditions contributing to death but not resulting in the underlying cause given in PART I

33. WAS AN AUTOPSY PERFORMED? ☐ Yes ☐ No

34. WERE AUTOPSY FINDINGS AVAILABLE TO COMPLETE THE CAUSE OF DEATH? ☐ Yes ☐ No

35. DID TOBACCO USE CONTRIBUTE TO DEATH? ☐ Yes ☐ Probably ☐ No ☐ Unknown

36. IF FEMALE:
☐ Not pregnant within past year
☐ Pregnant at time of death
☐ Not pregnant, but pregnant within 42 days of death
☐ Not pregnant, but pregnant 43 days to 1 year before death
☐ Unknown if pregnant within the past year

37. MANNER OF DEATH
☐ Natural ☐ Homicide
☐ Accident ☐ Pending Investigation
☐ Suicide ☐ Could not be determined

38. DATE OF INJURY (Mo/Day/Yr) (Spell Month) | 39. TIME OF INJURY | 40. PLACE OF INJURY (e.g., Decedent's home; construction site; restaurant; wooded area) | 41. INJURY AT WORK? ☐ Yes ☐ No

42. LOCATION OF INJURY: State: | City or Town: | Street & Number: | Apartment No.: | Zip Code:

43. DESCRIBE HOW INJURY OCCURRED:

44. IF TRANSPORTATION INJURY, SPECIFY: ☐ Driver/Operator ☐ Passenger ☐ Pedestrian ☐ Other (Specify)

45. CERTIFIER (Check only one):
☐ Certifying physician-To the best of my knowledge, death occurred due to the cause(s) and manner stated.
☐ Pronouncing & Certifying physician-To the best of my knowledge, death occurred at the time, date, and place, and due to the cause(s) and manner stated.
☐ Medical Examiner/Coroner-On the basis of examination, and/or investigation, in my opinion, death occurred at the time, date, and place, and due to the cause(s) and manner stated.
Signature of certifier: _____

46. NAME, ADDRESS, AND ZIP CODE OF PERSON COMPLETING CAUSE OF DEATH (Item 32)

47. TITLE OF CERTIFIER | 48. LICENSE NUMBER | 49. DATE CERTIFIED (Mo/Day/Yr) | 50. **FOR REGISTRAR ONLY**–DATE FILED (Mo/Day/Yr)

To Be Completed By: FUNERAL DIRECTOR

51. DECEDENT'S EDUCATION-Check the box that best describes the highest degree or level of school completed at the time of death.
☐ 8th grade or less
☐ 9th-12th grade; no diploma
☐ High school graduate or GED completed
☐ Some college credit, but no degree
☐ Associate degree (e.g., AA, AS)
☐ Bachelor's degree (e.g., BA, AB, BS)
☐ Master's degree (e.g., MA, MS, MEng, MEd, MSW, MBA)
☐ Doctorate (e.g., PhD, EdD) or Professional degree (e.g., MD, DDS, DVM, LLB, JD)

52. DECEDENT OF HISPANIC ORIGIN? Check the box that best describes whether the decedent is Spanish/Hispanic/Latino. Check the "No" box if decedent is not Spanish/Hispanic/Latino.
☐ No, not Spanish/Hispanic/Latino
☐ Yes, Mexican, Mexican American, Chicano
☐ Yes, Puerto Rican
☐ Yes, Cuban
☐ Yes, other Spanish/Hispanic/Latino (Specify) _____

53. DECEDENT'S RACE (Check one or more races to indicate what the decedent considered himself or herself to be)
☐ White
☐ Black or African American
☐ American Indian or Alaska Native (Name of the enrolled or principal tribe) _____
☐ Asian Indian
☐ Chinese
☐ Filipino
☐ Japanese
☐ Korean
☐ Vietnamese
☐ Other Asian (Specify) _____
☐ Native Hawaiian
☐ Guamanian or Chamorro
☐ Samoan
☐ Other Pacific Islander (Specify) _____
☐ Other (Specify) _____

54. DECEDENT'S USUAL OCCUPATION (Indicate type of work done during most of working life. DO NOT USE RETIRED).

55. KIND OF BUSINESS/INDUSTRY

SOURCE: "U.S. Standard Certificate of Death," Centers for Disease Control and Prevention, National Center for Health Statistics, rev. November 2003, http://www.cdc.gov/nchs/data/dvs/death11-03final-acc.pdf (accessed February 13, 2012)

these areas after the 1960s. For example, Edward H. Liston reports in "Education of Death and Dying: A Survey of American Medical Schools" (*Journal of Medical Education*, vol. 48, no. 6, June 1973) that in 1972 approximately half of U.S. medical schools included some formal teaching on death and dying. In "Characteristics of Death Education Curricula in American Medical Schools" (*Journal of Medical Education*, vol. 55, no. 10, October 1980), Marc D. Smith, Maryellen McSweeney, and Barry M. Katz indicate that the situation improved by the late 1970s. The researchers note that according to a survey conducted during the 1978–79 academic year, 92% of U.S. medical schools had "a structured death education curriculum." Nonetheless, the scope of this "structured" curriculum varied widely among medical schools. In most of these schools it consisted of a course or courses in which death and dying were only two of a variety of topics.

George E. Dickinson of the College of Charleston in Charleston, South Carolina, studied medical school offerings on end-of-life issues by mailing brief questionnaires to all accredited U.S. medical schools in 1975, 1980, 1985, 1990, 1995, 2000, and 2005 and published his findings in "Teaching End-of-Life Issues in US Medical Schools: 1975 to 2005" (*American Journal of Hospice and Palliative Medicine*, vol. 23, no. 3, June–July 2006). The percentage of medical schools that offered separate courses in death and dying fluctuated between 1975 and 2005, with a low of 7% of medical schools in 1975 to a high of 18% of medical schools in both 1990 and 2000. The percentage of lectures and short courses that incorporated death and dying information also fluctuated between 1975 and 2005, with a low of 70% of lectures and short courses incorporating death and dying topics in 1995 to a high of 87% in 2005. Nonetheless, the number of students enrolled in death and dying offerings increased during this period, growing slowly from 71% in 1975 to 77% in 1995. A jump then occurred, with medical schools reporting 96% of their students enrolled in death and dying offerings in both 2000 and 2005. On a more general note, Dickenson indicates that before 2000, approximately 70% of medical schools included "something" in their curriculum on death and dying, and by 2005, 100% did.

In both 2000 and 2005 palliative care training was not covered in separate courses in many U.S. medical schools, with only 11% of schools offering a separate course in 2000 and 8% in 2005. The most popular mode of palliative care training by medical schools was incorporating palliative care topics as modules of larger courses. This was the case in 41% of medical schools in 2000 and in 59% of medical schools in 2005. The percentage of schools that included palliative care training throughout the curriculum and in clerkships in which students are usually assigned patients decreased from 22% in 2000 to 12% in 2005.

In "Palliative Care in Medical School Curricula: A Survey of United States Medical Schools" (*Journal of Palliative Medicine*, vol. 11, no. 9, November 2008), Emily S. Van Aalst-Cohen, Raine Riggs, and Ira R. Byock provide an update on offerings in palliative care in U.S. medical schools. In 2007 the researchers conducted a survey of 128 medical schools and also used information from the Association of American Medical Colleges Curriculum Management and Information Tool database. They determine that palliative care was a required course in 30% of medical schools, was an elective in 15% of medical schools, and was integrated into required courses in 53% of medical schools.

One program in particular stands out in death and dying education. The Education in Palliative and End-of-Life Care (EPEC) Project is an ongoing training program developed in 1998 by the American Medical Association (AMA). The EPEC Project has a death and dying curriculum that emphasizes the development of skills and competence in the areas of communication, ethical decision making, palliative care, psychosocial issues, and pain and symptom management. The program became fully operational in 1999 and provides curricula to all leaders of medical societies, medical school deans, and major medical organizations. Between 1996 and 2003 the EPEC Project was supported with funding from the Robert Wood Johnson Foundation. After 2003 it was sponsored by and housed at Northwestern University's Feinberg School of Medicine in Chicago, Illinois, with a mission to educate all health care professionals on the essential clinical competencies in end-of-life care.

According to the EPEC Project (2012, http://www.epec.net/), it "has created a comprehensive, consensus-based, end-user friendly curriculum for the field of palliative care in the United States." By providing conferences and distance-learning opportunities for physicians and other health care workers from various disciplines, the EPEC Project intends "to educate all health care professionals in the essential clinical competencies of palliative care."

Contemporary Ethical Guidelines for Physicians

Physicians are trained to save lives, not to let people die. Advanced medical technology, with respirators and parenteral nutrition (artificial feeding devices that provide nutrition to an otherwise unconscious patient), can prolong the process of dying. Ira R. Byock, a well-known palliative care physician and a former president of the American Academy of Hospice and Palliative Medicine, admits in one of his early books, *Dying Well: The Prospect for Growth at the End of Life* (1997), that "a strong presumption throughout my medical career was that all seriously ill people required vigorous life-prolonging treatment, including those who were expected to die, even patients with advanced chronic illness such as wide spread cancer, end stage congestive heart failure, and kidney or liver failure. It even extended to patients who saw death as a relief from suffering caused by their illness."

However, more recent medical education has changed the focus from life-prolonging treatment for all patients to one of understanding the futility of prolonging the life and death of a terminally ill and actively dying patient. Medical ethics now recognizes the obligation of physicians to shift the intent of care for dying patients from that of futile procedures that may only increase patient distress to that of comfort and closure.

The AMA provides ethical guidelines to help educate and support physicians in such end-of-life care. The AMA's *Code of Medical Ethics: Principles, Opinions, and Reports* (2012, http://www.ama-assn.org/ama/pub/ physician-resources/medical-ethics/code-medical-ethics .shtml) provides end-of-life ethical guidelines in the following areas: 2.037 "Medical Futility in End-of-Life Care"; 2.20 "Withholding or Withdrawing Life-Sustaining Medical Treatment"; 2.201 "Sedation to Unconsciousness in End-of-Life Care"; 2.21 "Euthanasia"; 2.211 "Physician-Assisted Suicide"; 2.22 "Do-Not-Resuscitate Orders"; and 2.225 "Optimal Use of Orders-Not-to-Intervene and Advance Directives."

The American College of Physicians also provides clinical practice guidelines in end-of-life care. Examples of articles that provide such guidelines include Amir Qaseem et al.'s "Evidence-Based Interventions to Improve the Palliative Care of Pain, Dyspnea, and Depression at the End of Life: A Clinical Practice Guideline from the American College of Physicians" (*Annals of Internal Medicine*, vol. 148, no. 2, January 15, 2008) and Karl A. Lorenz et al.'s "Evidence for Improving Palliative Care at the End of Life: A Systematic Review" (*Annals of Internal Medicine*, vol. 148, no. 2, January 15, 2008).

PATIENT AUTONOMY

According to the principle of patient autonomy, competent patients have the right to self-rule—to choose among medically recommended treatments and to refuse any treatment they do not want. To be truly autonomous, patients have to be told about the nature of their illness, the prospects for recovery, the course of the illness, alternative treatments, and treatment consequences. After thoughtful consideration, a patient makes an informed choice and grants "informed consent" to treatment or decides to forgo treatment. Decisions about medical treatment may be influenced by the patient's psychological state, family history, culture, values, and religious beliefs.

Cultural Differences

Even though patient autonomy is a fundamental aspect of medical ethics, not all patients want to know about their illnesses or be involved in decisions about their terminal care. In "Cultural Diversity at the End of Life: Issues and Guidelines for Family Physicians" (*American Family Physician*, vol. 71, no. 3, February 1, 2005), the best study regarding multicultural approaches to death and dying as of April 2012, H. Russell Searight and Jennifer Gafford of the Forest Park Hospital Family Medicine Residency Program in St. Louis, Missouri, note that the concept of patient autonomy is not easily applied to members of some racial and ethnic groups. Searight and Gafford explain the three basic dimensions in end-of-life treatment that vary culturally: communication of bad news, locus of decision making, and attitudes toward advance directives and end-of-life care.

Members of some ethnic groups, such as many Africans and Japanese, soften bad news with terms that do not overtly state that a person has a potentially terminal condition. For example, the term *growth* or *blood disease* may be used rather than telling a person he or she has a cancerous tumor or leukemia. This concept is taken one step further in many Hispanic, Chinese, and Pakistani communities, in which the terminally ill are generally protected from knowledge of their condition. Many reasons exist for this type of behavior, such as viewing the discussion of serious illness and death as disrespectful or impolite, not wanting to cause anxiety or eliminate hope in the patient, or believing that speaking about a condition makes it real. Many people of Asian and European cultures believe it is cruel to inform a patient of a terminal diagnosis.

Another excellent study on multiculturalism in death and dying issues is Jessica Doolen and Nancy L. York's "Cultural Differences with End-of-Life Care in the Critical Care Unit" (*Dimensions of Critical Care Nursing*, vol. 26, no. 5, September–October 2007). In this study, the researchers add similar cultural scenarios in communication about death and dying to those outlined by Searight and Gafford. Doolen and York note that South Koreans generally do not talk about the dying process because it fosters sadness and because such discussions may quicken the dying process. Those in the Filipino culture believe discussions of death interfere with God's will and, as in the South Korean culture, may hasten death.

The phrase "locus of decision making" refers to those making the end-of-life decisions: the physician, the family, and/or the patient. Searight and Gafford explain that the locus of decision making varies among cultures. For example, in North America the patient typically decides for his or her own medical care. South Koreans and Mexicans often approach end-of-life decision making differently, abiding by a collective decision process in which relatives make treatment choices for a family member without that person's input. East Europeans and Russians often look to the physician as the expert in end-of-life decision making. In Asian, Indian, and Pakistani cultures, physicians and family members may share decision making. Doolen and York note that in the Afghan culture health care decisions are made by the head of the family, possibly in consultation with an educated younger family member.

An advance directive (often called a living will) is a written statement that explains a person's wishes about end-of-life medical care. Completion of advance directives varies among cultures. For example, Searight and Gafford note that approximately 40% of elderly whites have completed advance directives, whereas only 16% of elderly African-Americans have done the same. Doolen and York add that Mexican-Americans, African-Americans, Native Americans, and Asian-Americans do not share the typical American philosophy that end-of-life decisions are the individual's responsibility and are much less likely than the general American population to sign advance directives or do-not-resuscitate orders.

Because of differences among cultures regarding various facets of end-of-life decision making and preparedness, physicians need to understand that patient autonomy is far from a universally held ideal. There are differences of opinion not only among ethnic groups but also within each ethnic group, such as differences with age. People bring their cultural values to bear on decisions about terminal care.

Health Care Proxies and Surrogate Decision Makers

When a patient is incompetent to make informed decisions about his or her medical treatment, a proxy or a surrogate must make the decision for that patient. Some patients, in anticipation of being in a position of incompetence, will execute a durable power of attorney for health care by designating a proxy. Most people choose family members or close friends who will make all medical decisions, including the withholding or withdrawal of life-sustaining treatments.

When a proxy has not been named in advance, health care providers usually involve family members in medical decisions. Most states have laws that govern surrogate decision making. Some states designate family members, by order of kinship, to assume the role of surrogates.

THE DESIRE TO DIE: EUTHANASIA AND ASSISTED SUICIDE

Serious diseases such as acquired immunodeficiency syndrome (AIDS) and metastatic cancer have directed societal attention to end-of-life decision making because many patients who are suffering as they die would like their death to be hastened. In "Oregonians' Reasons for Requesting Physician Aid in Dying" (*Archives of Internal Medicine*, vol. 169, no. 5, March 9, 2009), Linda Ganzini, Elizabeth R. Goy, and Steven K. Dobscha discuss the reasons that terminally ill Oregonians gave for wanting a physician to aid them in dying. In Oregon dying patients may make such requests under the Oregon Death with Dignity Act (see Chapter 6). Of the 56 patients who were surveyed, the average age was 65.8 years and nearly half had

completed college. Slightly more were female (52%) than male (48%), and nearly all were white (98%). Nearly two-thirds (61%) were single, divorced, or widowed, and most (95%) lived independently. The terminal diagnosis for most (77%) of the patients was cancer, but 11% had amyotrophic lateral sclerosis (a degenerative neurologic condition commonly known as Lou Gehrig's disease), 9% had heart disease, and the remaining 4% had AIDS or hepatitis C. Thirty-six percent were enrolled in hospice care.

Ganzini, Goy, and Dobscha determine that the patients' most important reasons for wanting physician aid in dying included controlling the circumstances of their death and dying at home. Furthermore, the patients wanted to avoid a poor quality of life, pain, the inability to care for themselves, and a loss of independence. Other important reasons included the perception of themselves as being a burden, the loss of dignity, and the fear of a bad death. In "Why Oregon Patients Request Assisted Death: Family Members' Views" (*Journal of General Internal Medicine*, vol. 23, no. 2, February 2008), Ganzini, Goy, and Dobscha note that family members' views on why patients requested physician-assisted death paralleled the patients' reasons.

Molly L. Olsen, Keith M. Swetz, and Paul S. Mueller discuss palliative sedation in "Ethical Decision Making with End-of-Life Care: Palliative Sedation and Withholding or Withdrawing Life-Sustaining Treatments" (*Mayo Clinic Proceedings*, vol. 85, no. 10, October 2010). The researchers define palliative sedation as medications that "induce decreased or absent awareness in order to relieve otherwise intractable suffering at the end of life." Palliative sedation is legal but is not used frequently. Even so, it is an important medical tool for end-of-life care.

Olsen, Swetz, and Mueller discuss the differences among various end-of-life treatments, their use, the cause of death, and their legality. The five end-of-life treatments that they address are withholding life-sustaining treatment, withdrawing life-sustaining treatment, palliative sedation and analgesia (painkillers), physician-assisted suicide, and euthanasia. In the first, life-sustaining treatment is withheld if it is not already being used, and in the second, life-sustaining treatment is withdrawn if it is being used. For example, if a dying patient suffers a heart attack, nothing will be done to resuscitate him or her (withholding life-sustaining treatment). In another example, if a patient is on a ventilator, he or she will slowly be removed from the device (withdrawing life-sustaining treatment). The goal of both end-of-life treatments is to avoid life-saving interventions, and both are legal. The third treatment, providing palliative sedation and analgesia, is done to relieve patient symptoms and is legal as well. The patients' cause of death from all three end-of-life treatments is the underlying disease.

Physician-assisted suicide is legal only in Oregon, Washington, and Montana; it is illegal in the 47 remaining states. Its goal is to end the dying patient's life. In physician-assisted suicide, the physician sets up the drug in a way that the patient can administer it. Euthanasia is different in that the physician administers the drug. The goal of both is termination of the patient's life. Physician-assisted suicide is legal or illegal, depending on the state in which the patient lives, whereas euthanasia is illegal in all 50 states.

Jack Kevorkian (1928–2011) conducted physician-assisted suicides in the 1990s until he performed euthanasia on a terminally ill man in 1998, which he videotaped and gave the video to the CBS television show *60 Minutes* for broadcast. In 1999 he was tried and convicted for this death, and he served until 2007, when he was paroled. He died in 2011 at the age of 83 from a pulmonary thrombosis (blood clot). One of his famous quotes was "Dying is not a crime." Chapter 6 details more of Kevorkian's life.

CHAPTER 4
THE END OF LIFE: MEDICAL CONSIDERATIONS

TRENDS IN CAUSES OF DEATH

The primary causes of death in the United States have changed dramatically over the past two centuries. During the 1800s and early 1900s infectious (communicable) diseases such as influenza, tuberculosis, and diphtheria (a potentially deadly upper respiratory infection) were the leading causes of death. These have been replaced by chronic noninfectious diseases; that is, heart disease, malignant neoplasms (cancer), and chronic lower respiratory disease were the three leading causes of death in 2010. (See Table 4.1.)

In 2010 the age-adjusted death rate for heart disease, which accounts for changes in the age distribution of the population across time, was 178.5 deaths per 100,000 population, the age-adjusted death rate for cancer was 172.5 per 100,000 population, and the age-adjusted death rate for chronic lower respiratory diseases was 42.1 per 100,000 population. (See Table 4.1.) Together, these three diseases accounted for 53% of all deaths in the United States in 2010.

Many factors are involved in having a heart attack or developing cancer. For example, Norrina Allen et al. indicate in "Impact of Blood Pressure and Blood Pressure Change during Middle Age on the Remaining Lifetime Risk for Cardiovascular Disease: The Cardiovascular Lifetime Risk Pooling Project" (*Circulation*, vol. 125, no. 1, January 3, 2012) that changes in blood pressure in middle age have a significant bearing on the lifetime risk for cardiovascular disease (CVD). The researchers find that those who had normal blood pressure at middle age had the lowest risk for CVD, whereas those who developed hypertension (high blood pressure) in middle age raised their risk for CVD. Concerning cancer, the National Cancer Institute notes in the fact sheet "Obesity and Cancer Risk" (January 3, 2012, http://www.cancer.gov/cancer topics/factsheet/Risk/obesity) that cancer rates in general have decreased, but that cancer rates have increased for some less common types of cancer. The institute believes

that obesity is a major cause of these types of cancers, which include cancers of the esophagus, pancreas, colon and rectum, breast (after menopause), endometrium, kidney, thyroid, and gallbladder.

Not surprisingly, the leading causes of death vary by age. For those from birth to 34 years old, accidents and their adverse effects were the leading cause of death between 1999 and 2009. (See Table 4.2.) Accidents were also the leading cause of death for those aged 35 to 44 years between 2002 and 2009. For those aged 35 to 44 years, cancer was the leading cause of death between 1999 and 2001, with accidents and their adverse effects second and heart disease third. Cancer and heart disease caused the most deaths among those 45 years and older between 1999 and 2009.

The age group of 25 to 44 years is not shown as such in Table 4.3, but it is notable that the acquired immunodeficiency syndrome (AIDS) was the sixth-leading cause of death in this group in 2007, according to the Centers for Disease Control and Prevention's (CDC) National Center for Injury Prevention and Control (2012, http://webappa .cdc.gov/sasweb/ncipc/leadcaus10.html). Nonetheless, deaths from AIDS have fallen dramatically since the mid-1990s largely due to the growing use of antiretroviral drugs. In 1994 and 1995 AIDS was the leading cause of death in this age group in the United States. The CDC indicates in *HIV/AIDS Surveillance Report: U.S. HIV and AIDS Cases Reported through December 1997* (1997, http://www.cdc .gov/hiv/topics/surveillance/resources/reports/pdf/hivsur92 .pdf) that a decline occurred in U.S. AIDS deaths in 1996 for the first time since the disease was first recognized and tracked in 1981. According to the CDC, in *HIV/AIDS Surveillance Report: U.S. HIV and AIDS Cases Reported through December 1999* (1999, http://www.cdc.gov/hiv/ topics/surveillance/resources/reports/pdf/hasr1102.pdf), this downward trend in the annual number of deaths from AIDS continued through 1998, when AIDS dropped to being the fifth-leading cause of death among

TABLE 4.1

Death rates for the 15 leading causes of death, 2010, and percentage change, 2009–10

Rank[a]	Cause of death	Number	Death rate	Age-adjusted death rate[b]		
				2010	**2009**	**Percent change**
—	All causes	2,465,932	798.7	746.2	749.6	−0.5
1	Diseases of heart	595,444	192.9	178.5	182.8	−2.4
2	Malignant neoplasms	573,855	185.9	172.5	173.5	−0.6
3	Chronic lower respiratory diseases	137,789	44.6	42.1	42.7	−1.4
4	Cerebrovascular diseases	129,180	41.8	39.0	39.6	−1.5
5	Accidents (unintentional injuries)	118,043	38.2	37.1	37.5	−1.1
6	Alzheimer's disease	83,308	27.0	25.0	24.2	3.3
7	Diabetes mellitus	68,905	22.3	20.8	21.0	−1.0
8	Nephritis, nephrotic syndrome and nephrosis	50,472	16.3	15.3	15.1	1.3
9	Influenza and pneumonia	50,003	16.2	15.1	16.5	−8.5
10	Intentional self-harm (suicide)	37,793	12.2	11.9	11.8	0.8
11	Septicemia	34,843	11.3	10.6	11.0	−3.6
12	Chronic liver disease and cirrhosis	31,802	10.3	9.4	9.1	3.3
13	Essential hypertension and hypertensive renal disease	26,577	8.6	7.9	7.8	1.3
14	Parkinson's disease	21,963	7.1	6.8	6.5	4.6
15	Pneumonitis due to solids and liquids	17,001	5.5	5.1	4.9	4.1
—	All other causes	488,954	158.5	—	—	—

—Category not applicable.
[a]Rank based on number of deaths.
[b]Rates are per 100,000 population.
Notes: Data are subject to sampling and random variation. Data are based on a continuous file of records received from the states. Rates are per 100,000 population. Rates are based on populations enumerated in the 2010 census as of April 1 for 2010 and estimated as of July 1 for 2009. Figures for 2010 are based on weighted data rounded to the nearest individual, so categories may not add to totals.

SOURCE: Sherry L. Murphy, Jiaquan Xu, and Kenneth D. Kochanek, "Table B. Deaths and Death Rates for 2010 and Age-Adjusted Death Rates and Percent Changes in Age-Adjusted Rates From 2009 to 2010 for the 15 Leading Causes of Death in 2010: United States, Final 2009 and Preliminary 2010," in "Deaths: Preliminary Data for 2010," *National Vital Statistics Reports*, vol. 60, no. 4, January 11, 2012, http://www.cdc.gov/nchs/data/nvsr/nvsr60/nvsr60_04.pdf (accessed January 31, 2012)

people aged 25 to 44 years. As the downward trend continued, not only had AIDS dropped to being the sixth-leading cause of death in those aged 25 to 44 years by 2006 but also the number of deaths from AIDS reached an all-time low of 16,605 in 2008.

Between 2006 and 2008 most males with AIDS contracted the human immunodeficiency virus (HIV; the virus that leads to AIDS) via male-to-male sexual contact or injection drug use. (See Table 4.3.) Most females contracted the virus by heterosexual contact with high-risk partners or injection drug use. Children most often contracted the virus perinatally (immediately before and after birth) from infected mothers. The South and the Northeast, respectively, experienced more AIDS deaths during these years than other parts of the United States.

LIFE-SUSTAINING TREATMENTS

As people succumb to the chronic, noninfectious diseases that are the leading causes of death in the United States, life-sustaining (life support) treatments are often used. Such treatments are not controversial when a patient suffers from a treatable illness, because life support is a temporary measure that is used only until the body can function on its own. The ongoing debate is about using life-sustaining treatments with the incurably ill and permanently unconscious. Not only do these treatments prolong life but also they may prolong death and may even add to a patient's suffering.

Another side of the debate is expressed by Shan Mohammed and Elizabeth Peter in "Rituals, Death and the Moral Practice of Medical Futility" (*Nursing Ethics*, vol. 16, no. 3, May 2009). The researchers suggest that medical interventions with dying patients, which may be considered futile in a physiological sense, may not be futile in a psychological and social sense. They argue that providing life support technologies to dying patients "have significant ritualistic value and serve important social functions in the process of dying.... As moral practices, CPR and ICU [intensive care unit] care help to address the problem of being responsible for the patient's death, dissipate the sense of ambiguity between life and death, establish a social script for letting go, and realize a space where the grieving process can begin." Mohammed and Peter acknowledge, however, that physiological suffering may occur when life support is provided to dying patients and suggest that "ultimately, it may be possible to explore alternative practices of death and dying that result in less suffering and cost to both patients and the health care system."

The following sections describe the types of life-sustaining medical interventions that are often used in end-of-life care and that may help or hinder a terminal patient's progress toward a comfortable death.

TABLE 4.2

Death rates, by age, for the 15 leading causes of death, 1999–2009

Cause of death and year	All ages[a]	Under 1 year[b]	1–4 years	5–14 years	15–24 years	25–34 years	35–44 years	45–54 years	55–64 years	65–74 years	75–84 years	85 years and over	Age-adjusted rate
All causes													
2009	793.8	619.8	26.1	13.9	70.6	102.3	179.8	420.6	871.9	1,928.8	4,774.4	13,021.2	741.1
2008	813.0	650.5	28.3	14.1	75.6	103.3	179.7	420.4	879.2	1,995.6	5,017.7	13,015.1	758.3
2007	803.6	684.5	28.6	15.3	79.9	104.9	184.4	420.9	877.7	2,011.3	5,011.6	12,946.5	760.2
2006	810.4	690.7	28.4	15.2	82.2	106.3	190.2	427.5	890.9	2,062.1	5,115.0	13,253.1	776.5
2005	825.9	692.5	29.4	16.3	81.4	104.4	193.3	432.0	906.9	2,137.1	5,260.0	13,798.6	798.8
2004	816.5	685.2	29.9	16.8	80.1	102.1	193.5	427.0	910.3	2,164.6	5,275.1	13,823.5	800.8
2003	841.9	700.0	31.5	17.0	81.5	103.6	201.6	433.2	940.9	2,255.0	5,463.1	14,593.3	832.7
2002	847.3	695.0	31.2	17.4	81.4	103.6	202.9	430.1	952.4	2,314.7	5,556.9	14,828.3	845.3
2001	848.5	683.4	33.3	17.3	80.7	105.2	203.6	428.9	964.6	2,353.3	5,582.4	15,112.8	854.5
2000	854.0	736.7	32.4	18.0	79.9	101.4	198.9	425.6	992.2	2,399.1	5,666.5	15,524.4	869.0
1999	857.0	736.0	34.2	18.6	79.3	102.2	198.0	418.2	1,005.0	2,457.3	5,714.5	15,554.6	875.6
Diseases of heart													
2009	195.2	9.1	0.9	0.5	2.4	7.6	26.7	82.8	193.4	431.7	1,199.3	4,115.0	180.1
2008	202.9	9.2	1.1	0.6	2.5	7.9	26.7	85.4	198.0	449.8	1,276.7	4,175.7	186.5
2007	204.3	10.0	1.1	0.6	2.6	7.9	27.4	85.3	200.3	462.9	1,315.0	4,267.7	190.9
2006	211.0	8.4	1.0	0.6	2.5	8.2	28.3	88.0	207.3	490.3	1,383.1	4,480.8	200.2
2005	220.0	8.7	0.9	0.6	2.7	8.1	28.9	89.7	214.8	518.9	1,460.8	4,778.4	211.1
2004	222.2	10.3	1.2	0.6	2.5	7.9	29.3	90.2	218.8	541.6	1,506.3	4,895.9	217.0
2003	235.6	11.0	1.2	0.6	2.7	8.2	30.7	92.5	233.2	585.0	1,611.1	5,278.4	232.3
2002	241.7	12.4	1.1	0.6	2.5	7.9	30.5	93.7	241.5	615.9	1,677.2	5,466.8	240.8
2001	245.8	11.9	1.5	0.7	2.5	8.0	29.6	92.9	246.9	635.1	1,725.7	5,664.2	247.8
2000	252.6	13.0	1.2	0.7	2.6	7.4	29.2	94.2	261.2	665.6	1,780.3	5,926.1	257.6
1999	259.9	13.8	1.2	0.7	2.8	7.6	30.2	95.7	269.9	701.7	1,849.9	6,063.0	266.5
Malignant neoplasms													
2009	184.9	1.7	2.1	2.2	3.8	8.8	30.1	113.5	307.1	682.3	1,201.4	1,619.8	173.2
2008	186.0	1.6	2.4	2.2	3.9	8.6	29.9	113.6	309.0	701.5	1,235.8	1,566.1	175.3
2007	186.6	1.7	2.2	2.4	3.9	8.5	30.8	114.3	315.4	715.5	1,256.3	1,590.2	178.4
2006	187.0	1.8	2.3	2.2	3.9	9.0	31.9	116.3	321.2	727.2	1,263.8	1,606.1	180.7
2005	188.7	1.8	2.3	2.5	4.1	9.0	33.2	118.6	326.9	742.7	1,274.8	1,637.7	183.8
2004	188.6	1.8	2.5	2.5	4.1	9.1	33.4	119.0	333.4	755.1	1,280.4	1,653.3	185.8
2003	191.5	1.9	2.5	2.6	4.0	9.4	35.0	122.2	343.0	770.3	1,302.5	1,698.2	190.1
2002	193.2	1.8	2.6	2.6	4.3	9.7	35.8	123.8	351.1	792.1	1,311.9	1,723.9	193.5
2001	194.4	1.6	2.7	2.5	4.3	10.1	36.8	126.5	356.5	802.8	1,315.8	1,765.6	196.0
2000	196.5	2.4	2.7	2.5	4.4	9.8	36.6	127.5	366.7	816.3	1,335.6	1,819.4	199.6
1999	197.0	1.8	2.7	2.5	4.5	10.0	37.1	127.6	374.6	827.1	1,331.5	1,805.8	200.8
Chronic lower respiratory diseases													
2009	44.7	0.6	0.4	0.3	0.4	0.7	1.8	10.5	40.7	150.6	372.8	652.9	42.3
2008	46.4	0.7	0.3	0.3	0.4	0.6	1.9	9.9	41.7	158.9	396.9	656.2	44.0
2007	42.4	1.0	0.3	0.3	0.4	0.6	1.8	9.5	39.1	148.1	368.9	596.1	40.8
2006	41.6	0.7	0.3	0.3	0.4	0.6	1.9	9.1	39.2	149.3	363.4	589.1	40.5
2005	44.2	0.8	0.3	0.3	0.4	0.6	2.0	9.4	42.0	160.5	385.6	637.2	43.2
2004	41.5	0.9	0.3	0.3	0.4	0.6	2.0	8.4	40.4	153.8	366.7	601.7	41.1
2003	43.5	0.8	0.3	0.3	0.5	0.7	2.1	8.7	43.3	163.2	383.0	635.1	43.3
2002	43.3	1.0	0.4	0.3	0.5	0.8	2.2	8.7	42.4	163.0	386.7	637.6	43.5
2001	43.2	1.0	0.3	0.3	0.4	0.7	2.2	8.5	44.1	167.9	379.8	644.7	43.7
2000	43.4	0.9	0.3	0.3	0.5	0.7	2.1	8.6	44.2	169.4	386.1	648.6	44.2
1999	44.5	0.9	0.4	0.3	0.5	0.8	2.0	8.5	47.5	177.2	397.8	646.0	45.4
Cerebrovascular diseases													
2009	42.0	3.4	0.3	0.2	0.4	1.3	4.6	13.8	30.2	84.5	292.1	945.8	38.9
2008	44.1	3.3	0.4	0.2	0.4	1.3	4.8	13.8	31.0	88.9	314.5	972.6	40.7
2007	45.1	3.1	0.3	0.2	0.5	1.2	4.9	14.6	32.1	93.0	322.3	1,015.5	42.2
2006	45.8	3.4	0.3	0.2	0.5	1.3	5.1	14.7	33.3	96.3	335.1	1,039.6	43.6
2005	48.4	3.1	0.4	0.2	0.5	1.4	5.2	15.0	33.0	101.1	359.0	1,141.8	46.6
2004	51.1	3.1	0.3	0.2	0.5	1.4	5.4	14.9	34.3	107.8	386.2	1,245.9	50.0
2003	54.2	2.5	0.3	0.2	0.5	1.5	5.5	15.0	35.6	112.9	410.7	1,370.1	53.5
2002	56.4	2.9	0.3	0.2	0.4	1.4	5.4	15.1	37.2	120.3	431.0	1,445.9	56.2
2001	57.4	2.7	0.4	0.2	0.5	1.5	5.5	15.1	38.0	123.4	443.9	1,500.2	57.9
2000	59.6	3.3	0.3	0.2	0.5	1.5	5.8	16.0	41.0	128.6	461.3	1,589.2	60.9
1999	60.0	2.7	0.3	0.2	0.5	1.4	5.7	15.2	40.6	130.8	469.8	1,614.8	61.6

Cardiopulmonary Resuscitation

Traditional cardiopulmonary resuscitation (CPR) consists of two basic life-support skills that are administered in the event of cardiac or respiratory arrest: artificial circulation and artificial respiration. Cardiac arrest may be caused by a heart attack, which is an interruption of blood flow to the heart muscle. A coronary artery that is clogged with an accumulation of fatty deposits is a common cause of interrupted blood

TABLE 4.2

Death rates, by age, for the 15 leading causes of death, 1999–2009 [CONTINUED]

Cause of death and year	All ages[a]	Under 1 year[b]	1–4 years	5–14 years	15–24 years	25–34 years	35–44 years	45–54 years	55–64 years	65–74 years	75–84 years	85 years and over	Age-adjusted rate
Accidents (unintentional injuries)													
2009	38.4	27.7	8.6	4.2	28.9	33.8	36.4	44.8	37.2	43.0	102.5	296.4	37.3
2008	40.1	30.5	8.8	4.6	33.1	35.6	37.8	45.9	37.9	44.7	106.2	289.0	38.8
2007	41.0	30.2	9.6	5.5	37.4	36.9	39.2	46.3	37.3	45.2	105.5	286.7	40.0
2006	40.6	27.8	9.9	5.6	38.2	37.0	40.2	45.5	36.2	44.5	105.1	274.9	39.8
2005	39.7	26.4	10.3	6.0	37.4	34.9	38.6	43.2	35.8	46.3	106.1	279.5	39.1
2004	38.1	25.8	10.3	6.5	37.0	32.6	37.3	40.7	33.2	44.0	103.7	276.7	37.7
2003	37.6	23.6	10.9	6.4	37.1	31.5	37.8	38.8	32.9	44.1	101.9	278.9	37.3
2002	37.0	23.5	10.5	6.6	38.0	31.5	37.2	36.6	31.4	44.2	101.3	275.4	36.9
2001	35.7	24.2	11.2	6.9	36.1	29.9	35.4	34.1	30.3	42.8	100.9	276.4	35.7
2000	34.8	23.1	11.9	7.3	36.0	29.5	34.1	32.6	30.9	41.9	95.1	273.5	34.9
1999	35.1	22.3	12.4	7.6	35.3	29.6	33.8	31.8	30.6	44.6	100.5	282.4	35.3
Alzheimer's disease													
2009	25.7	*	*	*	*	*	*	0.3	2.1	19.8	177.4	901.0	23.5
2008	27.1	*	*	*	*	*	*	0.2	2.2	21.5	193.3	910.1	24.4
2007	24.7	*	*	*	*	*	*	0.2	2.2	20.6	176.7	849.1	22.7
2006	24.2	*	*	*	*	*	*	0.2	2.1	20.2	175.6	848.3	22.6
2005	24.2	*	*	*	*	*	*	0.2	2.1	20.5	177.3	861.6	22.9
2004	22.5	*	*	*	*	*	*	0.2	1.9	19.7	168.7	818.8	21.8
2003	21.8	*	*	*	*	*	*	0.2	2.0	20.9	164.4	802.4	21.4
2002	20.4	*	*	*	*	*	*	0.1	1.9	19.7	158.1	752.3	20.2
2001	18.9	*	*	*	*	*	*	0.2	2.1	18.7	147.5	710.3	19.1
2000	17.6	*	*	*	*	*	*	0.2	2.0	18.7	139.6	667.7	18.1
1999	16.0	*	*	*	*	*	*	0.2	1.9	17.4	129.5	601.3	16.5
Diabetes mellitus													
2009	22.4	*	*	0.1	0.4	1.5	4.5	12.8	32.7	71.1	144.4	269.4	20.9
2008	23.2	*	*	0.1	0.5	1.4	4.4	12.7	33.8	76.1	153.8	271.4	21.8
2007	23.7	*	*	0.1	0.4	1.5	4.6	13.1	34.6	78.1	162.7	276.2	22.5
2006	24.2	*	*	0.1	0.4	1.7	4.8	13.2	36.2	81.8	166.8	285.2	23.3
2005	25.3	*	*	0.1	0.5	1.5	4.7	13.4	37.2	86.8	177.2	312.1	24.6
2004	24.9	*	*	0.1	0.4	1.5	4.6	13.4	37.1	87.2	176.9	307.0	24.5
2003	25.5	*	*	0.1	0.4	1.6	4.6	13.9	38.5	90.8	181.1	317.5	25.3
2002	25.4	*	*	0.1	0.4	1.6	4.8	13.7	37.7	91.4	182.8	320.6	25.4
2001	25.1	*	*	0.1	0.4	1.5	4.3	13.6	37.8	91.4	181.4	321.8	25.3
2000	24.6	*	*	0.1	0.4	1.6	4.3	13.1	37.8	90.7	179.5	319.7	25.0
1999	24.5	*	*	0.1	0.4	1.4	4.3	12.9	38.3	91.8	178.0	317.2	25.0
Influenza and pneumonia													
2009[c]	17.5	5.9	0.9	0.6	1.0	1.9	3.2	6.5	11.9	30.1	105.9	413.5	16.2
2008	18.5	5.2	0.9	0.2	0.5	0.9	2.1	5.1	11.1	31.1	119.1	465.2	16.9
2007	17.5	5.2	0.7	0.3	0.4	0.8	1.8	4.4	9.6	28.7	114.1	463.2	16.2
2006	18.8	6.4	0.8	0.2	0.4	0.8	1.9	4.6	10.0	32.0	127.8	502.5	17.8
2005	21.3	6.5	0.7	0.3	0.4	0.9	2.1	5.1	11.3	35.5	142.2	593.9	20.3
2004	20.3	6.7	0.7	0.2	0.4	0.8	2.0	4.6	10.8	34.6	139.3	582.6	19.8
2003	22.4	8.0	1.0	0.4	0.5	0.9	2.2	5.2	11.2	37.3	151.1	666.1	22.0
2002	22.8	6.5	0.7	0.2	0.4	0.9	2.2	4.8	11.2	37.5	156.9	696.6	22.6
2001	21.8	7.4	0.7	0.2	0.5	0.9	2.2	4.6	10.7	36.3	148.5	685.6	22.0
2000	23.2	7.6	0.7	0.2	0.5	0.9	2.4	4.7	11.9	39.1	160.3	744.1	23.7
1999	22.8	8.4	0.8	0.2	0.5	0.8	2.4	4.6	11.0	37.2	157.0	751.8	23.5
Nephritis, nephrotic syndrome and nephrosis													
2009	15.9	2.6	*	*	0.2	0.6	2.0	5.3	13.8	39.5	114.0	306.3	14.9
2008	15.9	3.3	*	*	0.2	0.6	1.8	5.0	14.3	40.7	113.8	295.7	14.8
2007	15.4	3.4	0.1	0.1	0.2	0.6	1.7	5.1	13.6	40.1	113.0	290.6	14.5
2006	15.1	3.9	*	*	0.2	0.7	1.8	5.2	13.8	39.4	111.4	290.5	14.5
2005	14.8	3.9	*	0.1	0.2	0.7	1.7	4.8	13.6	39.3	110.3	288.3	14.3
2004	14.5	4.3	*	0.1	0.2	0.6	1.8	5.0	13.6	38.6	108.4	286.6	14.2
2003	14.6	4.5	*	0.1	0.2	0.7	1.8	4.9	13.6	40.1	109.5	293.1	14.4
2002	14.2	4.3	*	0.1	0.2	0.7	1.7	4.7	13.0	39.2	109.1	288.6	14.2
2001	13.9	3.3	*	0.0	0.2	0.6	1.7	4.6	13.0	40.2	104.2	287.7	14.0
2000	13.2	4.3	*	0.1	0.2	0.6	1.6	4.4	12.8	38.0	100.8	277.8	13.5
1999	12.7	4.4	*	0.1	0.2	0.6	1.6	4.0	12.0	37.1	97.6	268.9	13.0

flow to the heart. By contrast, respiratory arrest may be the result of an accident (such as drowning) or the final stages of a pulmonary disease (such as emphysema—a disease in which the alveoli [microscopic air sacs] of the lungs are destroyed).

In CPR, artificial circulation is accomplished by compressing the chest rhythmically to cause blood to flow sufficiently to give a person a chance for survival. Artificial respiration (rescue breathing) is accomplished by breathing into the victim's mouth. According to the

TABLE 4.2

Death rates, by age, for the 15 leading causes of death, 1999–2009 [CONTINUED]

Cause of death and year	All ages[a]	Under 1 year[b]	1–4 years	5–14 years	15–24 years	25–34 years	35–44 years	45–54 years	55–64 years	65–74 years	75–84 years	85 years and over	Age-adjusted rate
Intentional self-harm (suicide)													
2009	12.0	—	—	0.7	10.1	12.8	16.1	19.3	16.7	14.0	15.7	15.6	11.8
2008	11.9	—	—	0.6	10.1	12.9	15.8	18.7	16.2	13.9	16.2	14.9	11.6
2007	11.5	—	—	0.5	9.7	13.0	15.6	17.7	15.5	12.6	16.3	15.6	11.3
2006	11.1	—	—	0.5	9.9	12.3	15.1	17.2	14.5	12.6	15.9	15.9	10.9
2005	11.0	—	—	0.7	10.0	12.4	14.9	16.5	13.9	12.6	16.9	16.9	10.9
2004	11.0	—	—	0.7	10.3	12.7	15.0	16.6	13.8	12.3	16.3	16.4	10.9
2003	10.8	—	—	0.6	9.7	12.7	14.9	15.9	13.8	12.7	16.4	16.9	10.8
2002	11.0	—	—	0.6	9.9	12.6	15.3	15.7	13.6	13.5	17.7	18.0	10.9
2001[d]	10.8	—	—	0.7	9.9	12.8	14.7	15.2	13.1	13.3	17.4	17.5	10.7
2000	10.4	—	—	0.7	10.2	12.0	14.5	14.4	12.1	12.5	17.6	19.6	10.4
1999	10.5	—	—	0.6	10.1	12.7	14.3	13.9	12.2	13.4	18.1	19.3	10.5
Septicemia													
2009	11.6	5.2	0.4	0.2	0.3	0.9	2.2	5.5	13.3	32.0	78.4	173.8	10.9
2008	11.8	6.7	0.6	0.2	0.3	0.9	2.1	5.7	13.5	32.0	82.3	172.4	11.1
2007	11.5	6.6	0.5	0.2	0.4	0.7	2.1	5.5	12.9	32.8	79.9	174.4	11.0
2006	11.4	6.5	0.5	0.2	0.3	0.7	2.0	5.2	12.8	32.1	82.4	177.3	11.0
2005	11.5	7.4	0.5	0.2	0.4	0.8	1.9	5.2	12.9	32.6	81.4	187.3	11.2
2004	11.4	6.6	0.5	0.2	0.3	0.8	1.9	5.4	12.9	32.4	81.6	186.7	11.2
2003	11.7	6.9	0.5	0.2	0.4	0.8	2.1	5.3	13.1	32.6	85.0	202.5	11.6
2002	11.7	7.3	0.5	0.2	0.3	0.8	1.9	5.2	12.6	34.7	86.5	203.0	11.7
2001	11.3	7.7	0.7	0.2	0.3	0.7	1.8	5.0	12.3	32.8	82.3	205.9	11.4
2000	11.1	7.2	0.6	0.2	0.3	0.7	1.9	4.9	11.9	31.0	80.4	215.7	11.3
1999	11.0	7.5	0.6	0.2	0.3	0.7	1.8	4.6	11.4	31.2	79.4	220.7	11.3
Chronic liver disease and cirrhosis													
2009	10.0	*	*	*	0.1	1.1	6.0	18.8	26.3	25.9	26.9	20.1	9.2
2008	9.9	*	*	*	0.1	1.0	6.0	18.5	25.3	26.8	28.1	19.9	9.2
2007	9.7	*	*	*	0.1	0.9	6.0	18.7	24.5	26.7	28.4	19.8	9.1
2006	9.2	*	*	*	0.1	0.8	5.8	17.8	22.8	26.0	29.0	19.4	8.8
2005	9.3	*	*	*	0.1	0.8	6.1	17.7	23.5	27.2	29.0	19.7	9.0
2004	9.2	*	*	*	*	0.8	6.3	18.0	22.6	27.7	28.8	19.7	9.0
2003	9.5	*	*	*	*	0.9	6.8	18.3	23.0	29.5	30.0	20.1	9.3
2002	9.5	*	*	*	0.1	0.9	7.0	18.0	22.9	29.4	31.4	21.4	9.4
2001	9.5	*	*	*	0.1	1.0	7.4	18.5	22.7	30.0	30.2	22.2	9.5
2000	9.4	*	*	*	0.1	1.0	7.5	17.7	23.8	29.8	31.0	23.1	9.5
1999	9.4	*	*	*	0.1	1.0	7.3	17.4	23.7	30.6	31.9	23.2	9.6
Essential hypertension and hypertensive renal disease													
2009	8.4	*	*	*	0.1	0.3	1.0	3.1	7.2	16.6	50.5	198.3	7.7
2008	8.5	*	*	*	0.1	0.3	1.0	3.0	7.3	16.8	52.1	195.6	7.7
2007	7.9	*	*	*	0.1	0.2	0.9	2.8	6.5	16.2	49.5	191.1	7.4
2006	8.0	*	*	*	0.0	0.3	0.9	3.0	6.9	16.8	51.0	189.4	7.5
2005	8.4	*	*	*	0.1	0.2	0.9	2.7	6.4	17.7	55.6	210.0	8.0
2004	7.9	*	*	*	0.1	0.3	0.8	2.7	6.3	17.1	52.6	198.5	7.7
2003	7.5	*	*	*	0.1	0.2	0.8	2.5	6.3	16.9	51.7	188.9	7.4
2002	7.0	*	*	*	0.1	0.2	0.8	2.3	5.7	16.0	48.2	180.4	7.0
2001	6.8	*	*	*	0.1	0.3	0.7	2.4	5.8	15.5	47.7	171.9	6.8
2000	6.4	*	*	*	*	0.2	0.8	2.3	5.9	15.1	45.5	162.9	6.5
1999	6.1	*	*	*	*	0.2	0.7	2.2	5.5	15.2	43.6	152.1	6.2
Parkinson's disease													
2009	6.7	*	*	*	*	*	*	0.2	1.3	11.4	70.1	149.7	6.4
2008	6.7	*	*	*	*	*	*	0.2	1.2	12.5	71.4	142.9	6.4
2007	6.7	*	*	*	*	*	*	0.1	1.2	11.9	71.9	143.5	6.4
2006	6.5	*	*	*	*	*	*	0.2	1.3	12.2	69.8	144.8	6.3
2005	6.6	*	*	*	*	*	*	0.2	1.4	13.0	71.2	143.7	6.4
2004	6.1	*	*	*	*	*	*	0.2	1.2	12.0	67.5	135.8	6.1
2003	6.2	*	*	*	*	*	*	0.2	1.3	12.7	67.8	138.2	6.2
2002	5.9	*	*	*	*	*	*	0.1	1.2	12.2	63.9	135.2	5.9
2001	5.8	*	*	*	*	*	*	0.1	1.2	11.7	64.6	134.2	5.9
2000	5.6	*	*	*	*	*	*	0.1	1.1	11.5	61.9	131.9	5.7
1999	5.2	*	*	*	*	*	*	0.1	1.0	11.0	58.2	124.4	5.4

article "Changing the Rules on CPR for Cardiac Arrest" (*Harvard Women's Health Watch*, vol. 14, no. 10, June 2007), research indicates that in the case of cardiac arrest, providing chest compressions only is more effective than providing chest compressions and rescue breathing. Medical researchers have determined that taking the time to give rescue breaths to heart attack victims reduces the effectiveness of chest compressions, and effective chest

TABLE 4.2

Death rates, by age, for the 15 leading causes of death, 1999–2009 [CONTINUED]

Cause of death and year	All ages[a]	Under 1 year[b]	1–4 years	5–14 years	15–24 years	25–34 years	35–44 years	45–54 years	55–64 years	65–74 years	75–84 years	85 years and over	Age-adjusted rate
Assault (homicide)													
2009	5.5	7.4	2.2	0.8	11.3	10.2	6.7	4.6	2.9	2.3	2.0	2.2	5.5
2008	5.9	7.9	2.5	0.8	12.4	11.3	6.8	4.8	2.9	2.3	1.8	2.1	5.9
2007	6.1	8.3	2.4	0.9	13.1	11.7	7.1	4.9	3.0	2.1	2.1	1.5	6.1
2006	6.2	8.1	2.2	1.0	13.5	11.7	6.9	5.1	3.2	2.1	2.1	1.9	6.2
2005	6.1	7.5	2.3	0.8	13.0	11.8	7.1	4.8	2.8	2.4	2.2	2.1	6.1
2004	5.9	8.0	2.4	0.8	12.2	11.2	6.8	4.8	3.0	2.4	2.2	2.1	5.9
2003	6.1	8.5	2.4	0.8	13.0	11.3	7.0	4.9	2.8	2.4	2.5	2.2	6.0
2002	6.1	7.5	2.7	0.9	12.9	11.2	7.2	4.8	3.2	2.3	2.3	2.1	6.1
2001	7.1	8.2	2.7	0.8	13.3	13.1	9.5	6.3	4.0	2.9	2.5	2.4	7.1
2000	6.0	9.2	2.3	0.9	12.6	10.4	7.1	4.7	3.0	2.4	2.4	2.4	5.9
1999	6.1	8.7	2.5	1.1	12.9	10.5	7.1	4.6	3.0	2.6	2.5	2.4	6.0

*Figure does not meet standards of reliability or precision.
—Category not applicable.
[a]Figures for age not stated included in "All ages" but not distributed among age groups.
[b]Death rates for "Under 1 year" (based on population estimates) differ from infant mortality rates (based on live births).
[c]Influenza due to certain identified influenza virus was added to the category in 2009.
[d]Figures include September 11, 2001 related deaths for which death certificates were filed as of October 24, 2002.

SOURCE: "Table 9. Death Rates by Age and Age-Adjusted Death Rates for the 15 Leading Causes of Death in 2009: United States, 1999–2009," in "Death Final Data 2009," *National Vital Statistics Reports*, vol. 60, no. 3, 2012, http://www.cdc.gov/nchs/data/dvs/deaths_2009_release.pdf (accessed February 6, 2012)

compressions are vital in helping the heart retain its ability to beat on its own after being shocked with a defibrillator (a device that delivers an electrical shock to the heart). However, if the person experiences respiratory arrest, rescue breathing must be performed to keep the person alive until an ambulance arrives.

The article "Changing the Rules on CPR for Cardiac Arrest" indicates that people who have cardiac arrest away from a hospital have a survival rate of only 1% to 3%. Steven M. Bradley and Tom D. Rea suggest in "Improving Bystander Cardiopulmonary Resuscitation" (*Current Opinion in Critical Care*, vol. 17, no. 3, June 2011) that only a minority of cardiac arrest victims receive CPR from bystanders. However, chest compressions are easier for a bystander to administer (without rescue breathing) when he or she notices a person who is unconscious and not breathing normally. The goal of this change is to help those who become unconscious outside of a hospital setting receive CPR and thus increase their chances of survival.

REFUSAL OF CPR WITH A DO-NOT-RESUSCITATE ORDER. CPR is intended for generally healthy individuals who unexpectedly suffer a heart attack or other trauma, such as drowning. Usually, following CPR, survivors eventually resume a normal life. The outcome is quite different, however, for patients in the final stages of a terminal illness. In "Life-Support Interventions at the End of Life: Unintended Consequences" (*American Journal of Nursing*, vol. 110, no. 1, January 2010), Shirley A. Scott of the Orlando Regional Medical Center in Orlando, Florida, notes that "fewer than 5% of terminally ill patients survive

CPR to leave the hospital. Even if they do survive, they may require mechanical ventilation indefinitely. Depending on how long a patient's brain was deprived of oxygen, there may be brain damage significant enough to result in coma or leave the patient in a persistent vegetative state. Quality of life may be considerably diminished, and the prolonged dying process will likely add to the stress the family is already experiencing." Scott adds that during CPR, a dying patient may experience a broken rib or ribs, which can puncture the lungs and necessitate the insertion of a chest tube. The chest tube is usually uncomfortable and is a common site of infection. The CPR process may also result in a ruptured liver or spleen, which would require surgery.

A person not wishing to be resuscitated in case of cardiac or respiratory arrest may ask a physician to write a do-not-resuscitate (DNR) order on his or her chart. This written order instructs health care personnel not to initiate CPR, which can be very important because CPR is usually performed in an emergency. Even if a patient's living will includes refusal of CPR, emergency personnel rushing to a patient have no time to check the living will. A DNR order on a patient's chart is more accessible. A living will, also called an advance directive, is a written document stating how an individual wants medical decisions to be made if he or she loses the ability to make those decisions for him- or herself (see Chapter 7).

NONHOSPITAL DNR ORDERS. Outside the hospital setting, such as at home, people who do not want CPR performed in case of an emergency can request a nonhospital DNR order from their physician. Also called a prehospital

TABLE 4.3

Estimated numbers of deaths of persons with AIDS, by year of death and selected characteristics, 2006–08 and cumulative

	2006	Estimated[a]		2007	Estimated[a]		2008	Estimated[a]		Cumulative[b]	
	No.	No.	Rate	No.	No.	Rate	No.	No.	Rate	No.	Est. no.[a]
Age at death (yr)											
<13	12	13	0.0	6	7	0.0	4	5	0.0	5,158	5,198
13–14	5	5	0.1	9	11	0.1	0	0	0.0	292	299
15–19	46	49	0.2	36	41	0.2	36	44	0.2	1,231	1,264
20–24	176	190	0.9	146	168	0.8	135	168	0.8	9,497	9,674
25–29	455	492	2.4	429	493	2.3	384	497	2.3	46,742	47,442
30–34	895	972	4.9	778	891	4.5	654	833	4.2	101,311	102,864
35–39	1,934	2,098	9.9	1,676	1,920	9.0	1,270	1,622	7.7	125,560	128,050
40–44	3,171	3,437	15.2	2,713	3,092	14.0	2,184	2,771	12.8	114,403	117,431
45–49	3,382	3,667	16.0	2,987	3,401	14.7	2,586	3,273	14.2	82,189	84,982
50–54	2,686	2,897	14.0	2,557	2,905	13.7	2,311	2,889	13.3	51,358	53,423
55–59	1,686	1,822	9.9	1,574	1,784	9.7	1,700	2,117	11.3	29,574	30,838
60–64	883	955	7.0	884	1,005	6.8	940	1,176	7.7	16,873	17,580
≥65	966	1,044	2.8	893	1,012	2.6	968	1,212	3.1	17,227	17,979
Race/ethnicity											
American Indian/Alaska Native	73	80	—	65	76	—	63	79	—	1,745	1,813
Asian[c]	97	105	—	65	76	—	65	81	—	2,979	3,057
Black/African American	8,143	8,786	—	7,490	8,531	—	6,512	8,182	—	233,896	240,894
Hispanic/Latino[d]	2,983	3,224	—	2,581	2,884	—	2,469	3,029	—	108,590	111,438
Native Hawaiian/other Pacific Islander	6	7	—	9	10	—	11	13	—	341	351
White	4,597	5,017	—	4,090	4,722	—	3,686	4,769	—	248,083	253,473
Multiple races	396	421	—	388	431	—	364	449	—	5,628	5,841
Transmission category											
Male adult or adolescent											
Male-to-male sexual contact	4,865	6,190	—	4,485	6,080	—	3,868	5,959	—	266,985	289,672
Injection drug use	2,764	3,450	—	2,305	3,045	—	2,061	3,008	—	115,416	129,071
Male-to-male sexual contact and injection drug use	1,225	1,452	—	1,048	1,303	—	909	1,275	—	42,941	46,262
Heterosexual contact[e]	1,284	1,745	—	1,146	1,692	—	1,111	1,808	—	24,221	30,478
Other[f]	1,832	143	—	1,733	122	—	1,661	116	—	43,359	9,548
Subtotal	**11,970**	**12,979**	**10.7**	**10,717**	**12,243**	**9.9**	**9,610**	**12,166**	**9.8**	**492,922**	**505,031**
Female adult or adolescent											
Injection drug use	1,448	1,888	—	1,296	1,778	—	1,163	1,758	—	45,022	52,138
Heterosexual contact[e]	1,823	2,621	—	1,704	2,577	—	1,487	2,541	—	40,250	49,316
Other[f]	1,000	92	—	923	77	—	860	79	—	17,470	4,717
Subtotal	**4,271**	**4,601**	**3.6**	**3,923**	**4,432**	**3.4**	**3,510**	**4,377**	**3.4**	**102,742**	**106,171**
Child (<13 yrs at diagnosis)											
Perinatal	49	53		42	48		48	58		5,135	5,200
Other[g]	7	8	—	6	7	—	4	5	—	616	623
Subtotal	**56**	**61**	**0.1**	**48**	**55**	**0.1**	**52**	**62**	**0.1**	**5,751**	**5,823**
Region of residence											
Northeast	4,438	4,692	8.6	3,887	4,197	7.6	3,472	4,004	7.3	189,360	192,050
Midwest	1,451	1,641	2.5	1,311	1,614	2.4	1,201	1,656	2.5	57,457	59,734
South	7,536	8,123	7.5	7,131	8,149	7.4	6,424	8,332	7.4	214,701	221,508
West	2,337	2,562	3.7	1,934	2,267	3.2	1,657	2,096	3.0	118,413	121,204
U.S. dependent areas	535	623	14.4	425	504	11.6	418	517	11.9	21,484	22,528
Total[h]	**16,297**	**17,641**	**5.8**	**14,688**	**16,730**	**5.5**	**13,172**	**16,605**	**5.4**	**601,415**	**617,025**

Note. Deaths of persons with an AIDS diagnosis may be due to any cause.

[a]Estimated numbers resulted from statistical adjustment that accounted for reporting delays and missing risk-factor information, but not for incomplete reporting. Rates are per 100,000 population. Rates by race/ethnicity are not provided because U.S. census information is limited for U.S. dependent areas. Rates are not calculated by transmission category because of the lack of denominator data.

[b]From the beginning of the epidemic through 2008.

[c]Includes Asian/Pacific Islander legacy cases

[d]Hispanics/Latinos can be of any race.

[e]Heterosexual contact with a person known to have, or to be at high risk for, HIV infection.

[f]Includes hemophilia, blood transfusion, perinatal exposure, and risk factor not reported or not identified.

[g]Includes hemophilia, blood transfusion, and risk factor not reported or not identified.

[h]Includes persons of unknown race/ethnicity. Because column totals for estimated numbers were calculated independently of the values for the subpopulations, the values in each column may not sum to the column total.

SOURCE: "Table 12b. Deaths of Persons with an AIDS Diagnosis, by Year of Death and Selected Characteristics, 2006–2008 and Cumulative—United States and 5 U.S. Dependent Areas," in "Diagnoses of HIV Infection and AIDS in the United States and Dependent Areas, 2009," *HIV/AIDS Surveillance Report 2009*, vol. 21, U.S. Department of Health and Human Services, Centers for Disease Control and Prevention, February 2011, http://www.cdc.gov/hiv/surveillance/resources/reports/2009report/pdf/table12b.pdf (accessed January 31, 2012)

DNR order, it instructs emergency medical personnel to withhold CPR. The DNR order may be on a bracelet or necklace or on a wallet card. However, laypeople performing CPR on an individual with a nonhospital DNR order cannot be prosecuted by the law. Caring Connections (http://www.caringinfo.org/stateaddownload), a program of the National Hospice and Palliative Care Organization (NHPCO), provides information about each of the 50 states' advance directives, including information about laws authorizing nonhospital DNR orders.

Mechanical Ventilation

When a patient's lungs are not functioning properly, a ventilator (or respirator) breathes for the patient. Most ventilators are positive-pressure ventilators. That is, they deliver gas under pressure to the patient's lungs to support gas exchange. The pressure is relieved when gas is exhaled via an exhalation pathway. Negative-pressure ventilators (iron lungs) are rarely used because they are needed for patients with polio. Due to widespread vaccination for this disease, polio has been nearly eradicated.

In positive-pressure ventilators, oxygen is supplied to the lungs via a tube that is inserted through the mouth or nose into the windpipe. Mechanical ventilation is generally used to temporarily maintain normal breathing in those who have been in serious accidents or who suffer from a serious illness, such as pneumonia. In some cases, if the patient needs ventilation indefinitely, the physician might perform a tracheotomy to open a hole in the neck for placement of the breathing tube in the windpipe.

Ventilators are also used on terminally ill patients. In these cases the machine keeps the patient breathing but does nothing to cure the disease. Once ventilation is started, it raises the question of when ventilation will be stopped. Those preparing a living will are advised to give clear instructions about their desires regarding continued use of an artificial respirator that could prolong the process of dying.

Artificial Nutrition and Hydration

Artificial nutrition and hydration (ANH) is another technology that has further complicated the dying process. In the 21st century nutrients and fluids that are supplied intravenously or through a stomach or intestinal tube can indefinitely sustain the nutritional and hydration needs of comatose and terminally ill patients. ANH has a strong emotional impact because it relates to basic sustenance. In addition, the symbolism of feeding can be so powerful that families who know that their loved one would not want to be kept alive may still feel that not feeding is wrong. The NHPCO explains in "Artificial Nutrition (Food) and Hydration (Fluids) at the End of Life" (2009, http://www.caringinfo.org/files/public/brochures/ArtificialNutritionAndHydration.pdf) that appetite loss is common in dying patients and is not a significant

contributor to their suffering. It also explains that the withdrawal of ANH from a dying patient does not lead to a long and painful death. Moreover, the NHPCO suggests that avoiding ANH contributes to a more comfortable death.

ANH has traditionally been used in end-of-life care when patients experience a loss of appetite and difficulty swallowing. Health care practitioners use ANH to prolong life, prevent aspiration pneumonia (inflammation of the lungs due to inhaling food particles or fluid), maintain independence and physical function, and decrease suffering and discomfort. However, ANH does not always accomplish these goals, as the Hospice and Palliative Nurses Association (HPNA) notes in its position statement "Artificial Nutrition and Hydration in Advanced Illness" (October 2011, http://www.hpna.org/PicView.aspx?ID=1527). The HPNA indicates that "studies have shown that tube feeding does not appear to prolong life and complications from tube placement may increase mortality in certain populations. Furthermore, artificially-delivered nutrition does not protect against aspiration and in some patient populations may actually increase the risk of aspiration and its complications."

According to the Academy of Nutrition and Dietetics (formerly the American Dietetic Association), in the position statement "Ethical and Legal Issues in Nutrition, Hydration, and Feeding" (*Journal of the American Dietetic Association*, vol. 108, no. 5, May 2008), the "loss of appetite is common with terminally ill patients and does not reduce quality of life except for reducing the enjoyment of food." It notes that "withholding or minimizing hydration can have the desirable effect of reducing disturbing oral and bronchial secretions, need for frequent urination, and reduced cough from diminished pulmonary congestion. Withholding nutrition has been studied closely and the majority of reports indicate that physiological adaptation allows patients not to suffer from absence of food." In fact, the Academy of Nutrition and Dietetics indicates that dehydration of the dying patient causes metabolic changes that have a sedative effect on the brain prior to death. However, the academy emphasizes that "each patient is unique, and the plan of care should be constantly reassessed for each individual." The academy reports that it will publish a reaffirmed and updated position statement in 2012.

Many medically related organizations have position statements on ANH in dying patients, including the NHPCO, in "Commentary and Position Statement on Artificial Nutrition and Hydration" (September 12, 2010, http://www.nhpco.org/files/public/ANH_Statement_Commentary.pdf); the American Academy of Hospice and Palliative Medicine, in "Statement on Artificial Nutrition and Hydration Near the End of Life" (December 8, 2006, http://www.aahpm.org/positions/default/nutrition.html); and the American Academy of Neurology, in "Position Statement on Laws and Regulations Concerning Life-Sustaining Treatment,

Including Artificial Nutrition and Hydration, for Patients Lacking Decision-Making Capacity" (June 2006, http://www.aan.com/globals/axon/assets/2680.pdf).

Kidney Dialysis

Kidney dialysis is a medical procedure by which a machine takes over the function of the kidneys in removing waste products from the blood. Dialysis can be used when an illness or injury temporarily impairs kidney function. It may also be used by patients with irreversibly damaged kidneys awaiting organ transplantation.

Kidney failure may also occur as an end stage of a terminal illness. Even though dialysis may cleanse the body of waste products, it cannot cure the disease. Dialysis patients may also suffer from various side effects, including chemical imbalances in the body, low blood pressure, nausea and vomiting, headache, itching, and fatigue. The procedure must be done several times a week. People who wish to let their illness take its course may refuse dialysis. They will eventually lapse into a coma and die.

DISORDERS OF CONSCIOUSNESS

A coma is a deep state of unconsciousness that is caused by damage to the brain, often from illness or trauma. The patient is neither awake nor aware; his or her eyes are always closed. A coma rarely lasts for more than one month, and most people in a coma recover quickly, die, or progress to a vegetative state within that time.

Most often, patients who do not recover quickly from a coma progress to a vegetative/unresponsive state: they experience periods of wakefulness (eyes open) but without awareness (see Chapter 2). Those in a vegetative/unresponsive state for one month are then referred to as being in a persistent vegetative state, and after a longer period are referred to as being in a permanent vegetative state/unresponsive wakefulness state (PVS/UWS). The word *permanent* implies no chance of recovery.

Table 2.2 in Chapter 2 lists the criteria for the diagnosis of a PVS/UWS. PVS/UWS patients are unaware of themselves or their environment. They do not respond to stimuli, understand language, or have control of bowel and bladder functions. They intermittently open their eyes but are not conscious—a condition often referred to as eyes-open unconsciousness.

Some PVS/UWS patients may recover further to regain partial consciousness. This condition is called a minimally conscious state (MCS). The perception of the minimally conscious patient is severely altered, but the patient is awake and shows an awareness of self or the environment, exhibiting behaviors such as following simple commands and smiling or crying at appropriate times. Some patients emerge from an MCS and some remain in

TABLE 4.4

Criteria for a minimally conscious state (MCS)

Impaired responsiveness
Limited by perceptible awareness of surroundings or self evidenced by one or more of the following:

MC−	MC+
Following someone with the eyes	Following commands
Crying or smiling appropriately to emotional stimuli	Using words understandably
Localization of unpleasant stimuli	Non-functional communication

SOURCE: Adapted from Marie-Aurélie Bruno et al., "From Unresponsive Wakefulness to Minimally Conscious PLUS and Functional Locked-in Syndromes: Recent Advances in Our Understanding of Disorders of Consciousness," *Journal of Neurology*, vol. 258, no. 7, July 2011

an MCS permanently. Table 4.4 lists the criteria for the diagnosis of an MCS.

In "From Unresponsive Wakefulness to Minimally Conscious PLUS and Functional Locked-in Syndromes: Recent Advances in Our Understanding of Disorders of Consciousness" (*Journal of Neurology*, vol. 258, no. 7, July 2011), Marie-Aurélie Bruno et al. propose a splitting of the category of MCS into MC+ (high-level behavioral responses) and MC− (low-level behavioral responses). High-level behavioral responses include following commands and saying words that are understandable. (See Table 4.4.) Low-level behavioral responses include following someone with the eyes, or smiling or crying appropriately to emotional stimuli. The person with MC+ can exhibit lower-level behaviors as well as higher-level behaviors.

Another disorder of consciousness that rarely occurs after a coma is locked-in syndrome. The patient with locked-in syndrome is awake and has full consciousness, but all the voluntary muscles of the body are paralyzed except (usually) for those that control vertical eye movement and blinking. People with locked-in syndrome communicate primarily with eye or eyelid movements.

Treatment of PVS/UWS and MCS Patients

Cynda Hylton Rushton, Brett Daniel Kaylor, and Myra Christopher discuss in "Twenty Years since *Cruzan* and the Patient Self-Determination Act: Opportunities for Improving Care at the End of Life in Critical Care Settings" (*Ethics in Critical Care*, vol. 23, no 1, January–March 2012) the progress that has been made in decision making for critical care patients between 1990 and 2010, the 20-year anniversary since the U.S. Supreme Court ruled in *Cruzan v. Director* (497 U.S. 261 [1990]). The researchers suggest that two major decisions have occurred: the Patient Self-Determination Act (PSDA) and the hearing of *Cruzan* by the court. The PSDA allows patients to "choose or refuse treatment and to name someone to speak for them when they are no longer able to speak for themselves." However, problems have arisen in that a patient or nonpatient must make various decisions when a life-or-death situation is not facing them at the time. The result has been that many adults fail to create an advance directive or a living will. In addition, they do not decide who will speak for them if they should become incapacitated.

Nonetheless, advanced care planning (ACP) is something that is supposed to be a dialogue that takes place throughout a person's life. Young adults and pregnant women should be sure to have their directives in place. ACP is meant to be an ongoing process in which people discuss with one another what they want for end-of-life care.

ORGAN TRANSPLANTATION

People who have died as a result of brain injury and subsequent brain death usually have other body organs that are healthy and able to be successfully transplanted. Most organ and tissue donations are from traumatic brain injury victims. Once death is pronounced, the body is kept on mechanical support (if possible) to maintain the organs until it is determined whether the person will be a donor.

There are some organ and tissue donations that can come from living people. For example, it is possible to lead a healthy life with only one of the two kidneys that humans are born with, so people with two healthy kidneys will sometimes donate one to someone in need. Portions of the liver, lungs, and pancreas have also been donated, but this is less common. In most cases, living donors make their donations to help a family member or close friend.

Organ transplantation has come a long way since the first kidney was transplanted from one identical twin to another in 1954. The introduction in 1983 of cyclosporine, an immunosuppressant drug that helps prevent the body's immune system from rejecting a donated organ, made it possible to successfully transplant a variety of organs and tissues.

Figure 4.1 and Figure 4.2 show the organs and tissues that are transplantable with 21st-century immunosuppressant drugs and technologies. The organs that may be transplanted from people who have died are the heart, kidneys, intestine, pancreas, liver, and lungs. Tissues that may be transplanted from people who have died include bone, cartilage, cornea, heart valve, rotator cuff, skin, Achilles tendon, and blood vessels. Living people may donate a kidney; parts of a lung, liver, or pancreas; or bone marrow. Typically, donated organs must be transplanted within six to 48 hours of harvest, whereas some tissue may be stored for future use.

Soon after organ transplantation began, the demand for donor organs exceeded the supply. In 1984 Congress passed the National Organ Transplant Act to create "a centralized network to match scarce donated organs with critically ill patients." (For the process of matching organ

FIGURE 4.1

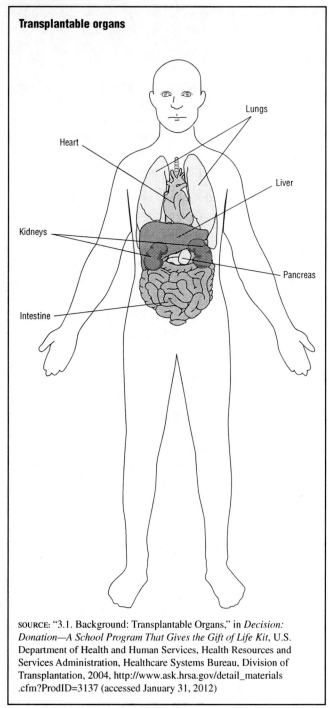

Transplantable organs

SOURCE: "3.1. Background: Transplantable Organs," in *Decision: Donation—A School Program That Gives the Gift of Life Kit*, U.S. Department of Health and Human Services, Health Resources and Services Administration, Healthcare Systems Bureau, Division of Transplantation, 2004, http://www.ask.hrsa.gov/detail_materials .cfm?ProdID=3137 (accessed January 31, 2012)

donors and recipients, see Figure 4.3.) In the 21st century organ transplant is an accepted medical treatment for end-stage illnesses.

The United Network for Organ Sharing (UNOS), a private company that is under contract with the Division of Transplantation of the U.S. Department of Health and Human Services, manages the national transplant waiting list. It maintains data on all clinical organ transplants and distributes organ donor cards. (See Figure 4.4.) It also assists in placing donated organs for transplantation by operating the donor-recipient computer matching process

FIGURE 4.2

Transplantable tissues

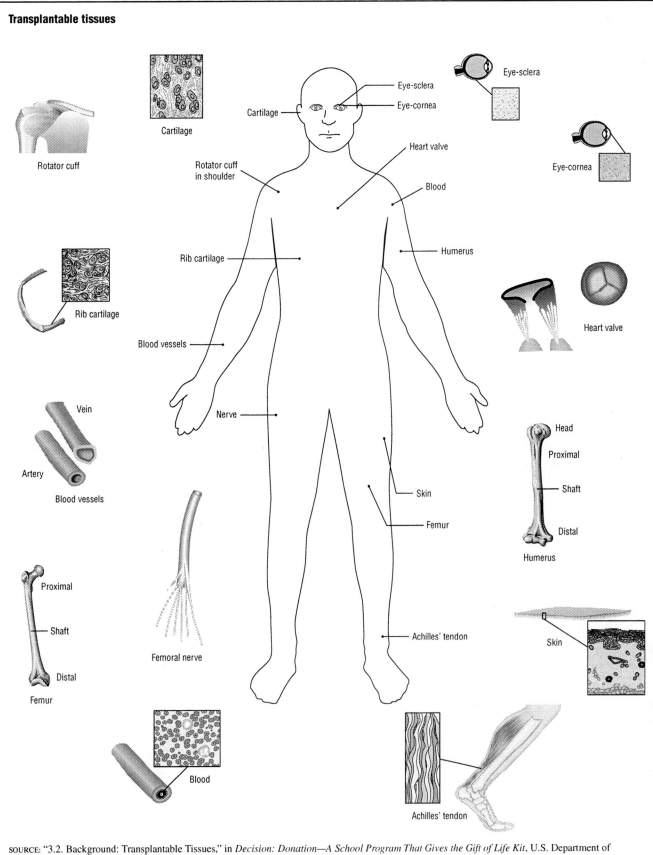

SOURCE: "3.2. Background: Transplantable Tissues," in *Decision: Donation—A School Program That Gives the Gift of Life Kit*, U.S. Department of Health and Human Services, Health Resources and Services Administration, Healthcare Systems Bureau, Division of Transplantation, 2004, http://www.ask.hrsa.gov/detail_materials.cfm?ProdID=3137 (accessed February 23, 2012)

FIGURE 4.3

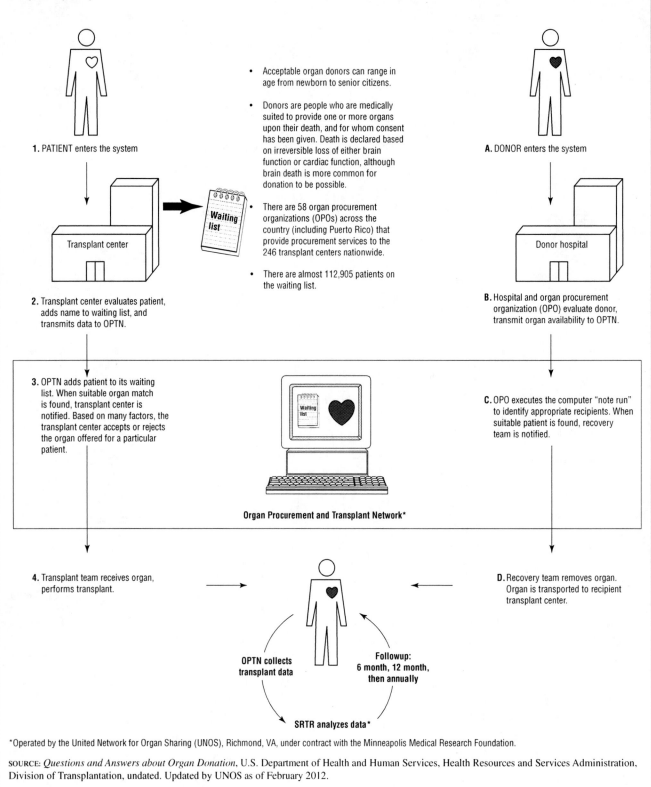

Matching donors and recipients: The Organ Procurement & Transplantation Network (OPTN) and the Scientific Registry of Transplant Recipients (SRTR)

1. PATIENT enters the system

2. Transplant center evaluates patient, adds name to waiting list, and transmits data to OPTN.

3. OPTN adds patient to its waiting list. When suitable organ match is found, transplant center is notified. Based on many factors, the transplant center accepts or rejects the organ offered for a particular patient.

4. Transplant team receives organ, performs transplant.

- Acceptable organ donors can range in age from newborn to senior citizens.

- Donors are people who are medically suited to provide one or more organs upon their death, and for whom consent has been given. Death is declared based on irreversible loss of either brain function or cardiac function, although brain death is more common for donation to be possible.

- There are 58 organ procurement organizations (OPOs) across the country (including Puerto Rico) that provide procurement services to the 246 transplant centers nationwide.

- There are almost 112,905 patients on the waiting list.

Waiting list

Organ Procurement and Transplant Network*

A. DONOR enters the system

Donor hospital

B. Hospital and organ procurement organization (OPO) evaluate donor, transmit organ availability to OPTN.

C. OPO executes the computer "note run" to identify appropriate recipients. When suitable patient is found, recovery team is notified.

D. Recovery team removes organ. Organ is transported to recipient transplant center.

OPTN collects transplant data

Followup: 6 month, 12 month, then annually

SRTR analyzes data*

*Operated by the United Network for Organ Sharing (UNOS), Richmond, VA, under contract with the Minneapolis Medical Research Foundation.

SOURCE: *Questions and Answers about Organ Donation*, U.S. Department of Health and Human Services, Health Resources and Services Administration, Division of Transplantation, undated. Updated by UNOS as of February 2012.

and helps with the transportation of donated organs for transplantation. As of April 3, 2012, the UNOS (http://www.unos.org/) reported that 113,736 people were waiting for a transplant in the United States. Between January and December 2011, 28,535 transplants had been performed in the United States.

Table 4.5 shows the waiting list for organs between 1999 and 2008. "Total registrations" refers to all the registrations from all the transplant centers for all organs. Therefore, this figure is larger than "total patients," which is the number of patients waiting for a transplant.

FIGURE 4.4

Organ/tissue donor card

Organ/Tissue Donor Card

Donate Life

I wish to donate my organs and tissues. I wish to give:

☐ **any needed organs and tissues** ☐ **only the following organs and tissues:**

____

Donor Signature ______________________ **Date** __________

Witness ______________________________

Witness ______________________________

SOURCE: Organ/Tissue Donor Card, U.S. Department of Health and Human Services, undated

An individual may show up as more than one registration in the "registrations" category because that individual may be registered at more than one transplant center or for more than one organ. However, individuals waiting for transplants are counted only once in the "total patients" category, but they may show up more than once in the listing of organ types under that heading if they need more than one organ.

The total number of patients waiting for an organ transplant grew 54.3% over nine years, from 65,204 in 1999 to 100,597 in 2008. (See Table 4.5.) The total number of registrations grew approximately the same percentage (56%), from 68,096 in 1999 to 106,245 in 2008. By contrast, the organ transplants during this same period grew by only 25%, from 21,826 in 1999 to 27,281 in 2008. (See Table 4.6.)

The kidney is the most frequently transplanted organ. In 2008 there were 16,067 (58.9%) kidney transplants out of a total of 27,281 organ transplants. (See Table 4.6.) There were also 5,817 (21.3%) liver, 2,085 (7.6%) heart, and 1,473 (5.4%) lung transplants.

The number of all donors rose by 30.8% between 1999 and 2008, from 10,862 to 14,203. (See Table 4.7.) The number of deceased donors increased by 37.1%, from 5,824 to 7,984, and the number of living donors

TABLE 4.5

United Network for Organ Sharing (UNOS) and Scientific Registry of Transplant Recipients (SRTR) national patient waiting list for organ transplant, end of year, 1999–2008

	Year									
	1999	**2000**	**2001**	**2002**	**2003**	**2004**	**2005**	**2006**	**2007**	**2008**
Total registrations	**68,096**	**74,728**	**80,105**	**81,759**	**85,221**	**89,636**	**92,790**	**97,147**	**101,804**	**106,245**
Organ type										
Heart-lung	227	203	207	195	187	169	136	133	105	91
Heart	3,933	3,945	3,885	3,717	3,440	3,177	2,908	2,766	2,646	2,722
Intestine	106	141	169	183	172	196	202	236	224	216
Kidney	43,632	47,230	50,337	53,178	56,522	61,020	65,029	70,078	75,834	80,972
Kidney-pancreas	2,135	2,450	2,472	2,506	2,435	2,427	2,496	2,378	2,307	2,310
Liver	14,165	16,426	18,243	17,034	17,247	17,302	17,374	17,102	16,939	16,450
Lung	3,371	3,564	3,722	3,752	3,837	3,859	3,141	2,847	2,230	2,029
Pancreas after kidney	277	457	678	784	929	981	981	1,003	933	870
Pancreas transplant alone	250	312	392	410	452	505	523	604	586	585
Total patients	**65,204**	**71,554**	**76,787**	**78,344**	**81,708**	**85,170**	**88,625**	**92,686**	**96,874**	**100,597**
Organ type										
Heart-lung	221	201	207	195	187	169	134	133	105	91
Heart	3,910	3,927	3,864	3,702	3,431	3,164	2,898	2,758	2,637	2,711
Intestine	101	133	164	180	167	191	200	232	220	212
Kidney	41,177	44,568	47,574	50,296	53,513	57,141	61,505	66,255	71,601	76,089
Kidney-pancreas	2,048	2,361	2,367	2,405	2,354	2,362	2,428	2,322	2,235	2,234
Liver	13,922	16,087	17,889	16,686	16,892	16,858	16,865	16,582	16,365	15,807
Lung	3,303	3,513	3,671	3,702	3,797	3,816	3,109	2,819	2,211	2,016
Pancreas after kidney	274	453	667	771	918	969	971	990	919	856
Pancreas transplant alone	248	311	384	407	449	500	515	595	581	581

SOURCE: "Table 1.3. Waiting List at End of Year, 1999 to 2008," in *2009 Annual Report of the U.S. Organ Procurement and Transplantation Network and the Scientific Registry of Transplant Recipients: Transplant Data 1999–2008*, U.S. Department of Health and Human Services, Health Resources and Services Administration, Healthcare Systems Bureau, Division of Transplantation, 2010, http://www.ustransplant.org/annual_reports/current/103_dh.pdf (accessed February 1, 2012). The data and analyses reported in the 2009 Annual Report of the U.S. Organ Procurement and Transplantation Network and the Scientific Registry of Transplant Recipients have been supplied by UNOS and Arbor Research under contract with HHS/HRSA. The authors alone are responsible for reporting and interpreting these data; the views expressed herein are those of the authors and not necessarily those of the U.S. Government.

TABLE 4.6

United Network for Organ Sharing (UNOS) and Scientific Registry of Transplant Recipients (SRTR) transplants, by organ and donor type, 1999–2008

Organ/donor type	Year									
	1999	2000	2001	2002	2003	2004	2005	2006	2007	2008
All organs										
Total	21,826	23,019	23,957	24,553	25,087	26,542	27,533	28,291	27,586	27,281
Deceased	16,818	17,097	17,366	17,935	18,273	19,553	20,633	21,561	21,279	21,065
Living	5,008	5,922	6,591	6,618	6,814	6,989	6,900	6,730	6,307	6,216
Heart-lung										
Total	51	46	27	32	28	38	34	31	31	26
Deceased	51	46	27	32	28	38	34	31	31	26
Living	—	—	—	—	—	—	—	—	—	—
Heart										
Total	2,157	2,167	2,171	2,112	2,026	1,960	2,062	2,146	2,143	2,085
Deceased	2,157	2,167	2,171	2,112	2,026	1,960	2,062	2,145	2,143	2,085
Living	—	—	—	—	—	—	—	1	—	—
Intestine										
Total	31	30	42	42	52	52	68	60	57	69
Deceased	29	27	42	41	48	46	63	57	57	69
Living	2	3	—	1	4	6	5	3	—	—
Kidney										
Total	12,633	13,450	14,106	14,526	14,857	15,672	16,076	16,644	16,120	16,067
Deceased	7,916	7,958	8,068	8,286	8,387	9,027	9,507	10,211	10,082	10,101
Living	4,717	5,492	6,038	6,240	6,470	6,645	6,569	6,433	6,038	5,966
Kidney-pancreas										
Total	937	914	889	902	869	880	896	914	848	825
Deceased	930	908	886	902	866	880	895	913	848	825
Living	7	6	3	—	3	—	1	1	—	—
Liver										
Total	4,604	4,808	4,988	5,060	5,364	5,781	5,999	6,135	5,890	5,817
Deceased	4,352	4,407	4,464	4,697	5,042	5,460	5,679	5,849	5,629	5,568
Living	252	401	524	363	322	321	320	286	261	249
Lung										
Total	892	958	1,059	1,041	1,080	1,168	1,403	1,401	1,461	1,473
Deceased	863	940	1,034	1,028	1,065	1,153	1,403	1,397	1,458	1,473
Living	29	18	25	13	15	15	1	4	3	—
Multi-organ										
Total	176	223	240	322	351	443	523	570	669	583
Deceased	175	222	240	322	351	441	520	568	664	583
Living	1	1	—	—	—	2	3	2	5	—
Pancreas after kidney										
Total	220	305	304	374	344	419	343	292	259	214
Deceased	220	305	304	374	344	419	342	292	259	213
Living	—	—	—	—	—	—	1	—	—	1
Pancreas transplant alone										
Total	125	118	131	142	116	129	129	98	108	122
Deceased	125	117	130	141	116	129	129	98	108	122
Living	—	1	1	1	—	—	—	—	—	—

Notes: — = None in category. An organ that is divided into segments (liver, lung, pancreas, intestine) is counted once per transplant. Kidney-pancreas and heart-lung transplants are counted as one transplant. Other multiple organ transplants are counted only in the multiple organ row.

SOURCE: "Table 1.7. Transplants by Organ and Donor Type, 1999 to 2008," in *2009 Annual Report of the U.S. Organ Procurement and Transplantation Network and the Scientific Registry of Transplant Recipients: Transplant Data 1998–2008*, U.S. Department of Health and Human Services, Health Resources and Services Administration, Healthcare Systems Bureau, Division of Transplantation, 2010, http://www.ustransplant.org/annual_reports/current/107_dh.pdf (accessed February 1, 2012). The data and analyses reported in the 2009 Annual Report of the U.S. Organ Procurement and Transplantation Network and the Scientific Registry of Transplant Recipients have been supplied by UNOS and Arbor Research under contract with HHS/HRSA. The authors alone are responsible for reporting and interpreting these data; the views expressed herein are those of the authors and not necessarily those of the U.S. Government.

increased by 23.4%, from 5,038 to 6,219. Most living donors provide kidneys. The donation of kidneys by living donors increased by 26.3%, from 4,725 in 1999 to 5,968 in 2008. Living donors may also contribute a portion of their liver; the donation of liver tissue by living donors stayed nearly static, from 253 in 1999 to 250

TABLE 4.7

United Network for Organ Sharing (UNOS) and Scientific Registry of Transplant Recipients (SRTR) organ donors, by organ and donor type, 1999–2008

	Year									
	1999	2000	2001	2002	2003	2004	2005	2006	2007	2008
All organs										
Total	**10,862**	**11,926**	**12,695**	**12,820**	**13,285**	**14,154**	**14,495**	**14,751**	**14,402**	**14,203**
Deceased	5,824	5,985	6,080	6,190	6,457	7,150	7,593	8,019	8,086	7,984
Living	5,038	5,941	6,615	6,630	6,828	7,004	6,902	6,732	6,316	6,219
Kidney										
Total	**10,111**	**10,988**	**11,569**	**11,878**	**12,226**	**12,972**	**13,271**	**13,613**	**13,285**	**13,153**
Deceased	5,386	5,489	5,528	5,638	5,753	6,325	6,700	7,178	7,241	7,185
Living	4,725	5,499	6,041	6,240	6,473	6,647	6,571	6,435	6,044	5,968
Pancreas										
Total	**1,635**	**1,705**	**1,821**	**1,874**	**1,774**	**2,019**	**2,045**	**2,032**	**1,932**	**1,831**
Deceased	1,628	1,698	1,817	1,873	1,771	2,019	2,043	2,031	1,932	1,830
Living	7	7	4	1	3	—	2	1	—	1
Liver										
Total	**5,200**	**5,399**	**5,630**	**5,657**	**6,004**	**6,642**	**7,016**	**7,305**	**7,204**	**6,995**
Deceased	4,947	4,997	5,106	5,294	5,682	6,319	6,693	7,017	6,938	6,745
Living	253	402	524	363	322	323	323	288	266	250
Intestine										
Total	**97**	**90**	**116**	**113**	**127**	**172**	**191**	**189**	**206**	**197**
Deceased	95	87	116	112	123	166	184	185	205	197
Living	2	3	—	1	4	6	7	4	1	—
Heart										
Total	**2,316**	**2,284**	**2,276**	**2,223**	**2,120**	**2,096**	**2,220**	**2,277**	**2,287**	**2,226**
Deceased	2,316	2,284	2,276	2,223	2,120	2,096	2,220	2,276	2,287	2,226
Living	—	—	—	—	—	—	—	1	—	—
Lung										
Total	**835**	**861**	**936**	**945**	**990**	**1,092**	**1,287**	**1,330**	**1,388**	**1,388**
Deceased	777	825	887	920	961	1,064	1,285	1,325	1,382	1,388
Living	58	36	49	25	29	28	2	5	6	—
Donation after cardiac death										
Total	**87**	**117**	**168**	**189**	**268**	**391**	**564**	**642**	**791**	**848**
Deceased	87	117	168	189	268	391	564	642	791	848

Notes: — = None in category Includes only organs recovered for transplant. The number of transplants using living donors may be different from the number of living donors. This is because there is a small number of multi-organ living donors and multiple donors for one transplant. For example, a living donor might donate a kidney and pancreas segment; or two living donors might each donate a lung lobe for one transplant procedure. A donor of an organ divided into segments (liver, lung, pancreas, intestine) is counted only once for that organ. A donor of multiple organs is counted once for each organ recovered. Donors after cardiac death are included in the deceased donor counts as well and are counted separately on the last line.

SOURCE: "Table 1.1. U.S. Organ Donors by Organ and Donor Type, 1999 to 2008," in *2009 Annual Report of the U.S. Organ Procurement and Transplantation Network and the Scientific Registry of Transplant Recipients: Transplant Data 1999–2008*, U.S. Department of Health and Human Services, Health Resources and Services Administration, Healthcare Systems Bureau, Division of Transplantation, 2010, http://www.ustransplant.org/annual_reports/current/101_dh.pdf (accessed February1, 2012). The data and analyses reported in the 2009 Annual Report of the U.S. Organ Procurement and Transplantation Network and the Scientific Registry of Transplant Recipients have been supplied by UNOS and Arbor Research under contract with HHS/HRSA. The authors alone are responsible for reporting and interpreting these data; the views expressed herein are those of the authors and not necessarily those of the U.S. Government.

in 2008. Living donors of pancreas, intestine, and lung tissue are few, with living donors dropping precipitously to only one donor in 2008 (of pancreatic tissue) from the 67 in 1999 (primarily lung tissue). Edward R. Garrity et al. suggest in "Heart and Lung Transplantation in the United States, 1996–2005" (*American Journal of Transplantation*, vol. 7, suppl. 1, May 2007) that the reason for this decrease in the demand for living donor lung transplantation was a system change in May 2005 for allocating lungs from deceased donors. This change resulted in a decrease in the number of people on lung transplant waiting lists and an increase in the ability to get patients transplanted sooner.

Organ Donation

The Uniform Anatomical Gift Act of 1968 gives a person the opportunity to sign a donor card indicating a desire to donate organs or tissue after death. People who wish to be donors should complete a donor card, which should be carried at all times. Alternatively, the wish to be a donor can be indicated on a driver's license or in a living will. Prospective donors should inform their family and physician of their decision. At the time of death, hospitals always ask for the family's consent, even if a donor has already indicated his or her wish to donate organs. Should the family refuse, doctors will not take the organs, despite the deceased's wish. In 2008 most organ donors whose cause of death was known died of a stroke (40%) or head trauma (34.9%), as might happen in a motor vehicle accident. (See Table 4.8.) Anoxia (lack of oxygen, as in drowning or choking) was the cause of death of 21.5% of organ donors.

TABLE 4.8

Causes of death of donors of any organ, 1998–2008

	Year									
	1999	2000	2001	2002	2003	2004	2005	2006	2007	2008
Total	5,824	5,985	6,080	6,190	6,457	7,150	7,593	8,019	8,086	7,984
Cause of death										
Anoxia	640	619	697	741	855	1,024	1,147	1,349	1,482	1,718
Cerebrovascular/stroke	2,508	2,612	2,631	2,635	2,767	3,127	3,336	3,356	3,307	3,191
Head trauma	2,430	2,520	2,545	2,610	2,617	2,794	2,908	3,058	3,022	2,786
CNS tumor	61	62	52	56	49	60	57	57	46	42
Other	171	171	154	148	169	144	145	199	229	247
Unknown	14	1	1	—	—	1	—	—	—	—
Cause of death (%)										
Anoxia	11.0%	10.3%	11.5%	12.0%	13.2%	14.3%	15.1%	16.8%	18.3%	21.5%
Cerebrovascular/stroke	43.1%	43.6%	43.3%	42.6%	42.9%	43.7%	43.9%	41.9%	40.9%	40.0%
Head trauma	41.7%	42.1%	41.9%	42.2%	40.5%	39.1%	38.3%	38.1%	37.4%	34.9%
CNS tumor	1.0%	1.0%	0.9%	0.9%	0.8%	0.8%	0.8%	0.7%	0.6%	0.5%
Other	2.9%	2.9%	2.5%	2.4%	2.6%	2.0%	1.9%	2.5%	2.8%	3.1%
Unknown	0.2%	0.0%	0.0%	—	—	0.0%	—	—	—	—

Notes: (%) = Percentages are calculated based on totals including missing and unknown cases.
— = None in category. CNS = Central nervous system.
Includes donors of organs recovered for transplant and not used, as well as those transplanted.
Not all recovered organs are actually transplanted.

SOURCE: Adapted from "Table 2.1. Deceased Donor Characteristics, 1999 to 2008 Deceased Donors of Any Organ," in *2009 Annual Report of the U.S. Organ Procurement and Transplantation Network and the Scientific Registry of Transplant Recipients: Transplant Data 1999–2008*, U.S. Department of Health and Human Services, Health Resources and Services Administration, Healthcare Systems Bureau, Division of Transplantation, 2010, http://www.ustransplant.org/annual_reports/current/201_dc.pdf (accessed February 1, 2012). The data and analyses reported in the 2009 Annual Report of the U.S. Organ Procurement and Transplantation Network and the Scientific Registry of Transplant Recipients have been supplied by UNOS and Arbor Research under contract with HHS/HRSA. The authors alone are responsible for reporting and interpreting these data; the views expressed herein are those of the authors and not necessarily those of the U.S. Government.

CHAPTER 5
SERIOUSLY ILL CHILDREN

What greater pain could mortals have than this: To see their children dead before their eyes?

—Euripides

To a parent, the death of a child is an affront to the proper order of things. Children are supposed to outlive their parents, not the other way around. When a child comes into the world irreparably ill, what is a parent to do: insist on continuous medical intervention, hoping against hope that the child survives, or let nature take its course and allow the newborn to die? When a five-year-old child has painful, life-threatening disabilities, the parent is faced with a similar agonizing decision. That decision is the parent's to make, preferably with the advice of a sensitive physician. However, what if the ailing child is an adolescent who refuses further treatment for a terminal illness? Does a parent honor that wish? This chapter focuses on infant and child death, the conditions that often cause mortality at young ages, and medical decision making for seriously ill children.

INFANT MORTALITY AND LIFE EXPECTANCY AT BIRTH

Marian F. MacDorman and T. J. Mathews of the National Center for Health Statistics indicate in *Recent Trends in Infant Mortality in the United States* (October 2008, http://www.cdc.gov/nchs/data/databriefs/db09.pdf) that between 1900 and 2000 the U.S. infant mortality rate declined dramatically. In 1900 the infant mortality rate was approximately 100 deaths per 1,000 live births, whereas in 2000 it was 6.9 deaths per 1,000 live births. With each decade, infant mortality declined significantly. However, between 2000 and 2006 the infant mortality rate remained relatively steady. (See Table 5.1.)

Table 5.1 shows the decline in infant mortality rates between 1983 and 2006, Table 5.2 shows figures between 2007 and 2008, and Table 5.3 shows figures for 2009 and preliminary figures for 2010. The data in these three tables are from different data sets so they cannot be

compared precisely, but the trend of a stabilization (and slight decrease) of infant mortality rates from 2000 onward appears to continue through 2010.

Advances in neonatology (the medical subspecialty that is concerned with the care of newborns, especially those at risk), which date back to the 1960s, have contributed to the huge drop in infant death rates from that time to 2000 and to the maintenance of lowered infant death rates since 2000. Infants born prematurely or with low birth weights, who were once likely to die, now can survive life-threatening conditions because of the development of neonatal intensive care units. However, the improvements are not consistent for newborns of all races.

African-American infants are more than twice as likely as non-Hispanic white and Hispanic infants to die before their first birthday. In 2009 and 2010 the national death rate for African-American infants was 12.6 and 11.6, respectively, per 1,000 live births, compared with 5.3 and 5.1, respectively, for non-Hispanic white infants and 5.4 and 5.5, respectively, for Hispanic infants. (See Table 5.3.) In 2006 the national death rate for African-American infants was slightly higher than in 2010, 12.9 falling to 11.6 per 1,000 live births, compared with 5.6 falling to 5.1 per 1,000 live births for non-Hispanic whites and 5.4 rising to 5.5 per 1,000 births for Hispanic infants. (See Table 5.1 and Table 5.3.)

Native American or Alaskan Native infants are about one and half times as likely as non-Hispanic white and Hispanic infants to die before their first birthday. In 2006 the national death rate for Native American or Alaskan Native infants was 8.3 per 1,000 live births, compared with 5.6 for non-Hispanic white infants and 5.4 for Hispanic infants. (See Table 5.1.)

When are infants dying? Table 5.1 and Table 5.2 show death rates during the neonatal period (under 28 days after birth) and the postneonatal period (from 28 days after birth to 11 months of age). The neonatal and postneonatal deaths

TABLE 5.1

Infant, neonatal, and postneonatal mortality rates, by race and Hispanic origin of mother, selected years 1983–2006

[Data are based on linked birth and death certificates for infants.]

Race and Hispanic origin of mother	1983[a]	1985[a]	1990[a]	1995[b]	2000[b]	2004[b]	2005[b]	2006[b]
	Infant[c] deaths per 1,000 live births							
All mothers	**10.9**	**10.4**	**8.9**	**7.6**	**6.9**	**6.8**	**6.9**	**6.7**
White	9.3	8.9	7.3	6.3	5.7	5.7	5.7	5.6
Black or African American	19.2	18.6	16.9	14.6	13.5	13.2	13.3	12.9
American Indian or Alaska Native	15.2	13.1	13.1	9.0	8.3	8.4	8.1	8.3
Asian or Pacific Islander[d]	8.3	7.8	6.6	5.3	4.9	4.7	4.9	4.5
Hispanic or Latina[e, f]	9.5	8.8	7.5	6.3	5.6	5.5	5.6	5.4
Mexican	9.1	8.5	7.2	6.0	5.4	5.5	5.5	5.3
Puerto Rican	12.9	11.2	9.9	8.9	8.2	7.8	8.3	8.0
Cuban	7.5	8.5	7.2	5.3	4.6	4.6	4.4	5.1
Central and South American	8.5	8.0	6.8	5.5	4.6	4.6	4.7	4.5
Other and unknown Hispanic or Latina	10.6	9.5	8.0	7.4	6.9	6.7	6.4	5.8
Not Hispanic or Latina:								
White[f]	9.2	8.6	7.2	6.3	5.7	5.7	5.8	5.6
Black or African American[f]	19.1	18.3	16.9	14.7	13.6	13.6	13.6	13.4
	Neonatal[c] deaths per 1,000 live births							
All mothers	**7.1**	**6.8**	**5.7**	**4.9**	**4.6**	**4.5**	**4.5**	**4.5**
White	6.1	5.8	4.6	4.1	3.8	3.8	3.8	3.7
Black or African American	12.5	12.3	11.1	9.6	9.1	8.9	8.9	8.7
American Indian or Alaska Native	7.5	6.1	6.1	4.0	4.4	4.3	4.0	4.3
Asian or Pacific Islander[d]	5.2	4.8	3.9	3.4	3.4	3.2	3.4	3.2
Hispanic or Latina[e, f]	6.2	5.7	4.8	4.1	3.8	3.8	3.9	3.7
Mexican	5.9	5.4	4.5	3.9	3.6	3.7	3.8	3.7
Puerto Rican	8.7	7.6	6.9	6.1	5.8	5.3	5.9	5.4
Cuban	5.0*	6.2	5.3	3.6*	3.2*	2.8*	3.1*	3.6
Central and South American	5.8	5.6	4.4	3.7	3.3	3.4	3.2	3.1
Other and unknown Hispanic or Latina	6.4	5.6	5.0	4.8	4.6	4.7	4.3	3.7
Not Hispanic or Latina:								
White[f]	5.9	5.6	4.5	4.0	3.8	3.7	3.7	3.6
Black or African American[f]	12.0	11.9	11.0	9.6	9.2	9.1	9.1	9.0
	Postneonatal[c] deaths per 1,000 live births							
All mothers	**3.8**	**3.6**	**3.2**	**2.6**	**2.3**	**2.3**	**2.3**	**2.2**
White	3.2	3.1	2.7	2.2	1.9	1.9	2.0	1.9
Black or African American	6.7	6.3	5.9	5.0	4.3	4.3	4.3	4.2
American Indian or Alaska Native	7.7	7.0	7.0	5.1	3.9	4.2	4.0	4.0
Asian or Pacific Islander[d]	3.1	2.9	2.7	1.9	1.4	1.5	1.5	1.4
Hispanic or Latina[e, f]	3.3	3.2	2.7	2.1	1.8	1.7	1.8	1.7
Mexican	3.2	3.2	2.7	2.1	1.8	1.7	1.7	1.6
Puerto Rican	4.2	3.5	3.0	2.8	2.4	2.5	2.4	2.6
Cuban	2.5*	2.3*	1.9*	1.7*	*	1.7*	1.4*	1.4*
Central and South American	2.6	2.4	2.4	1.9	1.4	1.2	1.5	1.4
Other and unknown Hispanic or Latina	4.2	3.9	3.0	2.6	2.3	2.0	2.1	2.1
Not Hispanic or Latina:								
White[f]	3.2	3.0	2.7	2.2	1.9	2.0	2.1	1.9
Black or African American[f]	7.0	6.4	5.9	5.0	4.4	4.5	4.5	4.4

*Estimates are considered unreliable. Rates preceded by an asterisk are based on fewer than 50 deaths in the numerator. Rates not shown are based on fewer than 20 deaths in the numerator.

[a]Rates based on unweighted birth cohort data.

[b]Rates based on a period file using weighted data.

[c]Infant (under 1 year of age), neonatal (under 28 days), and postneonatal (28 days–11 months).

[d]Starting with 2003 data, estimates are not available for Asian or Pacific Islander subgroups during the transition from single-race to multiple-race reporting.

[e]Persons of Hispanic origin may be of any race.

[f]Prior to 1995, data are shown only for states with an Hispanic-origin item on their birth certificates.

Notes: The race groups white, black, American Indian or Alaska Native, and Asian or Pacific Islander include persons of Hispanic and non-Hispanic origin. Starting with 2003 data, some states reported multiple-race data. The multiple-race data for these states were bridged to the single-race categories of the 1977 Office of Management and Budget standards for comparability with other states. National linked files do not exist for 1992–1994.

Neonatal = under 28 days. Death is usually associated with a prenatal problem. Postneonatal = 28 days to 11 months. Death is usually associated with something other than a prenatal problem.

SOURCE: "Table 15. Infant, Neonatal, and Postneonatal Mortality Rates, by Detailed Race and Hispanic Origin of Mother: United States, Selected Years 1983–2006," in *Health, United States, 2010: With Special Feature on Death and Dying*, Centers for Disease Control and Prevention, National Center for Health Statistics, 2011, http://www.cdc.gov/nchs/data/hus/hus10.pdf (accessed February 1, 2012)

together comprise the infant death rate. Of all infant deaths in 2008, about two-thirds (65%) occurred during the neonatal period. For example, 4.3 infants died per 1,000 live births of all mothers in 2008 during the neonatal period, compared with a total of 6.6 infant deaths per 1,000 live births of all mothers.

TABLE 5.2

Infant deaths and infant mortality rates, by age, race, and Hispanic origin, 2007–08

[Rates are infant (under 1 year), neonatal (under 28 days), and postneonatal (28 days–11 months) deaths per 1,000 live births in specified group]

Infant age and sex	2008 Number	2008 Rate	2007 Number	2007 Rate	Percent change* from 2007 to 2008
Infant					
Total	28,059	6.61	29,138	6.75	−2.1
Male	15,669	7.21	16,293	7.38	−2.3
Female	12,390	5.97	12,845	6.09	−2.0
Neonatal					
Total	18,211	4.29	19,058	4.42	−2.9
Male	10,144	4.67	10,587	4.79	−2.5
Female	8,067	3.89	8,471	4.02	−3.2
Postneonatal					
Total	9,848	2.32	10,080	2.34	−0.9
Male	5,525	2.54	5,706	2.58	−1.6
Female	4,323	2.08	4,374	2.07	0.5

*Based on a comparison of the 2008 and 2007 mortality rates.
Notes: Neonatal = under 28 days. Death is usually associated with a prenatal (prebirth) problem.
Postneonatal = 28 days to 11 months. Death is usually associated with something other than a prenatal problem.

SOURCE: Arialdi M. Miniño et al., "Table D. Number of Infant, Neonatal, and Postneonatal Deaths and Mortality Rates, by Sex: United States, 2007–2008," in "Deaths: Final Data for 2008," *National Vital Statistics Reports*, vol. 59, no. 10, December 7, 2011, http://www.cdc.gov/nchs/data/nvsr/nvsr59/nvsr59_10.pdf (accessed February 21, 2012)

Life expectancy is the age to which people born in a particular year in a particular location can anticipate living. Infants born in 2010 in the United States are expected to live an average of 78.7 years, up from 78.6 years in 2009. (See Table 5.4.) However, those in certain groups have slightly different life expectancies. Females have a longer life expectancy than males. Female infants born in 2010 are expected to live for 81.1 years, whereas males born in that same year are expected to live for 76.2 years.

CAUSES OF INFANT MORTALITY

Birth defects are the leading cause of infant mortality in the United States. Birth defects are abnormalities of structure, function, or metabolism present at birth. In 2010 these congenital problems accounted for 5,077 out of 24,548 total causes of infant deaths. (See Table 5.5.) Birth defects are listed in Table 5.5 as congenital malformations, deformations, and chromosomal abnormalities.

Some of the more serious birth defects are anencephaly (absence of the majority of the brain) and spina bifida (incomplete development of the back and spine). Down syndrome, a condition in which babies are born with an extra copy of chromosome 21 in their cells, results in anatomical and developmental problems along with cognitive deficits. Down syndrome children may be born with birth defects that are fatal, including defects of the heart, lungs, and gastrointestinal tract. However, many Down syndrome children live well into their 50s and beyond.

According to the Centers for Disease Control and Prevention (CDC), in "Birth Defects" (February 24, 2011, http://

www.cdc.gov/ncbddd/bd/default.htm), one out of every 33 babies born in the United States each year has a birth defect. The CDC notes that babies born with birth defects are more likely to have poor health and long-term disabilities than babies born without birth defects.

Disorders related to short gestation (premature birth) and low birth weight accounted for the second-leading cause of infant mortality in 2010—out of a total of 24,548 infant deaths, 4,130 babies died from these disorders. (See Table 5.5.) Other causes of infant deaths were sudden infant death syndrome, maternal complications of pregnancy, accidents, and complications of the placenta, umbilical cord, and membranes. These six leading causes of infant mortality accounted for 60% of the total infant deaths in all races in 2010.

BIRTH DEFECTS

The March of Dimes Foundation, a national volunteer organization that seeks to improve infant health by preventing birth defects and lowering infant mortality rates, reports in "Birth Defects" (2011, http://www.marchofdimes.com/pnhec/4439_1206.asp) that approximately 120,000 babies are born annually in the United States with birth defects. Some birth defects have genetic causes—inherited abnormalities such as Tay-Sachs disease (a fatal disease that generally affects children of east European Jewish ancestry) or chromosomal irregularities such as Down syndrome. Other birth defects result from environmental factors—infections during pregnancy, such as rubella (German measles), or drugs used by the pregnant woman. The specific causes of many birth defects are unknown, but scientists

TABLE 5.3

Infant deaths and infant mortality rates, by age, race, and Hispanic origin, 2009 and 2010

Age, race, and Hispanic origin	2010		2009	
	Number	Rate	Number	Rate
All races[a]				
Under 1 year	24,548	6.14	26,412	6.39
Under 28 days	16,167	4.04	17,255	4.18
28 days–11 months	8,381	2.10	9,157	2.22
Total white				
Under 1 year	15,933	5.19	16,817	5.30
Under 28 days	10,603	3.45	11,054	3.48
28 days–11 months	5,330	1.74	5,763	1.82
Non-Hispanic white				
Under 1 year	11,002	5.09	11,608	5.25
Under 28 days	7,199	3.33	7,562	3.42
28 days–11 months	3,803	1.76	4,046	1.83
Total black				
Under 1 year	7,388	11.61	8,312	12.64
Under 28 days	4,760	7.48	5,374	8.17
28 days–11 months	2,627	4.13	2,938	4.47
Hispanic[b]				
Under 1 year	5,167	5.46	5,424	5.43
Under 28 days	3,523	3.72	3,629	3.63
28 days–11 months	1,644	1.74	1,795	1.80

[a]Includes races other than white and black.
[b]Includes all persons of Hispanic origin of any race.
Notes: Data are subject to sampling or random variation.
Data are based on the continuous file of records received from the states. Rates per 1,000 live births. Figures for 2010 are based on weighted data rounded to the nearest individual, so categories may not add to totals. Race and Hispanic origin are reported separately on both the birth and death certificate. Rates for Hispanic origin should be interpreted with caution because of the inconsistencies between reporting Hispanic origin on birth and death certificates.

SOURCE: Sherry L. Murphy, Jiaquan Xu, and Kenneth D. Kochanek, "Table 4. Infant Deaths and Infant Mortality Rates, by Age, Race and Hispanic Origin: United States, Final 2009 and Preliminary 2010," in "Deaths: Preliminary Data for 2010," *National Vital Statistics Reports*, vol. 60, no. 4, January 11, 2012, http://www.cdc.gov/nchs/data/nvsr/nvsr60/nvsr60_04.pdf (accessed January 31, 2012)

think that many result from a combination of genetic and environmental factors. Even though many birth defects are impossible to prevent, some can be avoided, such as those that are caused by maternal alcohol and drug consumption during pregnancy.

Neural Tube Defects

Neural tube defects (NTDs) are abnormalities of the brain and spinal cord resulting from the failure of the neural tube to develop properly during early pregnancy. The neural tube is the embryonic nerve tissue that develops into the brain and the spinal cord. Folic acid is a B vitamin that helps prevent NTDs in the developing embryo and fetus. The CDC reports in "Racial/Ethnic Differences in the Birth Prevalence of Spina Bifida— United States, 1995–2005" (*Morbidity and Mortality Weekly Report*, vol. 57, no. 53, January 9, 2009) that in 1992 it instituted the recommendation that women of childbearing age take 400 micrograms of folic acid daily. In addition, the U.S. Food and Drug Administration man-

dated that by 1998 cereal manufacturers were to add folic acid to their enriched cereal grain products.

In "Facts about Folic Acid" (January 13, 2012, http://www.cdc.gov/ncbddd/folicacid/about.html), the CDC notes that folic acid can help prevent NTDs if women who are contemplating pregnancy consume sufficient amounts of folic acid before conception and then throughout their pregnancy. The two most common NTDs are anencephaly and spina bifida.

ANENCEPHALY. Anencephalic infants die before birth (in utero or stillborn) or shortly thereafter. T. J. Mathews of the National Center for Health Statistics indicates in *Trends in Spina Bifida and Anencephalus in the United States, 1991–2006* (April 2009, http://www.cdc.gov/nchs/data/hestat/spine_anen/spine_anen.pdf), the most recent report on this topic as of April 2012, that the incidence of anencephaly decreased significantly from 18.4 cases per 100,000 live births in 1991 to 9.4 cases per 100,000 live births in 2001. (See Figure 5.1 and Table 5.6.) The largest drop during this period was between 1991 and 1992. Between 1993 and 2001 the general trend was downward. Between 2002 and 2003 the rates increased from 9.6 cases per 100,000 live births to 11.1 cases per 100,000 live births. Since 2003 rates have stabilized somewhat and were 11.2 cases per 100,000 live births in 2006.

Issues of brain death and organ donation sometimes surround anencephalic infants. One case that gained national attention was that of Theresa Ann Campo in 1992. Before their daughter's birth, Theresa's parents discovered through prenatal testing that their baby would be born without a fully developed brain. They decided to carry the fetus to term and donate her organs for transplantation. When baby Theresa was born, her parents asked for her to be declared brain dead. However, Theresa's brain stem was still functioning, so the court ruled against the parents' request. Baby Theresa died 10 days later and her organs were not usable for transplant because they had deteriorated as a result of oxygen deprivation.

Some physicians and ethicists agree that even if anencephalic babies have a brain stem, they should be considered brain dead. Lacking a functioning higher brain, these babies can feel nothing and have no consciousness. Others fear that declaring anencephalic babies dead could be the start of a slippery slope that might eventually include babies with other birth defects in the same category. Other people are concerned that anencephalic babies may be kept alive for the purpose of harvesting their organs for transplant at a later date.

SPINA BIFIDA. Spina bifida, which literally means "divided spine," is caused by the failure of the vertebrae (backbone) to completely cover the spinal cord early in

TABLE 5.4

Deaths and life expectancy at birth, by race and sex, with infant deaths and mortality rates, by race, 2009 and 2010

[Data are based on a continuous file of records received from the states. Figures for 2010 are based on weighted data rounded to the nearest individual, so categories may not add to totals.]

Measure and sex	All races[a]		White[b]		Black[b]	
	2010	2009	2010	2009	2010	2009
All deaths	**2,465,936**	**2,437,163**	**2,112,458**	**2,086,355**	**286,800**	**286,623**
Male	1,231,215	1,217,379	1,050,382	1,037,475	145,731	146,239
Female	1,234,721	1,219,784	1,062,076	1,048,880	141,068	140,384
Age-adjusted death rate[c, d]	746.2	749.6	741.0	742.8	897.7	912.7
Male	886.2	890.9	877.5	880.5	1,103.4	1,123.1
Female	634.3	636.8	630.1	631.3	752.0	763.3
Life expectancy at birth (in years)[e]	78.7	78.6	79.0	78.8	75.1	74.7
Male	76.2	76.0	76.5	76.4	71.8	71.4
Female	81.1	80.9	81.3	81.2	78.0	77.7
All infant deaths	**24,548**	**26,412**	**15,933**	**16,817**	**7,388**	**8,312**
Infant mortality rate[f]	6.14	6.39	5.19	5.30	11.61	12.64

[a]Includes races other than white and black.

[b]Race categories are consistent with the 1977 Office of Management and Budget (OMB) standards. Multiple-race data were reported for deaths by 37 states and the District of Columbia in 2010 and by 34 states and the District of Columbia in 2009, and were reported for births (used as the denominator in computing infant mortality rates), by 38 states and the District of Columbia in 2010 and by 33 states and the District of Columbia in 2009. The multiple-race data for these reporting areas were bridged to the single-race categories of the 1977 OMB standards for comparability with other reporting areas.

[c]Rates for 2009 are revised and may differ from rates previously published.

[d]Age-adjusted death rates are per 100,000 U.S. standard population, based on the year 2000 standard.

[e]Life expectancies for 2009 have been updated and may differ from those previously published.

[f]Infant mortality rates are deaths under 1 year per 1,000 live births in specified group.

SOURCE: Sherry L. Murphy, Jiaquan Xu, and Kenneth D. Kochanek, "Table A. Deaths, Age-Adjusted Death Rates, and Life Expectancy at Birth, by Race and Sex; and Infant Deaths and Mortality Rates, by Race: United States, Final 2009 and Preliminary 2010," in "Deaths: Preliminary Data for 2010," *National Vital Statistics Reports*, vol. 60, no. 4, January 11, 2012, http://www.cdc.gov/nchs/data/nvsr/nvsr60/nvsr60_04.pdf (accessed January 31, 2012)

TABLE 5.5

Ten leading causes of infant deaths and infant mortality rates, by race and Hispanic origin, 2010

[Data are based on a continuous file of records received from the states. Rates are per 100,000 live births. Figures are based on weighted data rounded to the nearest individual, so categories may not add to totals or subtotals.]

Rank*	Cause of death	Number	Rate
. . .	All causes	24,548	613.7
1	Congenital malformations, deformations and chromosomal abnormalities	5,077	126.9
2	Disorders related to short gestation and low birthweight, not elsewhere classified	4,130	103.2
3	Sudden infant death syndrome	1,890	47.2
4	Newborn affected by maternal complications of pregnancy	1,555	38.9
5	Accidents (unintentional injuries)	1,043	26.1
6	Newborn affected by complications of placenta, cord and membranes	1,030	25.7
7	Bacterial sepsis of newborn	569	14.2
8	Diseases of the circulatory system	499	12.5
9	Respiratory distress of newborn	496	12.4
10	Necrotizing enterocolitis of newborn	470	11.7
. . .	All other causes (residual)	7,789	194.7

. . .Category not applicable.

*Rank based on number of deaths.

Note: For certain causes of death such as unintentional injuries, homicides, suicides, and sudden infant death syndrome, preliminary and final data differ because of the truncated nature of the preliminary file. Data are subject to sampling or random variation. The infant mortality rate is the preferred indicator of the risk of dying during the first year of life.

SOURCE: Sherry L. Murphy, Jiaquan Xu, and Kenneth D. Kochanek, "Table 8. Infant Deaths and Infant Mortality Rates for the 10 Leading Causes of Infant Death: United States, Preliminary 2010," in "Deaths: Preliminary Data for 2010," *National Vital Statistics Reports*, vol. 60, no. 4, January 11, 2012, http://www.cdc.gov/nchs/data/nvsr/nvsr60/nvsr60_04.pdf (accessed January 31, 2012)

fetal development, leaving the spinal cord exposed. Depending on the amount of nerve tissue that is exposed, spina bifida defects range from minor developmental disabilities to paralysis.

Before the advent of antibiotics during the 1950s, most babies with severe spina bifida died soon after birth. With antibiotics and many medical advances, some of these newborns can be saved.

FIGURE 5.1

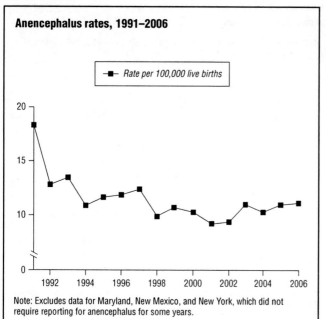

Anencephalus rates, 1991–2006

Note: Excludes data for Maryland, New Mexico, and New York, which did not require reporting for anencephalus for some years.

SOURCE: Adapted from T. J. Mathews, "Figure 2. Anencephalus Rates, 1991–2006," in *Trends in Spina Bifida and Anencephalus in the United States, 1991–2006*, Health E-Stats, Centers for Disease Control and Prevention, National Center for Health Statistics, April 2009, http://www.cdc.gov/nchs/data/hestat/spine_anen/spine_anen.pdf (accessed February 1, 2012)

TABLE 5.6

Number of live births, anencephalus cases, and anencephalus rates, 1991–2006

	Anencephalus cases	Total live births	Rate
2006	436	3,890,949	11.21
2005	432	3,887,109	11.11
2004	401	3,860,720	10.39
2003	441	3,715,577	11.14
2002	348	3,645,770	9.55
2001	343	3,640,555	9.42
2000	376	3,640,376	10.33
1999	382	3,533,565	10.81
1998	349	3,519,240	9.92
1997	434	3,469,667	12.51
1996	416	3,478,723	11.96
1995	408	3,484,539	11.71
1994	387	3,527,482	10.97
1993	481	3,562,723	13.50
1992	457	3,572,890	12.79
1991	655	3,564,453	18.38

Note: Excludes data for Maryland, New Mexico, and New York, which did not require reporting for anencephalus for some years.

SOURCE: Adapted from T. J. Mathews, "Table 2. Number of Live Births with Anencephalus and Rates per 100,000 Live Births: United States, 1991–2006," in *Trends in Spina Bifida and Anencephalus in the United States, 1991–2006*, Health E-Stats, Centers for Disease Control and Prevention, National Center for Health Statistics, April 2009, http://www.cdc.gov/nchs/data/hestat/spine_anen/spine_anen.pdf (accessed February 1, 2012)

The treatment of newborns with spina bifida can pose serious ethical problems. Should an infant with a milder form of the disease be treated actively and another with severe defects be left untreated? In severe cases, should the newborn be sedated and not be given nutrition and hydration until death occurs? Or should this seriously disabled infant be cared for while suffering from bladder and bowel malfunctions, infections, and paralysis? What if infants who have been left to die unexpectedly survive? Would they be more disabled than if they had been treated right away?

The development of fetal surgery to correct spina bifida before birth added another dimension to the debate. There are risks for both the mother and the fetus during and after fetal surgery, but techniques have improved since the first successful surgery of this type in 1997. In 2003 the National Institute of Child Health and Human Development began funding the Management of Myelomeningocele Study (MOMS; http://www.spinabifidamoms.com/english/index.html) to compare the progress between babies who have had prenatal (prebirth) surgery and those who have had postnatal (after birth) surgery. MOMS sought to enroll 200 participants, and as of April 2012, enrollment was closed. MOMS also began follow-up with the children of enrollees to compare the outcomes of the prenatal and postnatal surgery groups. As of April 2012, results had not been published.

According to Mathews, in *Trends in Spina Bifida and Anencephalus in the United States, 1991–2006*, spina bifida rates increased from 22.8 cases per 100,000 live births in 1992 to 28 cases per 100,000 live births in 1995, but after 1995 the rates declined to 18 cases per 100,000 live births in 2005 and 2006—the lowest spina bifida rates ever reported. (See Figure 5.2 and Table 5.7.) The CDC notes in "Racial/Ethnic Differences in the Birth Prevalence of Spina Bifida" that "from October 1995–December 1996 (before the folic acid fortification mandate) to October 1998–December 1999 (after the January 2008 mandate deadline), the prevalence of spina bifida decreased from 2.62 to 2.02 per 10,000 live births, a decrease of 22.9%." The CDC also analyzes racial and ethnic differences of the decline and reports that the prevalence of spina bifida in infants of non-Hispanic African-American mothers fell 19.8% during this period, which was well above the average percent decline. In contrast, the prevalence of spina bifida in infants of non-Hispanic white and Hispanic mothers remained nearly constant. The CDC suggests that "future public health efforts to reduce the prevalence of spina bifida should focus on subgroups of women with known risk factors for an NTD-affected pregnancy, such as obesity, Hispanic ethnicity, and certain genetic factors."

Using 2002 CDC data, Mikyong Shin et al. estimate in "Prevalence of Spina Bifida Among Children and Adolescents in 10 Regions in the United States" (*Pediatrics*, vol. 126, no. 2, August 2010) the prevalence of spina bifida among those aged birth to 19 years in 10 diverse regions of

FIGURE 5.2

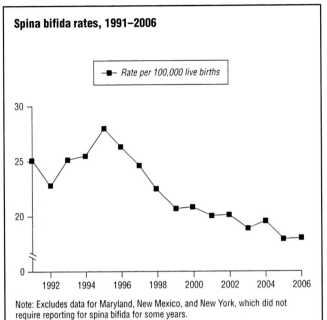

Spina bifida rates, 1991–2006

Note: Excludes data for Maryland, New Mexico, and New York, which did not require reporting for spina bifida for some years.

SOURCE: Adapted from T. J. Mathews, "Figure 1. Spina Bifida Rates, 1991–2006," in *Trends in Spina Bifida and Anencephalus in the United States, 1991–2006*, Health E-Stats, Centers for Disease Control and Prevention, National Center for Health Statistics, April 2009, http://www.cdc.gov/nchs/data/hestat/spine_anen/spine_anen.pdf (accessed February 1, 2012)

TABLE 5.7

Number of live births, spina bifida cases, and spina bifida rates, 1991–2006

	Spina bifida cases	Total live births	Rate
2006	700	3,890,949	17.99
2005	698	3,887,109	17.96
2004	755	3,860,720	19.56
2003	702	3,715,577	18.89
2002	734	3,645,770	20.13
2001	730	3,640,555	20.05
2000	759	3,640,376	20.85
1999	732	3,533,565	20.72
1998	790	3,519,240	22.45
1997	857	3,469,667	24.70
1996	917	3,478,723	26.36
1995	975	3,484,539	27.98
1994	900	3,527,482	25.51
1993	896	3,562,723	25.15
1992	816	3,572,890	22.84
1991	887	3,564,453	24.88

Note: Excludes data for Maryland, New Mexico, and New York, which did not require reporting for spina bifida for some years.

SOURCE: Adapted from T. J. Mathews, "Table 1. Number of Live Births with Spina Bifida and Rates per 100,000 Live Births: United States, 1991–2006," in *Trends in Spina Bifida and Anencephalus in the United States, 1991–2006*, Health E-Stats, Centers for Disease Control and Prevention, National Center for Health Statistics, April 2009, http://www.cdc.gov/nchs/data/hestat/spine_anen/spine_anen.pdf (accessed February 1, 2012)

the United States. The researchers determine that the prevalence of spina bifida varied across ages, race, ethnicity, and gender. Shin et al. believe that there are about 3.1 cases per 10,000 population, with lower rates among males and non-Hispanic African-Americans.

Down Syndrome

Down syndrome is a condition caused by chromosomal irregularities that occur during cell division of either the egg (primarily) or the sperm (occasionally) before conception. Instead of the normal 46 chromosomes, Down syndrome newborns have an extra copy of chromosome 21, giving them a total of 47 chromosomes. Along with having certain anatomical differences from non–Down syndrome children, Down children have varying degrees of intellectual disability (formerly called mental retardation) and approximately 40% have congenital heart diseases.

In "Facts about Down Syndrome" (June 8, 2011, http://www.cdc.gov/ncbddd/birthdefects/DownSyndrome.html), the CDC estimates the prevalence of Down syndrome as approximately one out of every 691 live births. The occurrence of this genetic condition rises with increasing maternal age, with a marked increase seen in children of women over 35 years of age.

Robert Barnhart and Barbara Connolly report in "Aging and Down Syndrome: Implications for Physical Therapy" (*Physical Therapy*, vol. 87, no. 10, October 2007) that the life expectancy of people with Down syndrome has increased over the decades, from an average of nine years of age in 1929 to 55 years in 2007. Except for the most severe heart defects, many other problems that accompany Down syndrome may be corrected by surgery and helped with exercise, strength training, and a healthy diet. Depending on the degree of intellectual disability, many people with Down syndrome are able to hold jobs and live independently.

Now that people with Down syndrome are growing older, researchers are able to document which diseases affect people with Down syndrome more than people without the syndrome. For example, in "Health Conditions Associated with Aging and End of Life of Adults with Down Syndrome" (*International Review of Research in Mental Retardation*, vol. 39, 2010), Anna J. Esbensen of the Cincinnati Children's Hospital Medical Center in Cincinnati, Ohio, determines that adults with Down syndrome have an "increased risk for skin and hair changes, early onset menopause, visual and hearing impairments, adult onset seizure disorder, thyroid dysfunction, diabetes, obesity, sleep apnea and musculoskeletal problems." She also finds that adults with Down syndrome are less likely to succumb to various solid-tumor cancers, heart disease, and hypertension.

Birth Defects and National Laws

In April 1998 President Bill Clinton (1946–) signed into law the Birth Defects Prevention Act, which authorized a nationwide network of birth defects research and prevention programs and called for a nationwide information clearinghouse on birth defects. The Children's Health Act of 2000 authorized expanded research and services for a variety of childhood health problems. In addition, it created the National Center on Birth Defects and Developmental Disabilities (NCBDDD) at the CDC, which was officially established in 2001.

Developmental disabilities are conditions that impair day-to-day functioning, such as difficulties with communication, learning, behavior, and motor skills. They are chronic conditions that initially appear in people aged 18 years and younger. The NCBDDD works with state health departments, academic institutions, and other public health partners to monitor birth defects and developmental disabilities and to support research to identify their causes or risk factors. In addition, the center develops strategies and promotes programs to prevent birth defects and developmental disabilities.

The Economic Cost of Long-Term Care for Birth Defects and Developmental Disabilities

In "Health of Children 3 to 17 Years of Age with Down Syndrome in the 1997–2005 National Health Interview Survey" (*Pediatrics*, vol. 123, no. 2, February 2009), Laura A. Schieve et al. compare the medical conditions, the developmental disorders, and the impact on health and health care needs in children aged three to 17 years with and without Down syndrome. The children with Down syndrome were found to have a higher frequency of food allergies, colds, and developmental disabilities (in addition to intellectual disability, which is common in Down syndrome). The researchers note that ">25% of children with Down syndrome needed help with personal care, regularly took prescription medications, had recently seen a medical specialist, and received physical therapy or related therapy." A control group of children with intellectual disability but not Down syndrome also had "multiple serious disabilities" and "high rates of medical conditions and high levels of health impact and service use." In their conclusion, Schieve et al. state that "current medical costs are estimated to be 12 to 14 times higher for children with DS [Down syndrome] than for those without DS."

The Schieve et al. study helps show how some people with birth defects and/or developmental disabilities require long-term care or medical services that result in increased medical costs. Sophie Mitra, Patricia A. Findley, and Usha Sambamoorthi conducted a retrospective analysis of the Medical Expenditure Panel Survey and published their results in "Health Care Expenditures of Living with a Disability: Total Expenditures, Out-of-Pocket Expenses, and Burden, 1996 to 2004" (*Archives of Physical Medicine and Rehabilitation*, vol. 90, no. 9, September 2009). The researchers determine that between 1996 and 2004 people with disabilities had significantly higher health

expenditures overall when compared with people without disabilities.

In "Health Disparities among Adults with Physical Disabilities or Cognitive Limitations Compared to Individuals with No Disabilities in the United States" (*Disability and Health Journal*, vol. 4, no. 2, 2011), another retrospective analysis of the Medical Expenditure Panel Survey, Amanda Reichard, Hayley Stolzle, and Michael H. Fox determine whether "adults with either physical disability or cognitive limitations experience significant health disparities in comparison to those with no disability." The researchers find that people with cognitive limitations or physical disabilities "had significantly higher prevalence rates for 7 chronic diseases" than people without these disabilities. They also determine that the disabilities group was less likely to receive types of preventive care that the nondisabilities group received. Reichard, Stolzle, and Fox comment that people with disabilities need as many public health interventions (if not more) to help prevent the development of costly chronic diseases and conditions, which may affect this group more than the nondisabilities group.

LOW BIRTH WEIGHT AND PREMATURITY

The usual length of human pregnancy is 40 weeks. Infants born before 37 weeks of pregnancy are considered to be premature. A premature infant does not have fully formed organ systems. If the premature infant is born with a birth weight that is comparable to a full-term baby and has organ systems only slightly underdeveloped, the chances of survival are great. Conversely, premature infants of very low birth weight are susceptible to many risks and are less likely to survive. If they survive, they may suffer from intellectual disability and other abnormalities of the nervous system.

A severe medical condition called respiratory distress syndrome (RDS) commonly affects premature infants born before 35 weeks of pregnancy. In RDS immature lungs do not function properly and may cause infant death within hours after birth. Intensive care includes the use of a mechanical ventilator to facilitate breathing. Premature infants also commonly have immature gastrointestinal systems, which preclude them from taking in nourishment properly. Unable to suck and swallow, they must be fed through a stomach tube.

Joyce A. Martin et al. of the CDC note in "Births: Final Data for 2008" (*National Vital Statistics Reports*, vol. 59, no. 1, December 8, 2010) that of the nearly 4.3 million live births in 2008, 523,033 (12.3%) were preterm (less than 37 weeks gestation) infants. Of this percentage, non-Hispanic African-American (17.5%) mothers were about one-third more likely than non-Hispanic white (11.1%) and Hispanic (12.1%) mothers to have a preterm birth in 2008. (See Figure 5.3.) According to Figure 5.4, the overall rates of preterm births have declined slightly since about 2006.

FIGURE 5.3

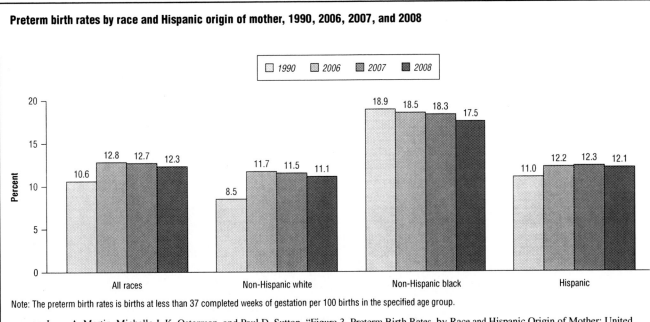

Preterm birth rates by race and Hispanic origin of mother, 1990, 2006, 2007, and 2008

□ 1990   ▨ 2006   ▨ 2007   ■ 2008

Note: The preterm birth rates is births at less than 37 completed weeks of gestation per 100 births in the specified age group.

SOURCE: Joyce A. Martin, Michelle J. K. Osterman, and Paul D. Sutton, "Figure 3. Preterm Birth Rates, by Race and Hispanic Origin of Mother: United States, 1990 and 2006 Final and 2007 and 2008 Preliminary," in "Are Preterm Births on the Decline in the United States? Recent Data from the National Vital Statistics System," in *NCHS Data Brief*, no. 39, May 2010, http://www.cdc.gov/nchs/data/databriefs/db39.pdf (accessed February 2, 2012)

FIGURE 5.4

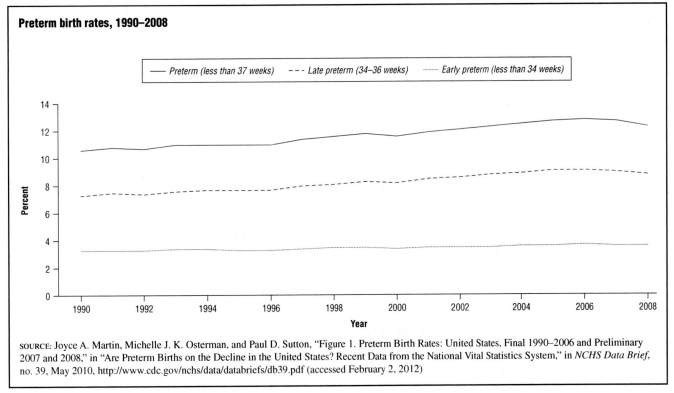

Preterm birth rates, 1990–2008

— Preterm (less than 37 weeks)   - - - Late preterm (34–36 weeks)   ⋯⋯ Early preterm (less than 34 weeks)

SOURCE: Joyce A. Martin, Michelle J. K. Osterman, and Paul D. Sutton, "Figure 1. Preterm Birth Rates: United States, Final 1990–2006 and Preliminary 2007 and 2008," in "Are Preterm Births on the Decline in the United States? Recent Data from the National Vital Statistics System," in *NCHS Data Brief*, no. 39, May 2010, http://www.cdc.gov/nchs/data/databriefs/db39.pdf (accessed February 2, 2012)

Prematurity may result from various causes, including poor maternal nutrition, teen pregnancy, drug and alcohol use, smoking, or sexually transmitted diseases. Joyce A. Martin, Michelle J. K. Osterman, and Paul D. Sutton of the CDC indicate in "Are Preterm Births on the Decline in the United States? Recent Data from the National Vital Statistics System" (*NCHS Data Brief*, no. 39, May 2010) that in 2008 teens had a higher percentage of preterm births than women between the ages of 20 and 39 years. (See Figure 5.5.)

FIGURE 5.5

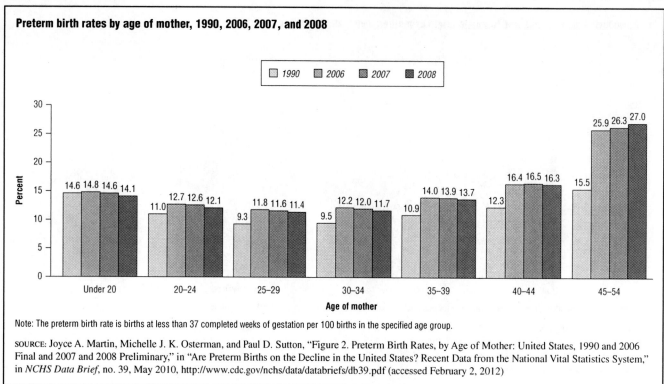

Preterm birth rates by age of mother, 1990, 2006, 2007, and 2008

Note: The preterm birth rate is births at less than 37 completed weeks of gestation per 100 births in the specified age group.

SOURCE: Joyce A. Martin, Michelle J. K. Osterman, and Paul D. Sutton, "Figure 2. Preterm Birth Rates, by Age of Mother: United States, 1990 and 2006 Final and 2007 and 2008 Preliminary," in "Are Preterm Births on the Decline in the United States? Recent Data from the National Vital Statistics System," in *NCHS Data Brief*, no. 39, May 2010, http://www.cdc.gov/nchs/data/databriefs/db39.pdf (accessed February 2, 2012)

Infants who weigh less than 5 pounds, 8 ounces (2,500 g) at birth are considered to be of low birth weight. Those born weighing less than 3 pounds, 4 ounces (1,500 g) have very low birth weight. In "Birth Weight and Health and Developmental Outcomes in US Children, 1997–2005" (*Maternal and Child Health Journal*, vol. 15, no. 7, October 2011), Sheree L. Boulet, Laura A. Schieve, and Coleen A. Boyle of the CDC note that children born with low birth weights are more likely to die within their first year or have long-term disabilities than babies born with a normal birth weight of between 5 pounds, 8 ounces and 8 pounds, 13 ounces (2,500 and 4,000 g). In addition, the researchers find that children born with low-normal birth weights (5 pounds, 8 ounces to 6 pounds, 10 ounces [2,500 to 2,999 g]) are more likely than those with birth weights of 7 pounds, 11 ounces to 8 pounds, 13 ounces (3,500 to 4,000 g) to have intellectual disability, cerebral palsy, learning disabilities, attention deficit hyperactivity disorder, or other developmental delays and to receive special education services.

According to the National Center for Health Statistics, in *Health, United States, 2010* (2011, http://www.cdc.gov/nchs/data/hus/hus10.pdf), in 2007 and 2008 cigarette smokers had a higher percentage of low-birth-weight babies than non-smokers (11.9% versus 7.4% in 2007 and 11.9% versus 7.3% in 2008) and a higher percentage of very-low-birth-weight babies (1.8% versus 1.3% in 2007 and 1.8% versus 1.3% in 2008). (See Table 5.8.)

According to Martin et al., 1.5% of the babies born in 2009 were very-low-birth-weight infants. The proportion of

very-low-birth-weight babies has been increasing since the 1980s, rising to 1.3% in 1990 and to 1.4% in 2000, although the rates stabilized somewhat between 2005 and 2009. (See Table 5.8 and Table 5.9.) Martin et al. report that the birth weight distribution in general has shifted toward lower birth weights since the early 1990s. The researchers explain that the shift is likely influenced by a variety of factors, including obstetric intervention earlier in pregnancy, such as induction of labor and cesarean delivery, older maternal age at child bearing, and increased use of infertility therapies. In 2008 the highest percentage of preterm babies (27%) was with women between the ages of 45 to 54 years. (See Figure 5.5.)

Alice Yuen Loke and Chung Fan Poon explain in "The Health Concerns and Behaviours of Primigravida: Comparing Advanced Age Pregnant Women with their Younger Counterparts" (*Journal of Clinical Nursing*, vol. 20, nos. 7–8, April 2011) that even though advanced-age pregnant women (over the age of 35 years) are more attuned to various healthy behaviors such as prenatal care, eating nutritiously, and getting sufficient exercise, they are also balancing their careers with taking care of aging parents and worrying about the health of their infants. It is well documented in scientific literature that there are increasing concerns regarding the health of the fetus/baby in women over the age of 35 years. Loke and Poon conclude that an educational program should be launched in the mass media to inform people of the concerns of becoming pregnant later in life.

TABLE 5.8

Low-birthweight live births, by mother's race, Hispanic origin, and smoking status, selected years 1970–2008

[Data are based on birth certificates]

Birthweight, race and Hispanic origin of mother, and smoking status of mother	1970	1975	1980	1985	1990	1995	2000	2005	2006	2007	2008
Low birthweight (less than 2,500 grams)					Percent of live births[a]						
All races	7.93	7.38	6.84	6.75	6.97	7.32	7.57	8.19	8.26	8.22	8.18
White	6.85	6.27	5.72	5.65	5.70	6.22	6.55	7.16	7.21	7.16	7.13
Black or African American	13.90	13.19	12.69	12.65	13.25	13.13	12.99	13.59	13.59	13.55	13.39
American Indian or Alaska Native	7.97	6.41	6.44	5.86	6.11	6.61	6.76	7.36	7.52	7.46	7.40
Asian or Pacific Islander[b]	—	—	6.68	6.16	6.45	6.90	7.31	7.98	8.12	8.10	8.18
Hispanic or Latina[c]	—	—	6.12	6.16	6.06	6.29	6.41	6.88	6.99	6.93	6.96
Mexican	—	—	5.62	5.77	5.55	5.81	6.01	6.49	6.58	6.50	6.49
Puerto Rican	—	—	8.95	8.69	8.99	9.41	9.30	9.92	10.14	9.83	9.86
Cuban	—	—	5.62	6.02	5.67	6.50	6.49	7.64	7.14	7.66	7.83
Central and South American	—	—	5.76	5.68	5.84	6.20	6.34	6.78	6.81	6.71	6.70
Other and unknown Hispanic or Latina	—	—	6.96	6.83	6.87	7.55	7.84	8.27	8.54	8.61	8.24
Not Hispanic or Latina:[c]											
White	—	—	5.69	5.61	5.61	6.20	6.60	7.29	7.32	7.28	7.22
Black or African American	—	—	12.71	12.62	13.32	13.21	13.13	14.02	13.97	13.90	13.71
									21 reporting areas		
Cigarette smoker[d]	—	—	—	—	A	A	A	A	12.02	11.85	11.85
Nonsmoker[d]	—	—	—	—	A	A	A	A	7.69	7.36	7.32
Very low birthweight (less than 1,500 grams)											
All races	1.17	1.16	1.15	1.21	1.27	1.35	1.43	1.49	1.49	1.49	1.46
White	0.95	0.92	0.90	0.94	0.95	1.06	1.14	1.20	1.20	1.19	1.18
Black or African American	2.40	2.40	2.48	2.71	2.92	2.97	3.07	3.15	3.05	3.11	2.93
American Indian or Alaska Native	0.98	0.95	0.92	1.01	1.01	1.10	1.16	1.17	1.28	1.27	1.28
Asian or Pacific Islander[b]	—	—	0.92	0.85	0.87	0.91	1.05	1.14	1.12	1.14	1.16
Hispanic or Latina[c]	—	—	0.98	1.01	1.03	1.11	1.14	1.20	1.19	1.21	1.20
Mexican	—	—	0.92	0.97	0.92	1.01	1.03	1.12	1.12	1.13	1.11
Puerto Rican	—	—	1.29	1.30	1.62	1.79	1.93	1.87	1.91	1.89	1.93
Cuban	—	—	1.02	1.18	1.20	1.19	1.21	1.50	1.28	1.27	1.43
Central and South American	—	—	0.99	1.01	1.05	1.13	1.20	1.19	1.13	1.15	1.13
Other and unknown Hispanic or Latina	—	—	1.01	0.96	1.09	1.28	1.42	1.36	1.36	1.44	1.34
Not Hispanic or Latina:[c]											
White	—	—	0.87	0.91	0.93	1.04	1.14	1.21	1.20	1.19	1.18
Black or African American	—	—	2.47	2.67	2.93	2.98	3.10	3.27	3.15	3.20	3.01
									21 reporting areas		
Cigarette smoker[d]	—	—	—	—	*	*	*	*	1.73	1.80	1.79
Nonsmoker[d]	—	—	—	—	*	*	*	*	1.41	1.32	1.29

—Data not available.

*Data not shown. Due to a change in reporting, data are not comparable to other years.

[a]Excludes live births with unknown birthweight. Percent based on live births with known birthweight.

[b]Starting with 2003 data, estimates are not available for Asian or Pacific Islander subgroups during the transition from single-race to multiple-race reporting.

[c]Prior to 1993, data from states lacking an Hispanic-origin item on the birth certificate were excluded. Data for non-Hispanic white and non-Hispanic black women for years prior to 1989 are not nationally representative and are provided for comparison with Hispanic data.

[d]Percent based on live births with known smoking status of mother and known birthweight.

Only reporting areas that have implemented the 2003 revision of the U.S. Standard Certificate of Live Birth are shown because maternal tobacco use data based on the 2003 revision are not comparable with data based on the 1989 or earlier revisions to the U.S. Standard Certificate of Live Birth. Data are for the 21 reporting areas that used the 2003 revision of the U.S. Standard Certificate of Live Birth for data on smoking in 2007 and 2008.

Notes: The race groups, white, black, American Indian or Alaska Native, and Asian or Pacific Islander, include persons of Hispanic and non-Hispanic origin. Persons of Hispanic origin may be of any race. Starting with 2003 data, some states reported multiple-race data.

The multiple-race data for these states were bridged to the single-race categories of the 1977 Office of Management and Budget standards for comparability with other states.

Interpretation of trend data should take into consideration expansion of reporting areas and immigration.

SOURCE: "Table 9. Low-Birthweight Live Births, by Detailed Race, Hispanic Origin, and Smoking Status of Mother: United States, Selected Years 1970–2008," in *Health, United States, 2010: With Special Feature on Death and Dying*, Centers for Disease Control and Prevention, National Center for Health Statistics, 2011, http://www.cdc.gov/nchs/data/hus/2010/009.pdf (accessed February 22, 2012)

WHO MAKES MEDICAL DECISIONS FOR INFANTS?

Before the 1980s courts in the United States were supportive of biological parents making decisions regarding the medical care of their newborns. Parents often made these decisions in consultation with pediatricians. Beginning in the 1980s medical advancements allowed for the survival of infants who would have not had a chance for survival before that time. Parents' and physicians' decisions became more challenging and complex.

The history of federal and state laws pertaining to the medical care of infants began in 1982 with the Baby Doe regulations. These regulations created a standard of medical care for infants: the possibility of future handicaps

TABLE 5.9

Percentage of births with selected medical or health characteristics, by race and Hispanic origin of mother, 2009

| | | Origin of mother | | | | | | | | |
| | | Hispanic | | | | | | Non-Hispanic | | |
Characteristic	All origins[a]	Total	Mexican	Puerto Rican	Cuban	Central and South American	Other and unknown Hispanic	Total[b]	White	Black
All births										
Mother						Percent				
Diabetes during pregancy	4.8	5.0	5.1	5.5	4.9	4.7	4.2	4.7	4.4	4.2
Weight gain of less than 11 lbs	8.0	9.2	9.5	8.9	5.5	8.2	9.1	7.7	6.5	12.6
Weight gain of more than 40 lbs	20.8	16.1	15.0	22.0	24.5	14.5	19.8	22.2	23.5	20.5
Induction of Labor	23.2	17.5	16.9	20.2	19.5	15.7	20.6	25.0	27.0	21.1
CNM delivery[c]	7.6	8.1	7.8	9.8	4.1	9.6	7.4	7.4	7.5	6.9
Cesarean delivery	32.9	31.6	30.3	34.3	48.8	32.6	33.2	33.3	32.8	35.4
Infant										
Gestational age										
Preterm[d]	12.2	12.0	11.5	13.8	13.2	12.0	13.4	12.2	10.9	17.5
Early preterm[e]	3.5	3.3	3.1	4.3	3.7	3.2	3.9	3.6	2.9	6.2
Late preterm[f]	8.7	8.6	8.3	9.5	9.5	8.8	9.5	8.7	8.0	11.2
Birthweight										
Very low birthweight[g]	1.5	1.2	1.1	1.9	1.5	1.1	1.4	1.5	1.2	3.1
Low birthweight[h]	8.2	6.9	6.5	9.6	7.5	6.6	8.3	8.5	7.2	13.6
4,000 grams or more[i]	7.6	7.1	7.5	5.8	6.9	6.9	5.8	7.8	9.1	4.1
Low 5 minute apgar[j]	1.8	1.3	1.3	1.5	1.4	1.1	1.7	1.9	1.7	3.0
Twin births[k]	33.2	22.5	20.6	29.6	34.8	23.4	25.5	36.5	37.0	38.0
Triplet/+ births[l]	153.5	83.5	67.9	127.0	162.2	85.4	129.5	174.8	201.4	105.6

[a]Includes origin not stated.
[b]Includes races other than white and black.
[c]Births delivered by certified nurse midwives (CNM).
[d]Born prior to 37 completed weeks of gestation.
[e]Born prior to 34 completed weeks of gestation.
[f]Born between 34 and 36 completed weeks of gestation.
[g]Less than 1,500 grams (3 lb 4 oz).
[h]Less than 2,500 grams (5 lb 8 oz).
[i]Equivalent to 8 lb 14 oz.
[j]Score of less than 7 on a 10 point scale.
[k]Live births in twin deliveries per 1,000 live births.
[l]Live births in triplet and other higher-order multiple deliveries per 100,000 live births.
Notes: Race and Hispanic origin are reported separately on birth certificates. Race categories are consistent with 1977 Office of Management and Budget Standards. Persons of Hispanic origin may be of any race.

SOURCE: Joyce A. Martin et al., "Table 19. Selected Medical or Health Characteristics of Births, by Hispanic Origin of Mother and by Race for Mothers of Non-Hispanic Origin: United States, 2009," in "Births: Final Data for 2009," *National Vital Statistics Reports*, vol. 60, no. 1, November 2011, http://www.cdc.gov/nchs/data/nvsr/nvsr60/nvsr60_01.pdf (accessed February 2, 2012)

in a child should play no role in his or her medical treatment decisions.

The Baby Doe Rules

In April 1982 an infant with Down syndrome was born at Bloomington Hospital in Indiana. The infant also had esophageal atresia, an obstruction in the esophagus that prevents the passage of food from the mouth to the stomach. Following their obstetrician's recommendation, the parents decided to forgo surgery to repair the baby's esophagus. The baby would be kept pain-free with medication and allowed to die.

Disagreeing with the parents' decision, the hospital took the parents to the county court. The judge ruled that the parents had the legal right to their decision, which was based on a valid medical recommendation. The Indiana Supreme Court refused to hear the appeal. Before the county prosecutor could present the case to the U.S. Supreme Court, the six-day-old baby died.

The public outcry following the death of "Baby Doe" (the infant's court-designated name) brought immediate reaction from the administration of President Ronald Reagan (1911–2004). The U.S. Department of Health and Human Services (HHS) informed all hospitals receiving federal funding that discrimination against handicapped newborns would violate section 504 of the Rehabilitation Act of 1973. This section (nondiscrimination under federal grants and programs) states: "No otherwise qualified individual with a disability in the United States...shall, solely by reason of her or his disability, be excluded from participation in, be denied the benefits of, or be subjected to discrimination under any program, service or activity receiving Federal financial assistance."

Furthermore, all hospitals receiving federal aid were required to post signs that read: "Discriminatory failure to feed and care for handicapped infants in this facility is prohibited by Federal law." The signs listed a toll-free hotline for anonymous reports of failure to comply.

Even though government investigators (called Baby Doe squads) were summoned to many hospitals to verify claims of mistreatment (the hotline had 500 calls in its first three weeks alone), no violation of the law could be found. On the contrary, the investigators found doctors resuscitating babies who were beyond treatment because they feared legal actions. Finally, a group led by the American Academy of Pediatrics filed suit in March 1983 to have the Baby Doe rules overturned because they believed them to be harsh, unreasonably intrusive, and not necessarily in the best interests of the child. After various legal battles, in 1986 the U.S. Supreme Court ruled that the HHS did not have the authority to require such regulations and invalidated them.

Child Abuse Amendments and Their Legacy

As the Baby Doe regulations were being fought in the courts, Congress enacted and President Reagan signed the Child Abuse Amendments (CAA) of 1984. The CAA extended and improved the provisions of the Child Abuse Prevention and Treatment Act (1974) and the Child Abuse Prevention and Treatment and Adoption Reform Act of 1978. The CAA established that states' child protection services systems would respond to complaints of medical neglect of children, including instances of withholding medically indicated treatment from disabled infants with life-threatening conditions. It noted that parents were the ones to make medical decisions for their disabled infants based on the advice of their physicians. These laws have been amended many times over the years, most recently by the Keeping Children and Families Safe Act of 2003, without voiding the states' and parents' responsibilities to disabled infants.

Born-Alive Infants Protection Act

The Born-Alive Infants Protection Act (BAIPA) was signed by President George W. Bush (1946–) in August 2002. The purpose of the law was to ensure that all infants born alive, whether developmentally able to survive long term or not, were given legal protection as people under federal law. The law did not prohibit or require medical care for newly born infants who were below a certain weight or developmental age, nor did it address gestational age. David Boyle et al. of the American Academy of Pediatrics Neonatal Resuscitation Program Steering Committee supported this point of view in "Born-Alive Infants Protection Act of 2001, Public Law No. 107-207" (*Pediatrics*, vol. 111, no. 3, March 1, 2003), stating that the law:

> Should not in any way affect the approach that physicians currently follow with respect to the extremely premature infant. . . . At the time of delivery, and regardless of the circumstances of the delivery, the medical condition and prognosis of the newly born infant should be assessed. At

that point decisions about withholding or discontinuing medical treatment that is considered futile may be considered by the medical care providers in conjunction with the parents acting in the best interest of their child. Those newly born infants who are deemed appropriate to not resuscitate or to have medical support withdrawn should be treated with dignity and respect, and provided with "comfort care" measures.

By 2005, however, the opinion that the BAIPA should not affect physicians' approach to their care of premature infants was questioned. Sadath A. Sayeed of the University of California, San Francisco, notes in "Baby Doe Redux? The Department of Health and Human Services and the Born-Alive Infants Protection Act of 2002: A Cautionary Note on Normative Neonatal Practice" (*Pediatrics*, vol. 116, no 4, October 1, 2005) that in 2005 the HHS announced that it would investigate circumstances in which medical care had been withheld from any born-alive infant. The agency also suggested, as with the Baby Doe regulations, that individuals in health care facilities should report any infractions of the law that they might notice.

Sayeed criticizes the law's "all-encompassing definition of born alive," reporting that it includes any fetus "'at any stage of development . . . regardless of whether the expulsion or extraction occurs as a result of natural or induced labor, cesarean section, or induced abortion,' and it makes no reference to standards of care or best interests, nor does it specifically protect a parent's decision-making authority. Under the law's strict logic, an 18-week miscarried fetus with a detectable heart beat after delivery is entitled to the full protections of the law as determined by 'any Act of Congress, or any ruling, regulation, or interpretation of the various administrative bureaus and agencies.'"

In "Resuscitation of Likely Nonviable Newborns: Would Neonatology Practices in California Change If the Born-Alive Infants Protection Act Were Enforced?" (*Pediatrics*, vol. 123, no. 4, April 2009), J. Colin Partridge et al. of the University of California, San Francisco, address the effects of the BAIPA. The researchers note that in 2005 they conducted a survey of neonatologists in active practice in California. More than half of the respondents had neither heard of the BAIPA nor its enforcement guidelines. The physicians admitted rarely assessing the medical condition and prognosis of any fetus less than 23 weeks of gestation; 23 weeks of gestation appears to be the threshold for a fetus to have a chance of survival outside of the womb. Only 6% of the responding neonatologists thought the law should be enforced. Partridge et al. conclude that "until outcomes for infants of <24 weeks' gestation improve, legislation that changes resuscitation practices for extreme prematurity seems an unjustifiable restriction of physician practice and parental rights."

Michael H. Malloy of the University of Texas Medical Branch in Galveston, Texas, discusses in "The Born-Alive Infant Protection Act: Impact on Fetal and Live Birth Mortality" (*American Journal of Perinatology*, vol. 28, no. 5, May 2011) whether the BAIPA has resulted in a decline in the fetal death rate or an increase in the live-born death rate at previable gestational ages of 17 to 22 weeks. Using fetal death files, Malloy determines that the fetal death rate has declined slightly and the live-birth mortality rate has increased slightly. He concludes that "the change appears to be isolated to only the most immature at 17 weeks gestation."

MEDICAL DECISION MAKING FOR CHILDREN

Under U.S. law, children under the age of 18 years cannot provide legally binding consent regarding their health care. Parents or guardians legally provide that consent, and, in most situations, physicians and the courts give parents wide latitude in the medical decisions they make for their children.

Religious Beliefs and Medical Treatment

Some parents refuse medical treatment for their children because of religious reasons. When such refusal means death or undue suffering for a child, the government may step in. Even though the U.S. Constitution prohibits government interference with religious practices and guarantees freedom of religion, the government concurrently has a responsibility to safeguard the health and well-being of its citizens.

Bruce Patsner of the University of Houston Law Center explains in "Faith versus Medicine: When a Parent Refuses a Child's Medical Care" (June 2009, http://www.law.uh .edu/Healthlaw/perspectives/2009/(BP)%20Faith.pdf) that the power of the government to intervene in the medical affairs of its citizens has limits, which are partly based on whether the intervention meets a "public health justification" criterion. For example, Patsner notes that the government's responsibility to protect the public health is the basis on which the government can implement mandatory vaccination programs. However, what happens in situations that involve individual children and circumstances that do not threaten public health?

Patsner suggests that such cases fall under the jurisdiction of state family laws, rather than federal laws, and that state family laws are not specific as to what decisions parents can or cannot make for their children regarding their medical care. Nonetheless, Patsner explains, "while parents may be entitled to believe whatever they want to believe from a religious point of view, denials of life-saving medical care to their children quickly cross over from mere belief into conduct, and this is not protected to the same degree. Put another way, parents are generally not allowed to sacrifice the lives of their children whose health interests they are supposed to protect before the children are legally old enough to be able to make their own decisions."

WISCONSIN COURT CASE. In 2009 two cases came to state courts that tested governmental limits to intervene in the medical decisions for a minor child when the parents refused medical treatment. The first case concerned 11-year-old Kara Neumann, who died in March 2008 from diabetic ketoacidosis, a complication of her undiagnosed and untreated type 1 diabetes. Dirk Johnson reports in "Trials for Parents Who Chose Faith over Medicine" (*New York Times*, January 20, 2009) that even though Kara "had grown so weak that she could not walk or speak," her parents refused to obtain medical care for her and instead relied on prayer to heal her. About a month after her death, Jill Falstad, the state attorney of Marathon County, Wisconsin, filed charges of reckless endangerment against Kara's parents. Each stood trial separately, and each faced up to 25 years in prison if convicted.

In "Prayer Death Case Headed to State Supreme Court, Experts Say" (*Capital Times* [Madison, WI], March 19, 2010), Jessica Vanegeren notes that both parents were found guilty of second-degree reckless homicide in 2009 and both appealed the decision. According to Vanegeren, the basis for their appeals was an inconsistency in Wisconsin's criminal codes. Wisconsin state law allows a religious exemption in child abuse and neglect cases but not in homicide cases. The Neumanns were convicted of this crime and sentenced to six months' prison time and ten years' probation. However, in February 2011 they asked a judge for a new trial. Two months later, in April 2011, Judge Vincent Howard denied their request.

MINNESOTA COURT CASE. The second case concerned 13-year-old Daniel Hauser, who had developed Hodgkin's lymphoma (a cancer of the immune system). Maura Lerner explains in "Sleepy Eye Parents, Teen Fight to Refuse Chemo" (*Star Tribune* [Minneapolis, MN], May 7, 2009) that in January 2009 Daniel was diagnosed with the cancer, and his physicians recommended six rounds of chemotherapy and radiation. Daniel underwent the first round of chemotherapy to treat the tumor in his chest, but the treatment made him temporarily sick. His parents responded by refusing any more treatments and chose instead to treat him themselves by changing his diet. Daniel and his parents belonged to the Nemenhah, an obscure Native American religious organization that favors natural healing processes over medical intervention. They cited religious reasons for their decision, and Daniel even claimed to be a medicine man within the organization.

James Olson, the attorney for Brown County, Minnesota, learned of Daniel's refusal and filed a petition against Daniel's parents, citing child neglect and endangerment. Olson asked the judge to order the boy into treatment for his highly curable cancer. Agreeing with the petition, the judge ordered the parents to have their son continue his chemotherapy and radiation treatments.

According to the article "Politics, Courts Dominate 2009 Minnesota Headlines" (Associated Press, December 25, 2009), in May 2009 Daniel's mother took him to California to avoid the judge's order but returned a week later. In November 2009 the judge closed the case after the court-ordered chemotherapy and radiation treatments put Daniel's cancer into remission (signs and symptoms disappeared).

End-of-Life Decisions for Adolescents

The United Nations defines adolescents as people between the ages of 10 and 19 years. Early adolescence is from 10 to 14 years, and late adolescence is from 15 to 19 years.

Caprice Knapp et al. indicate in "Adolescents with Life-Threatening Illnesses" (*American Journal of Hospice and Palliative Care*, vol. 27, no. 2, March 2010) that over 3,000 U.S. adolescents die each year from life-threatening illnesses such as cancer, heart disease, acquired immuno-deficiency syndrome (AIDS), and metabolic disorders. Even though many laws concerning adolescents have changed, such as allowing adolescents to seek medical treatment for reproductive health and birth control services without parental consent, most states have no laws for end-of-life decisions by adolescents.

Knapp et al. note that even though U.S. laws do not consider adolescents under the age of 18 years to be competent to make their own health care decisions, health care practitioners often do. The researchers note that "as children age, they develop a deeper understanding of their illness and its effect on their life." In a review of available studies, the researchers add, however, that a debate exists among practitioners from various medical fields as to the risks and benefits of adolescents making life-altering decisions. For example, imaging studies "suggest that adolescents do not have the capacity to make long-term decisions considering their stage of development," resulting in those under the age of 19 years being more likely "to make decisions based on emotions rather than facts." Conversely, behaviorists note that "a portfolio of evidence suggests that adolescents are capable of consenting to procedures and have the capacity to make decisions."

CHAPTER 6
SUICIDE, EUTHANASIA, AND PHYSICIAN-ASSISTED SUICIDE

BACKGROUND

Merriam-Webster's Dictionary (2012) defines the term *euthanasia*, which derives from the Greek for "easy death," as "the act or practice of killing or permitting the death of hopelessly sick or injured individuals . . . in a relatively painless way for reasons of mercy." This present-day definition differs from that of the classical Greeks, who considered euthanasia as simply "one mode of dying." To the Greeks, euthanasia was a rational act by people who deemed their life no longer useful. That these individuals sought the help of others to end their life was considered morally acceptable.

The movement to legalize euthanasia in England began in 1935 with the founding of the Voluntary Euthanasia Society by well-known figures such as the playwright George Bernard Shaw (1856–1950), the mathematician Bertrand Russell (1872–1970), and the novelist H. G. Wells (1866–1946). In 1936 the House of Lords (one of the houses of the English Parliament) defeated a bill that would have permitted euthanasia in cases of terminal illness. Nonetheless, it was common knowledge that physicians practiced euthanasia. That same year it was rumored that King George V (1865–1936), who had been seriously ill for several years, was "relieved of his sufferings" by his physician, with the approval of his wife, Queen Mary (1867–1953).

The Euthanasia Society of America was established in 1938. In 1967 this group prepared the first living will. Renamed the Society for the Right to Die in 1974, it merged in 1991 with another organization called Concern for Dying, and the two became Choice in Dying (CID). Even though the CID took no position on physician-assisted suicide, it "advocated for the rights of dying patients." It also educated the public about the importance of advance directives and end-of-life issues. In 2000 the CID dissolved, although many of its staff remained to found the Partnership for Caring, which continued the CID's programs. The organization's goal was to guarantee that Americans have access to quality end-of-life care. In early 2004 the Partnership for Caring merged with Last Acts, a coalition of professional and consumer organizations that work to improve end-of-life care. The merged organization was named the Last Acts Partnership, and its mission was to provide education, service, and counseling to people who needed accurate and reliable information about end-of-life care. The Last Acts Partnership was also an advocate for policy reform in end-of-life issues. In 2005 the Last Acts Partnership ceased its activities and all rights and copyrights to material produced by the Partnership for Caring, Last Acts, and the Last Acts Partnership were legally obtained by the National Hospice and Palliative Care Organization (NHPCO; http://www.nhpco.org/). As of April 2012, the NHPCO was still operating.

Euthanasia and the Nazis

The Nazis' version of euthanasia was a bizarre interpretation of an idea espoused by two German professors, the psychiatrist Alfred Hoche (1865–1943) and the jurist Karl Binding (1841–1920), in their 1920 book *Die Freigabe der Vernichtung lebensunwerten Lebens* (*The Permission to Destroy Life Unworthy of Life*). While initially advocating that it was ethical for physicians to assist in the death of those who requested an end to their suffering, the authors later argued that it was also permissible to end the lives of the mentally retarded and the mentally ill.

Some contemporary opponents of euthanasia fear that a society that allows physician-assisted suicide may eventually follow the path of the euthanasia program that was designed by the Nazi dictator Adolf Hitler (1889–1945) and his followers. That program began with the killing of physically and mentally impaired individuals and culminated in the annihilation of entire religious and ethnic groups considered by the Nazis to be unworthy of life. However, those supporting euthanasia argue that unlike the murderous Nazi euthanasia program, 21st-century proposals are based on voluntary requests by individuals in situations of physical suffering and would be sanctioned by laws passed by democratic governments.

Distinguishing between Euthanasia and Physician-Assisted Suicide

In the United States the debate over euthanasia distinguishes between active and passive euthanasia. Active euthanasia, also called voluntary active euthanasia by those who distinguish it from the kind of euthanasia that was practiced by the Nazis, involves the hastening of death through the administration of lethal drugs, as requested by the patient or another competent individual who represents the patient's wishes.

By contrast, passive euthanasia involves forgoing medical treatment, knowing that such a decision will result in death. This action is not considered to be illegal because the underlying illness, which is permitted to run its natural course, will ultimately cause death. It is generally accepted in the United States that terminally ill individuals have a right to refuse medical treatment, as do those who are sick but not terminally ill. However, some people think that allowing patients to forgo medical treatment is a practice tantamount to enabling suicide and is therefore morally reprehensible.

The debate about euthanasia in the United States has been expanded to include the question of whether a competent, terminally ill patient has the right to physician-assisted suicide, in which a physician provides the means (such as lethal drugs) for the patient to self-administer and commit suicide. The distinction between the two actions, euthanasia and physician-assisted suicide, is at times difficult to define. For example, a patient in the latter stages of amyotrophic lateral sclerosis (ALS; a degenerative neurologic condition commonly known as Lou Gehrig's disease) is physically unable to kill him- or herself; therefore, a physician who aids in such a person's suicide would technically be performing euthanasia.

SUICIDE

Different Cultures and Religions

Different religions and cultures have viewed suicide in different ways. Ancient Romans who dishonored themselves or their families were expected to commit suicide to maintain their dignity and, frequently, the family property. Early Christians were quick to embrace martyrdom as a guarantee of eternal salvation, but during the fourth century St. Augustine of Hippo (354–430) discouraged the practice. He and later theologians were concerned that many Christians who were suffering in this world would see suicide as a reasonable and legitimate way to depart to a better place in the hereafter. The view of the Christian theologian St. Thomas Aquinas (c. 1225–1274) is reflected in *Catechism of the Catholic Church* (August 23, 2002,

http://www.vatican.va/archive/ccc_css/archive/catechism/ccc_toc.htm) by the Vatican, which states that "suicide contradicts the natural inclination of the human being to preserve and perpetuate his life [and] is contrary to love for the living God."

Islam and Judaism also condemn the taking of one's own life. By contrast, Buddhist monks and nuns have been known to commit suicide by self-immolation (burning themselves alive) as a form of social protest. In a ritual called suttee, which is now outlawed, widows in India showed devotion to their deceased husbands by being cremated with them, sometimes throwing themselves on the funeral pyres, although it was not always voluntary. Widowers (men whose wives had died), however, did not follow this custom.

Quasi-religious reasons sometimes motivate mass suicide. In 1978 more than 900 members of a group known as the People's Temple killed themselves in Jonestown, Guyana. In 1997 a group called Heaven's Gate committed mass suicide in California. The devastating September 11, 2001, terrorist attacks against the United States were the result of a suicidal plot enacted by a religious extremist group. Suicide bombings in other parts of the world have also been attributed to extremist groups that have twisted or misinterpreted the fundamental tenets of Islam to further their political objectives.

The Japanese people have traditionally associated a certain idealism with suicide. During the 12th century samurai warriors practiced voluntary *seppuku* (ritual self-disembowelment) to avoid dishonor at the hands of their enemies. Some samurai committed this form of slow suicide to atone for wrongdoing or to express devotion to a superior who had died. As recently as 1970 the novelist Kimitake Hiraoka (1925–1970) publicly committed *seppuku*. During World War II (1939–1945) Japanese kamikaze pilots inflicted serious casualties by purposely crashing their planes into enemy ships, killing themselves along with enemy troops.

The article "Japan's Suicides Dip but Still among World's Highest" (Associated Press, March 3, 2011) notes that in 2010 Japan's suicide rate had dropped, but was still high. The Japan National Police Force indicated that 31,690 people committed suicide in 2010, which was a decrease of 3.5% from the year before. Regardless, it was the 13th consecutive year in which the number of people who committed suicide was over 30,000. At 24.4 suicides per 100,000 people in 2009, Japan had the second-highest suicide rate in the world, coming in just after Russia, a country with a suicide rate of 30.1 per 100,000 people. Both Japan and the United States have about the same number of suicides each year, but Japan has half the population.

According to the article "Suicides in Japan Spiked after Earthquake" (Agence France-Presse, March 9, 2012), in March 2011 the northern part of Japan was devastated with an earthquake and tsunami. National officials noted that in May, 20% more people took their lives than in that month in the year prior, explaining that this increase "was likely attributable at least in part to the widespread anxiety Japanese society felt in the aftermath of the catastrophe." The Japan National Police Force reported that 30,651 people committed suicide in Japan in 2011, making it "the 14th consecutive year the figure has exceeded 30,000."

Joe Chen, Yun Jeong Choi, and Yasuyuki Sawada of the University of Tokyo note in "How Is Suicide Different in Japan?" (*Japan and the World Economy*, vol. 21, no. 2, March 2009) that the suicide rate in Japan is more sensitive to economic factors (such as the gross domestic product [the total value of all the goods and services that are produced by a nation in a given year] per capita and the growth of the gross domestic product per capita) than to social factors (such as the divorce rate, birth rate, female labor force participation rate, and alcohol consumption). Nonetheless, both economic and social factors appear to have a greater effect on the suicide rate in Japan than they do in other developed countries.

Suicide in the United States

Except for certain desperate medical situations, suicide in the United States is generally considered to be an unacceptable act, the result of irrationality or severe depression. It is often referred to as a permanent solution to a short-term problem.

In spite of this generally held belief, suicide was the 10th-leading cause of death in the United States in 2009 and 2010. (See Table 4.1 in Chapter 4.) There were approximately 1.9 times as many suicides as homicides that year. Nevertheless, after 1950 the age-adjusted national suicide rate, which accounts for changes in the age distribution of the population across time, dropped from 13.2 suicides per 100,000 population in 1950 to 11.3 per 100,000 in 2007. (See Table 6.1.) However, the 2007 rate was up from a low of 10.4 suicides per 100,000 population in 2000.

GENDER AND RACIAL DIFFERENCES. In 2007 the suicide death rate for men (18.4 suicides per 100,000 population) was 3.9 times that for women (4.7 suicides per 100,000). (See Table 6.1.) Over the decades, the male suicide rate has ranged from 3.5 to 4.5 times as high as the female suicide rate, except for 1970. In that year the female suicide rate was up, resulting in the male suicide rate being only 2.7 times that of the female suicide rate.

The racial group with the lowest suicide death rate in 2007 was African-American females (1.7 suicides per 100,000 population), followed closely by Hispanic females (1.9 suicides per 100,000 population). (See Table 6.1.) In addition, adults aged 20 to 24 years had the lowest suicide death rate of all age groups 20 years and older. However, those in the age group 25 to 34 years had lower suicide rates than those 20 to 24 years as shown in Table 6.1 for 2000

and 2006. Suicide rates of teenagers and young children were lower than adult suicide rates.

DEMOGRAPHICS OF SUICIDE. Table 6.2 shows data that were collected from the National Survey on Drug Use and Health between 2008 and 2009. Even though Table 6.1 shows that more males than females died from suicide, Table 6.2 shows that slightly more females than males thought about, planned, and attempted suicide. The age group that had the highest percentage thinking about, planning, and attempting suicide was the 18- to 29-year-old group. Non-Hispanic African-American males attempted suicide the most, but according to Table 6.1, they were not the group that died in the greatest numbers. White males had the largest number of deaths, at a rate of 20.2 per 100,000 population, followed closely by Native American or Alaskan Native males, at a rate of 18.1 per 100,000 population.

Table 6.2 shows that attempting suicide decreases with the level of education. Those with less than a high school education attempted suicide the most, whereas those who had graduated from college attempted suicide the least. Likewise, those who were unemployed had the highest suicide attempt rate, whereas full-time workers had the lowest rate. There was very little distinction among those who lived in large metropolitan areas, small metropolitan areas, or nonmetropolitan areas.

Suicide among Young People

Suicide death rates among young people aged 15 to 24 years nearly tripled between 1950 and 1990, from 4.5 suicides per 100,000 population to 13.2 suicides per 100,000 population. (See Table 6.1.) Rates among young adults aged 25 to 34 years increased as well, but not as dramatically; they increased 1.8 times, from 9.1 suicides per 100,000 population in 1950 to 16 suicides per 100,000 population in 1980. However, the young adult rates were higher than the suicide rates among young people. For those aged 15 to 24 years, the suicide rates dropped from 1990 to 2000 and then continued to drop slightly through 2007. For those aged 25 to 44 years, suicide rates dropped between 1990 and 2000, and then rose slightly in 2006 and 2007. In 2007 suicide was the third-leading cause of death among people aged 15 to 24 years (accidents were first and homicides were second) and the second-leading cause of death among people aged 25 to 34 years (accidents were first and homicides were third). (See Table 4.2 in Chapter 4.)

ATTEMPTED SUICIDE AMONG YOUNG PEOPLE. Males of all races and ages are more likely to die from suicide attempts than are females of the same race and age. (See Table 6.1.) However, among high school students, females are more likely than males to attempt suicide. As shown in Table 6.3, 9.3% of female high school students attempted suicide in 2007, compared with 4.6% of male high school students. More female (18.7%) than male (10.3%) high

TABLE 6.1

Death rates for suicide, by sex, race, Hispanic origin, and age, selected years 1950–2007

[Data are based on death certificates]

Sex, race, Hispanic origin, and age	1950[a]	1960[a]	1970	1980	1990	2000	2006	2007
All persons				Deaths per 100,000 resident population				
All ages, age-adjusted[b]	13.2	12.5	13.1	12.2	12.5	10.4	10.9	11.3
All ages, crude	11.4	10.6	11.6	11.9	12.4	10.4	11.1	11.5
Under 1 year	—	—	—	—	—	—	—	—
1–4 years	—	—	—	—	—	—	—	—
5–14 years	0.2	0.3	0.3	0.4	0.8	0.7	0.5	0.5
15–24 years	4.5	5.2	8.8	12.3	13.2	10.2	9.9	9.7
15–19 years	2.7	3.6	5.9	8.5	11.1	8.0	7.3	6.9
20–24 years	6.2	7.1	12.2	16.1	15.1	12.5	12.5	12.6
25–44 years	11.6	12.2	15.4	15.6	15.2	13.4	13.8	14.3
25–34 years	9.1	10.0	14.1	16.0	15.2	12.0	12.3	13.0
35–44 years	14.3	14.2	16.9	15.4	15.3	14.5	15.1	15.6
45–64 years	23.5	22.0	20.6	15.9	15.3	13.5	16.0	16.8
45–54 years	20.9	20.7	20.0	15.9	14.8	14.4	17.2	17.7
55–64 years	26.8	23.7	21.4	15.9	16.0	12.1	14.5	15.5
65 years and over	30.0	24.5	20.8	17.6	20.5	15.2	14.2	14.3
65–74 years	29.6	23.0	20.8	16.9	17.9	12.5	12.6	12.6
75–84 years	31.1	27.9	21.2	19.1	24.9	17.6	15.9	16.3
85 years and over	28.8	26.0	19.0	19.2	22.2	19.6	15.9	15.6
Male								
All ages, age-adjusted[b]	21.2	20.0	19.8	19.9	21.5	17.7	18.0	18.4
All ages, crude	17.8	16.5	16.8	18.6	20.4	17.1	17.8	18.3
Under 1 year	—	—	—	—	—	—	—	—
1–4 years	—	—	—	—	—	—	—	—
5–14 years	0.3	0.4	0.5	0.6	1.1	1.2	0.7	0.6
15–24 years	6.5	8.2	13.5	20.2	22.0	17.1	16.2	15.9
15–19 years	3.5	5.6	8.8	13.8	18.1	13.0	11.5	11.1
20–24 years	9.3	11.5	19.3	26.8	25.7	21.4	20.8	20.8
25–44 years	17.2	17.9	20.9	24.0	24.4	21.3	21.5	22.3
25–34 years	13.4	14.7	19.8	25.0	24.8	19.6	19.7	20.7
35–44 years	21.3	21.0	22.1	22.5	23.9	22.8	23.2	23.8
45–64 years	37.1	34.4	30.0	23.7	24.3	21.3	24.8	25.8
45–54 years	32.0	31.6	27.9	22.9	23.2	22.4	26.2	27.0
55–64 years	43.6	38.1	32.7	24.5	25.7	19.4	22.7	24.3
65 years and over	52.8	44.0	38.4	35.0	41.6	31.1	28.5	28.6
65–74 years	50.5	39.6	36.0	30.4	32.2	22.7	22.7	22.5
75–84 years	58.3	52.5	42.8	42.3	56.1	38.6	33.3	34.3
85 years and over	58.3	57.4	42.4	50.6	65.9	57.5	43.2	41.8
Female								
All ages, age-adjusted[b]	5.6	5.6	7.4	5.7	4.8	4.0	4.5	4.7
All ages, crude	5.1	4.9	6.6	5.5	4.8	4.0	4.6	4.8
Under 1 year	—	—	—	—	—	—	—	—
1–4 years	—	—	—	—	—	—	—	—
5–14 years	0.1	0.1	0.2	0.2	0.4	0.3	0.3	0.3
15–24 years	2.6	2.2	4.2	4.3	3.9	3.0	3.2	3.2
15–19 years	1.8	1.6	2.9	3.0	3.7	2.7	2.8	2.5
20–24 years	3.3	2.9	5.7	5.5	4.1	3.2	3.6	3.9
25–44 years	6.2	6.6	10.2	7.7	6.2	5.4	5.9	6.2
25–34 years	4.9	5.5	8.6	7.1	5.6	4.3	4.7	5.0
35–44 years	7.5	7.7	11.9	8.5	6.8	6.4	7.0	7.3
45–64 years	9.9	10.2	12.0	8.9	7.1	6.2	7.7	8.2
45–54 years	9.9	10.2	12.6	9.4	6.9	6.7	8.4	8.8
55–64 years	9.9	10.2	11.4	8.4	7.3	5.4	6.8	7.3
65 years and over	9.4	8.4	8.1	6.1	6.4	4.0	3.9	3.9
65–74 years	10.1	8.4	9.0	6.5	6.7	4.0	4.1	4.2
75–84 years	8.1	8.9	7.0	5.5	6.3	4.0	4.0	3.8
85 years and over	8.2	6.0	5.9	5.5	5.4	4.2	3.1	3.1

school students seriously considered suicide. Also, more female (2.4%) than male (1.5%) high school students injured themselves in their suicide attempts. However, in 2007 the rate of suicide deaths of females aged 15 to 19 years was 2.5 suicides per 100,000 population, compared with 11.1 suicides per 100,000 population for males of the same age group. (See Table 6.1.)

Even though death rates from suicide declined among young adults aged 15 to 19 years between 1990 and 2007, the percentage of high school students who attempted suicide increased from 7.3% in 1991 to 8.4% in 2005, peaking at 8.8% in 2001. (See Table 6.1 and Table 6.3.) However, the percentage of students who attempted suicide dropped dramatically in 2007 to 6.9%. The percentage of students

TABLE 6.1

Death rates for suicide, by sex, race, Hispanic origin, and age, selected years 1950–2007 [CONTINUED]

[Data are based on death certificates]

Sex, race, Hispanic origin, and age	1950[a]	1960[a]	1970	1980	1990	2000	2006	2007
				Deaths per 100,000 resident population				
White male[c]								
All ages, age-adjusted[b]	22.3	21.1	20.8	20.9	22.8	19.1	19.6	20.2
All ages, crude	19.0	17.6	18.0	19.9	22.0	18.8	19.8	20.5
15–24 years	6.6	8.6	13.9	21.4	23.2	17.9	17.1	16.9
25–44 years	17.9	18.5	21.5	24.6	25.4	22.9	23.5	24.5
45–64 years	39.3	36.5	31.9	25.0	26.0	23.2	27.4	28.8
65 years and over	55.8	46.7	41.1	37.2	44.2	33.3	30.9	31.1
65–74 years	53.2	42.0	38.7	32.5	34.2	24.3	24.7	24.7
75–84 years	61.9	55.7	45.5	45.5	60.2	41.1	36.0	36.9
85 years and over	61.9	61.3	45.8	52.8	70.3	61.6	46.1	45.4
Black or African American male[c]								
All ages, age-adjusted[b]	7.5	8.4	10.0	11.4	12.8	10.0	9.4	8.8
All ages, crude	6.3	6.4	8.0	10.3	12.0	9.4	8.8	8.4
15–24 years	4.9	4.1	10.5	12.3	15.1	14.2	10.6	10.3
25–44 years	9.8	12.6	16.1	19.2	19.6	14.3	14.3	13.7
45–64 years	12.7	13.0	12.4	11.8	13.1	9.9	9.9	9.4
65 years and over	9.0	9.9	8.7	11.4	14.9	11.5	10.4	8.7
65–74 years	10.0	11.3	8.7	11.1	14.7	11.1	8.8	8.3
75–84 years[d]	*	*	*	10.5	14.4	12.1	11.6	11.2
85 years and over	. . .	*	*	*	*	*	*	*
American Indian or Alaska Native male[c]								
All ages, age-adjusted[b]	. . .	. . .	. . .	19.3	20.1	16.0	18.3	18.1
All ages, crude	. . .	. . .	. . .	20.9	20.9	15.9	19.3	19.2
15–24 years	. . .	. . .	. . .	45.3	49.1	26.2	35.9	32.3
25–44 years	. . .	. . .	. . .	31.2	27.8	24.5	26.0	28.6
45–64 years	. . .	. . .	. . .	*	*	15.4	18.0	15.9
65 years and over	. . .	. . .	. . .	*	*	*	*	*
Asian or Pacific Islander male[c]								
All ages, age-adjusted[b]	. . .	. . .	. . .	10.7	9.6	8.6	7.9	9.0
All ages, crude	. . .	. . .	. . .	8.8	8.7	7.9	8.0	8.7
15–24 years	. . .	. . .	. . .	10.8	13.5	9.1	12.0	13.4
25–44 years	. . .	. . .	. . .	11.0	10.6	9.9	9.2	9.8
45–64 years	. . .	. . .	. . .	13.0	9.7	9.7	9.7	10.7
65 years and over	. . .	. . .	. . .	18.6	16.8	15.4	10.6	12.9
Hispanic or Latino male[c, e]								
All ages, age-adjusted[b]	. . .	. . .	. . .	. . .	13.7	10.3	8.8	10.1
All ages, crude	. . .	. . .	. . .	. . .	11.4	8.4	7.9	8.8
15–24 years	. . .	. . .	. . .	. . .	14.7	10.9	11.6	11.5
25–44 years	. . .	. . .	. . .	. . .	16.2	11.2	10.8	11.9
45–64 years	. . .	. . .	. . .	. . .	16.1	12.0	10.3	12.9
65 years and over	. . .	. . .	. . .	. . .	23.4	19.5	12.1	15.9
White, not Hispanic or Latino male[e]								
All ages, age-adjusted[b]	. . .	. . .	. . .	. . .	23.5	20.2	21.4	21.9
All ages, crude	. . .	. . .	. . .	. . .	23.1	20.4	22.3	22.9
15–24 years	. . .	. . .	. . .	. . .	24.4	19.5	18.5	18.2
25–44 years	. . .	. . .	. . .	. . .	26.4	25.1	26.9	28.0
45–64 years	. . .	. . .	. . .	. . .	26.8	24.0	29.3	30.6
65 years and over	. . .	. . .	. . .	. . .	45.4	33.9	32.3	32.2
White female[c]								
All ages, age-adjusted[b]	6.0	5.9	7.9	6.1	5.2	4.3	5.1	5.2
All ages, crude	5.5	5.3	7.1	5.9	5.3	4.4	5.2	5.4
15–24 years	2.7	2.3	4.2	4.6	4.2	3.1	3.4	3.4
25–44 years	6.6	7.0	11.0	8.1	6.6	6.0	6.8	7.0
45–64 years	10.6	10.9	13.0	9.6	7.7	6.9	8.8	9.3
65 years and over	9.9	8.8	8.5	6.4	6.8	4.3	4.1	4.2
Black or African American female[c]								
All ages, age-adjusted[b]	1.8	2.0	2.9	2.4	2.4	1.8	1.4	1.7
All ages, crude	1.5	1.6	2.6	2.2	2.3	1.7	1.4	1.7
15–24 years	1.8	*	3.8	2.3	2.3	2.2	1.8	1.6
25–44 years	2.3	3.0	4.8	4.3	3.8	2.6	2.0	2.7
45–64 years	2.7	3.1	2.9	2.5	2.9	2.1	1.9	2.3
65 years and over	*	*	2.6	*	1.9	1.3	*	*

TABLE 6.1

Death rates for suicide, by sex, race, Hispanic origin, and age, selected years 1950–2007 [CONTINUED]

[Data are based on death certificates]

Sex, race, Hispanic origin, and age	1950[a]	1960[a]	1970	1980	1990	2000	2006	2007
American Indian or Alaska Native female[c]				Deaths per 100,000 resident population				
All ages, age-adjusted[b]	. . .	. . .	. . .	4.7	3.6	3.8	5.1	4.9
All ages, crude	. . .	. . .	. . .	4.7	3.7	4.0	5.4	5.1
15–24 years	. . .	. . .	. . .	*	*	*	8.9	7.8
25–44 years	. . .	. . .	. . .	10.7	*	7.2	8.0	6.9
45–64 years	. . .	. . .	. . .	*	*	*	*	*
65 years and over	. . .	. . .	. . .	*	*	*	*	*
Asian or Pacific Islander female[c]								
All ages, age-adjusted[b]	. . .	. . .	. . .	5.5	4.1	2.8	3.4	3.5
All ages, crude	. . .	. . .	. . .	4.7	3.4	2.7	3.3	3.6
15–24 years	. . .	. . .	. . .	*	3.9	2.7	4.0	3.8
25–44 years	. . .	. . .	. . .	5.4	3.8	3.3	3.3	4.6
45–64 years	. . .	. . .	. . .	7.9	5.0	3.2	4.2	4.0
65 years and over	. . .	. . .	. . .	*	8.5	5.2	6.9	5.2
Hispanic or Latina female[c, e]								
All ages, age-adjusted[b]	. . .	. . .	. . .	. . .	2.3	1.7	1.8	1.9
All ages, crude	. . .	. . .	. . .	. . .	2.2	1.5	1.7	1.8
15–24 years	. . .	. . .	. . .	. . .	3.1	2.0	2.6	2.2
25–44 years	. . .	. . .	. . .	. . .	3.1	2.1	2.3	2.7
45–64 years	. . .	. . .	. . .	. . .	2.5	2.5	2.4	2.8
65 years and over	. . .	. . .	. . .	. . .	*	*	1.7	*
White, not Hispanic or Latina female[e]								
All ages, age-adjusted[b]	. . .	. . .	. . .	. . .	5.4	4.7	5.6	5.7
All ages, crude	. . .	. . .	. . .	. . .	5.6	4.9	5.9	6.1
15–24 years	. . .	. . .	. . .	. . .	4.3	3.3	3.5	3.7
25–44 years	. . .	. . .	. . .	. . .	7.0	6.7	7.8	8.0
45–64 years	. . .	. . .	. . .	. . .	8.0	7.3	9.5	10.0
65 years and over	. . .	. . .	. . .	. . .	7.0	4.4	4.3	4.4

—Category not applicable.

*Rates based on fewer than 20 deaths are considered unreliable and are not shown.

. . .Data not available.

[a]Includes deaths of persons who were not residents of the 50 states and the District of Columbia (D.C.).

[b]Age-adjusted rates are calculated using the year 2000 standard population. Prior to 2003, age-adjusted rates were calculated using standard million proportions based on rounded population numbers. Starting with 2003 data, unrounded population numbers are used to calculate age-adjusted rates.

[c]The race groups, white, black, Asian or Pacific Islander, and American Indian or Alaska Native, include persons of Hispanic and non-Hispanic origin. Persons of Hispanic origin may be of any race. Death rates for the American Indian or Alaska Native and Asian or Pacific Islander populations are known to be underestimated.

[d]In 1950, rate is for the age group 75 years and over.

[e]Prior to 1997, excludes data from states lacking an Hispanic-origin item on the death certificate.

Notes: Starting with *Health, United States, 2003*, rates for 1991–1999 were revised using intercensal population estimates based on the 2000 census. Rates for 2000 were revised based on 2000 census counts. Rates for 2001 and later years were computed using 2000-based postcensal estimates. Figures for 2001 include September 11-related deaths for which death certificates were filed as of October 24, 2002.

Age groups were selected to minimize the presentation of unstable age-specific death rates based on small numbers of deaths and for consistency among comparison groups. Starting with 2003 data, some states allowed the reporting of more than one race on the death certificate. The multiple-race data for these states were bridged to the single-race categories of the 1977 Office of Management and Budget standards for comparability with other states.

SOURCE: "Table 39. Death Rates for Suicide, by Sex, Race, Hispanic Origin, and Age: United States, Selected Years 1950–2007," in *Health, United States, 2010: With Special Feature on Death and Dying*, Centers for Disease Control and Prevention, National Center for Health Statistics, 2011, http://www.cdc.gov/nchs/data/hus/hus10.pdf (accessed February 1, 2012)

who were injured during a suicide attempt also rose from 1.7% in 1991 to 2.9% in 2003, with a decline to 2.3% in 2005 and to 2% in 2007.

The percentage of high school students who attempted suicide in 2009 was highest among ninth (7.3%) and 10th graders (6.9%), and decreased with the rising grade level. (See Table 6.4.) The percentage of suicide attempts requiring medical attention followed a similar pattern: a higher percentage of the suicide attempts of ninth, 10th, and 11th graders required medical attention than did those of seniors. Hispanic students were the most likely to attempt suicide and non-Hispanic African-American students were the most

likely to have their suicide attempt treated by a doctor or a nurse. Non-Hispanic white students were the least likely to attempt suicide and to have their attempt treated by a doctor or a nurse. In addition, suicide attempts were the highest among high school students living in Hawaii (12.8%), Arkansas (12%), Louisiana (10.9%), South Carolina (10.8%), Alabama (10.7%), and West Virginia (10.7%). (See Table 6.5.)

In "Youth Risk Behavior Surveillance—United States, 2009" (*Morbidity and Mortality Weekly Report*, vol. 59, no. SS-5, June 4, 2010), Danice K. Eaton et al. of the CDC provide data on the percentage of high school

TABLE 6.2

Average annual number and percentage of adults aged 18 years and older who had suicidal thoughts, made a plan, or attempted suicide during the previous year, 2008–09

[In thousands]

Characteristic	Thought		Plan		Attempt	
	No.	%	No.	%	No.	%
Sex						
Male	3,789	3.5	1,045	1.0	442	0.4
Female	4,571	3.9	1,218	1.0	616	0.5
Age group (yrs)						
18–29	2,865	5.7	821	1.6	477	1.0
≥30	5,494	3.1	1,442	0.8	581	0.3
Race/ethnicity						
White, non-Hispanic	6,044	3.9	1,616	1.0	663	0.4
Black, non-Hispanic	911	3.5	262	1.0	182	0.7
Hispanic[a]	933	3.0	267	0.9	144	0.5
Asian, non-Hispanic	208	2.1	37	0.4	23	0.2
Education						
Less than high school	1,373	4.0	429	1.2	247	0.7
High school graduate[b]	2,823	4.0	730	1.0	393	0.6
Some college	2,359	4.1	672	1.2	304	0.5
College graduate or higher	1,805	2.8	433	0.7	113	0.2
Current employment						
Full-time	3,679	3.1	844	0.7	351	0.3
Part-time	1,380	4.5	405	1.3	200	0.6
Unemployed	768	6.5	244	2.1	118	1.0
Other[c]	2,532	3.9	770	1.2	389	0.6
County type						
Large metropolitan area[d]	4,353	3.6	1,148	1.0	559	0.5
Small metropolitan area[e]	2,692	3.9	777	1.1	351	0.5
Nonmetropolitan area[f]	1,315	3.5	338	0.9	148	0.4
Total[g]	**8,359**	**3.7**	**2,263**	**1.0**	**1,058**	**0.5**

Abbreviations: Thought = had serious thoughts of suicide; plan = made any suicide plan; attempt = attempted suicide.
Note: Estimates are based only on responses to suicide items in the Mental Health module. Respondents with unknown suicide information were excluded.
[a]Persons of Hispanic origin can be of any race.
[b]Includes persons with a general education diploma.
[c]Includes retired persons, disabled persons, homemakers, students, or other persons not in the labor force.
[d]Area with a population of ≥1 million persons.
[e]Area with a population of <1 million persons.
[f]Area that is outside of a metropolitan statistical area; includes urbanized counties with a population of ≥20,000 persons in urbanized areas, less urbanized counties with a population of ≥2,500 persons but <20,000 persons in urbanized areas, and completely rural counties with a population of <2,500 persons in urbanized areas.
[g]Totals exclude persons with missing or unknown race and ethnicity. Totals might vary due to rounding.

students who feel sad or hopeless, who seriously consider attempting suicide, and who make a suicide plan. In 2009, 26.1% of high school students in all grades felt sad or hopeless. (See Table 6.6.) Approximately 13.8% seriously considered attempting suicide and 10.9% made a suicide plan. (See Table 6.7.) In 2009 the states in which more than 30% of high school students felt sad or hopeless were Arizona (34.9%), Louisiana (31.2%), Hawaii (30.6%), and Nevada (30.3%). (See Table 6.8.)

Table 6.9 shows trends among high school students who seriously considered attempting suicide, made a plan about how to attempt suicide, attempted suicide one or more times, and resultant injuries, poisonings, or over-

doses that had to be treated by a medical practitioner between 1991 and 2009. During this period the percentage of high school students who seriously considered attempting suicide declined from 29% in 1991 to 13.8% in 2009, a decrease of 52.4%. Those who made a plan about how they would attempt suicide declined as well, from 18.6% in 1991 to 10.9% in 2009, a decrease of 41.4%. Those high school students who attempted suicide one or more times experienced a drop between 2001 and 2009, from 8.8% to 6.3%, a decrease of 28.4%. Finally, students whose suicide attempt resulted in an injury, poisoning, or an overdose that had to be treated by a doctor or nurse dropped from 2.9% in 2003 to 1.9% in 2009, a decrease of 34.5%. None of the behavior changes resulted in a statistically significant change between 2007 and 2009.

The use of firearms was the method most often used to commit suicide in 2008, with hanging/suffocation second and poisoning third. (See Table 6.10.) The rate of death by firearms (6 suicides per 100,000 population) was more than twice that of suffocation (2.8 suicides per 100,000 population), and suffocation was used slightly over 1.3 times as much as poisoning (2.1 suicides per 100,000 population). Other methods were used much less frequently.

The statistics in this section underscore the urgent need for prevention, education, and support programs to help teens and young adults who are at risk. The National Center for Injury Prevention and Control (NCIPC) sponsors initiatives to raise public awareness of suicide and strategies to reduce suicide deaths. Along with supporting research about risk factors for suicide in the general population, the NCIPC develops programs for high-risk populations.

SUICIDE AMONG LESBIAN, GAY, BISEXUAL, AND TRANSGENDER ADOLESCENTS. Adolescence (the transition to adulthood) is often a difficult period. For lesbian, gay, bisexual, and transgender (LGBT) adolescents this transition is compounded by having to come to terms with their sexuality in a society that has been generally unaccepting of homosexuality, but that is becoming somewhat more accustomed to and accepting of it.

During this period in their life, when the need to confide in and gain acceptance from friends and family may be crucial, LGBT adolescents are often torn between choices that do not necessarily meet these needs. Those who are open about their sexual orientation risk disappointing or even alienating their families and facing the hostility of their peers. Teens who choose not to disclose their sexual orientation may suffer emotional distress because they have nowhere to turn for emotional support. In either scenario, despair, isolation, anger, guilt, and overwhelming depression may promote suicidal thoughts or actual suicide attempts.

TABLE 6.3

Suicidal ideation and suicide attempts and injuries among students in grades 9–12, by sex, grade level, race, and Hispanic origin, selected years 1991–2007

[Data are based on a national sample of high school students, grades 9–12]

Sex, grade level, race, and Hispanic origin	1991	1993	1995	1997	1999	2001	2003	2005	2007
				Percent of students who seriously considered suicide[a]					
Total	**29.0**	**24.1**	**24.1**	**20.5**	**19.3**	**19.0**	**16.9**	**16.9**	**14.5**
Male									
Total	**20.8**	**18.8**	**18.3**	**15.1**	**13.7**	**14.2**	**12.8**	**12.0**	**10.3**
9th grade	17.6	17.7	18.2	16.1	11.9	14.7	11.9	12.2	10.8
10th grade	19.5	18.0	16.7	14.5	13.7	13.8	13.2	11.9	9.3
11th grade	25.3	20.6	21.7	16.6	13.7	14.1	12.9	11.9	10.7
12th grade	20.7	18.3	16.3	13.5	15.6	13.7	13.2	11.6	10.2
Not Hispanic or Latino:									
White	21.7	19.1	19.1	14.4	12.5	14.9	12.0	12.4	10.2
Black or African American	13.3	15.4	16.7	10.6	11.7	9.2	10.3	7.0	8.5
Hispanic or Latino	18.0	17.9	15.7	17.1	13.6	12.2	12.9	11.9	10.7
Female									
Total	**37.2**	**29.6**	**30.4**	**27.1**	**24.9**	**23.6**	**21.3**	**21.8**	**18.7**
9th grade	40.3	30.9	34.4	28.9	24.4	26.2	22.2	23.9	19.0
10th grade	39.7	31.6	32.8	30.0	30.1	24.1	23.8	23.0	22.0
11th grade	38.4	28.9	31.1	26.2	23.0	23.6	20.0	21.6	16.3
12th grade	30.7	27.3	23.9	23.6	21.2	18.9	18.0	18.0	16.7
Not Hispanic or Latina:									
White	38.6	29.7	31.6	26.1	23.2	24.2	21.2	21.5	17.8
Black or African American	29.4	24.5	22.2	22.0	18.8	17.2	14.7	17.1	18.0
Hispanic or Latina	34.6	34.1	34.1	30.3	26.1	26.5	23.4	24.2	21.1
				Percent of students who attempted suicide[a]					
Total	**7.3**	**8.6**	**8.7**	**7.7**	**8.3**	**8.8**	**8.5**	**8.4**	**6.9**
Male									
Total	**3.9**	**5.0**	**5.6**	**4.5**	**5.7**	**6.2**	**5.4**	**6.0**	**4.6**
9th grade	4.5	5.8	6.8	6.3	6.1	8.2	5.8	6.8	5.3
10th grade	3.3	5.9	5.4	3.8	6.2	6.7	5.5	7.6	4.9
11th grade	4.1	3.4	5.8	4.4	4.8	4.9	4.6	4.5	3.7
12th grade	3.8	4.5	4.7	3.7	5.4	4.4	5.2	4.3	4.2
Not Hispanic or Latino:									
White	3.3	4.4	5.2	3.2	4.5	5.3	3.7	5.2	3.4
Black or African American	3.3	5.4	7.0	5.6	7.1	7.5	7.7	5.2	5.5
Hispanic or Latino	3.7	7.4	5.8	7.2	6.6	8.0	6.1	7.8	6.3
Female									
Total	**10.7**	**12.5**	**11.9**	**11.6**	**10.9**	**11.2**	**11.5**	**10.8**	**9.3**
9th grade	13.8	14.4	14.9	15.1	14.0	13.2	14.7	14.1	10.5
10th grade	12.2	13.1	15.1	14.3	14.8	12.2	12.7	10.8	11.2
11th grade	8.7	13.6	11.4	11.3	7.5	11.5	10.0	11.0	7.8
12th grade	7.8	9.1	6.6	6.2	5.8	6.5	6.9	6.5	6.5
Not Hispanic or Latina:									
White	10.4	11.3	10.4	10.3	9.0	10.3	10.3	9.3	7.7
Black or African American	9.4	11.2	10.8	9.0	7.5	9.8	9.0	9.8	9.9
Hispanic or Latina	11.6	19.7	21.0	14.9	18.9	15.9	15.0	14.9	14.0
				Percent of students with an injurious suicide attempt[a, b]					
Total	**1.7**	**2.7**	**2.8**	**2.6**	**2.6**	**2.6**	**2.9**	**2.3**	**2.0**
Male									
Total	**1.0**	**1.6**	**2.2**	**2.0**	**2.1**	**2.1**	**2.4**	**1.8**	**1.5**
9th grade	1.0	2.1	2.3	3.2	2.6	2.6	3.1	2.1	1.9
10th grade	0.5	1.3	2.4	1.4	1.8	2.5	2.1	2.2	1.0
11th grade	1.5	1.1	2.0	2.6	2.1	1.6	2.0	1.4	1.4
12th grade	0.9	1.5	2.2	1.0	1.7	1.5	1.8	1.0	1.5
Not Hispanic or Latino:									
White	1.0	1.4	2.1	1.5	1.6	1.7	1.1	1.5	0.9
Black or African American	0.4	2.0	2.8	1.8	3.4	3.6	5.2	1.4	2.5
Hispanic or Latino	0.5	2.0	2.9	2.1	1.4	2.5	4.2	2.8	1.8

In 2007 the American Society for Suicide Prevention, the Suicide Prevention Resource Center, and the Gay and Lesbian Medical Association convened a meeting to address suicide concerns among the LGBT population. Together, the extensive panel headed by Ann P. Haas developed the paper "Suicide and Suicide Risk in Lesbian, Gay, Bisexual, and

TABLE 6.3

Suicidal ideation and suicide attempts and injuries among students in grades 9–12, by sex, grade level, race, and Hispanic origin, selected years 1991–2007 [CONTINUED]

[Data are based on a national sample of high school students, grades 9–12]

Sex, grade level, race, and Hispanic origin	1991	1993	1995	1997	1999	2001	2003	2005	2007
Female									
Total	**2.5**	**3.8**	**3.4**	**3.3**	**3.1**	**3.1**	**3.2**	**2.9**	**2.4**
9th grade	2.8	3.5	6.3	5.0	3.8	3.8	3.9	4.0	2.6
10th grade	2.6	5.1	3.8	3.7	4.0	3.6	3.2	2.4	3.1
11th grade	2.1	3.9	2.9	2.8	2.8	2.8	2.9	2.9	1.7
12th grade	2.4	2.9	1.3	2.0	1.3	1.7	2.2	2.2	1.8
Not Hispanic or Latina:									
White	2.3	3.6	2.9	2.6	2.3	2.9	2.4	2.7	2.1
Black or African American	2.9	4.0	3.6	3.0	2.4	3.1	2.2	2.6	2.1
Hispanic or Latina	2.7	5.5	6.6	3.8	4.6	4.2	5.7	3.7	3.9

ᵃResponse is for the 12 months preceding the survey.
ᵇA suicide attempt that required medical attention.
Notes: Only youths attending school participated in the survey. Persons of Hispanic origin may be of any race.

SOURCE: "Table 59. Suicidal Ideation, Suicide Attempts, and Injurious Suicide Attempts among Students in Grades 9–12, by Sex, Grade Level, Race, and Hispanic Origin: United States, Selected Years 1991–2007," in *Health, United States, 2009: With Special Feature on Medical Technology*, Centers for Disease Control and Prevention, National Center for Health Statistics, 2010, http://www.cdc.gov/nchs/data/hus/hus09.pdf (accessed February 24, 2012)

TABLE 6.4

Percentage of high school students who attempted suicide and whose suicide attempt required medical attention, by sex, race/ethnicity, and grade, 2009

Category	Attempted suicide			Suicide attempt treated by a doctor or nurse		
	Female %	Male %	Total %	Female %	Male %	Total %
Race/ethnicity						
White*	6.5	3.8	5.0	2.0	1.2	1.6
Black*	10.4	5.4	7.9	2.5	2.5	2.5
Hispanic	11.1	5.1	8.1	2.7	1.8	2.2
Grade						
9	10.3	4.5	7.3	2.8	1.4	2.1
10	8.8	5.2	6.9	2.3	2.0	2.2
11	7.8	4.7	6.3	2.6	1.7	2.1
12	4.6	3.8	4.2	1.0	1.4	1.2
Total	8.1	4.6	6.3	2.3	1.6	1.9

*Non-Hispanic.
Notes: Attempted suicide refers to one or more attempts during the 12 months before the survey.

SOURCE: Adapted from Danice K. Eaton et al., "Table 24. Percentage of High School Students Who Attempted Suicide and Whose Suicide Attempt Resulted in an Injury, Poisoning, or an Overdose That Had to Be Treated by a Doctor or Nurse, by Sex, Race/Ethnicity, and Grade—United States, Youth Risk Behavior Survey, 2009," in "Youth Risk Behavior Surveillance—United States, 2009," *Morbidity and Mortality Weekly Report*, vol. 59, no. SS-5, June 4, 2010, http://www.cdc.gov/mmwr/pdf/ss/ss5905.pdf (accessed February 2, 2012)

Transgender Populations: Review and Recommendations" (*Journal of Homosexuality*, vol. 58, vol. 1, 2011), which discusses what is known about suicide in the LGBT population and what can be done to help curb it.

Haas et al. note that among large-scale surveys, approximately 2.5% of men and 1.4% of women have had same-sex sexual partners during the past year. Regarding mental health issues, which is the single largest risk factor for suicide, lesbian women infrequently have such issues, whereas gay men often do. Studies cited in this report indicate that gay men have from three to six times as many suicide attempts as do straight men, and those with rejecting parents have about eight times as many attempts.

In addition, about four out of 10 (42%) married gay men and just over a quarter (28%) of married lesbian women have the same health coverage that married straight men and women have, and they often have to pay federal income tax on the benefits they receive.

TABLE 6.5

Percentage of high school students who attempted suicide and whose suicide attempt required medical attention, by sex and selected U.S. sites, 2009

Site	Attempted suicide			Suicide attempt treated by a doctor or nurse		
	Female %	Male %	Total %	Female %	Male %	Total %
State surveys						
Alabama	12.2	9.0	10.7	2.9	3.9	3.4
Alaska	11.5	5.1	8.5	3.0	2.3	2.6
Arizona	11.1	7.6	9.5	3.4	3.7	3.6
Arkansas	11.3	12.7	12.0	4.3	5.4	4.8
Colorado	9.3	5.6	7.6	3.5	2.4	3.1
Connecticut	7.3	7.5	7.4	2.5	3.0	2.7
Delaware	10.8	5.0	8.2	3.0	1.4	2.4
Florida	7.5	5.5	6.5	2.2	2.3	2.3
Georgia	10.1	6.4	8.3	3.6	2.7	3.2
Hawaii	13.9	11.5	12.8	4.7	4.3	4.5
Idaho	8.2	5.4	6.9	2.4	1.7	2.0
Illinois	9.1	8.6	8.9	2.9	2.8	2.9
Indiana	11.7	6.8	9.3	4.3	2.9	3.6
Kansas	7.9	4.5	6.1	2.5	1.2	1.8
Kentucky	9.1	8.4	8.8	3.2	3.8	3.5
Louisiana	11.1	10.3	10.9	4.9	5.0	4.9
Maine	7.7	8.1	7.9	—	—	—
Maryland	9.4	11.2	10.4	2.7	4.4	3.5
Massachusetts	7.0	6.6	6.8	2.2	2.9	2.6
Michigan	11.1	7.2	9.3	3.3	2.6	3.0
Mississippi	11.9	6.4	9.3	3.5	1.8	2.7
Missouri	7.9	5.0	6.4	3.3	1.6	2.5
Montana	7.9	7.4	7.7	3.0	2.6	2.8
Nevada	11.6	8.7	10.2	4.3	2.9	3.6
New Hampshire	5.1	4.2	4.7	1.6	1.6	1.6
New Jersey	—	—	—	—	—	—
New Mexico	11.7	7.6	9.7	3.7	2.6	3.2
New York	7.3	7.1	7.4	2.6	2.9	2.8
North Carolina	9.7	9.9	9.9	—	—	—
North Dakota	5.9	5.4	5.7	1.8	2.8	2.3
Oklahoma	8.9	5.2	7.0	3.4	1.9	2.6
Pennsylvania	8.4	3.1	5.7	1.8	1.6	1.7
Rhode Island	8.3	7.1	7.7	3.1	3.5	3.3
South Carolina	9.7	11.7	10.8	3.0	4.6	3.9
South Dakota	7.0	6.3	6.7	1.1	2.5	1.9
Tennessee	9.3	4.8	7.1	2.4	2.0	2.2
Texas	10.4	4.3	7.4	2.7	1.4	2.1
Utah	8.0	6.4	7.2	3.2	3.0	3.2
Vermont	5.1	3.4	4.3	1.8	1.3	1.6
West Virginia	11.7	9.8	10.7	4.0	4.9	4.6
Wisconsin	7.1	4.6	5.8	2.0	1.4	1.7
Wyoming	10.9	7.9	9.4	4.1	3.9	4.0
Median	9.3	6.8	7.9	3.0	2.7	2.8
Range	5.1–13.9	3.1–12.7	4.3–12.8	1.1–4.9	1.2–5.4	1.6–4.9
Local surveys						
Boston, MA	11.6	9.6	10.8	3.1	4.1	3.7
Broward County, FL	8.0	4.7	6.4	2.8	3.1	2.9
Charlotte-Mecklenburg, NC	13.0	13.9	13.5	—	—	—
Chicago, IL	10.7	15.4	13.3	3.3	8.1	5.9
Clark County, NV	11.9	8.0	10.0	4.1	2.3	3.2
Dallas, TX	13.8	10.1	12.0	5.1	3.9	4.5
Detroit, MI	15.6	12.9	14.3	4.4	5.7	5.0
Duval County, FL	9.3	10.2	10.0	3.2	3.4	3.4
Los Angeles, CA	7.4	10.2	8.8	2.3	4.2	3.2
Memphis, TN	10.4	6.4	8.7	2.0	3.1	2.6
Miami-Dade County, FL	8.1	6.4	7.3	2.7	2.4	2.6
Milwaukee, WI	13.7	11.0	12.4	4.8	4.4	4.6
New York City, NY	10.7	9.0	9.9	3.4	3.4	3.4
Orange County, FL	9.5	4.9	7.3	2.5	1.9	2.3
Palm Beach County, FL	9.4	5.8	7.8	2.6	2.2	2.6
Philadelphia, PA	14.7	8.8	12.0	4.4	4.7	4.5
San Bernardino, CA	10.2	8.5	9.4	3.1	2.5	2.8
San Diego, CA	7.9	4.1	6.0	1.9	1.3	1.6
San Francisco, CA	9.0	9.3	9.1	3.7	3.9	3.8

Haas et al. conclude with this message: "Over the last two decades, an increasing body of empirical research in the United States and other countries has pointed to significantly elevated suicide risk among LGBT compared to heterosexual people. Although many questions are as yet unanswered, there appears to be little doubt that a broad

TABLE 6.5

Percentage of high school students who attempted suicide and whose suicide attempt required medical attention, by sex and selected U.S. sites, 2009 [CONTINUED]

	Attempted suicide			Suicide attempt treated by a doctor or nurse		
Site	Female %	Male %	Total %	Female %	Male %	Total %
Seattle, WA	8.3	8.5	8.6	3.6	4.6	4.1
Median	10.3	8.9	9.6	3.2	3.4	3.4
Range	7.4–15.6	4.1–15.4	6.0–14.3	1.9–5.1	1.3–8.1	1.6–5.9

—Not available.
Notes: Time period refers the 12 months before the survey. Frequency is attempted one or more times.

SOURCE: Adapted from Danice K. Eaton et al., "Table 25. Percentage of High School Students Who Attempted Suicide and Whose Suicide Attempt Resulted in an Injury, Poisoning, or Overdose That Had to Be Treated by a Doctor or Nurse, by Sex—Selected U.S. Sites, Youth Risk Behavior Survey, 2009," in "Youth Risk Behavior Surveillance—United States, 2009," *Morbidity and Mortality Weekly Report*, vol. 59, no. SS-5, June 4, 2010, http://www.cdc.gov/mmwr/pdf/ss/ss5905.pdf (accessed February 2, 2012)

TABLE 6.6

Percentage of high school students who felt sad or hopeless, by sex, race/ethnicity, and grade, 2009

Category	Female %	Male %	Total %
Race/ethnicity			
White*	31.1	17.2	23.7
Black*	37.5	17.9	27.7
Hispanic	39.7	23.6	31.6
Grade			
9	35.8	18.6	26.6
10	34.7	18.2	26.1
11	35.5	19.6	27.3
12	28.9	19.8	24.3
Total	**33.9**	**19.1**	**26.1**

*Non-Hispanic.
Notes: Percentage of students who were sad or felt hopeless almost every day for 2 or more weeks in a row so that they stopped doing some usual activities during the 12 months before the survey.

SOURCE: Adapted from Danice K. Eaton et al., "Table 20. Percentage of High School Students Who Felt Sad or Hopeless, by Sex, Race/Ethnicity, and Grade—United States, Youth Risk Behavior Survey, 2009," in "Youth Risk Behavior Surveillance—United States, 2009," *Morbidity and Mortality Weekly Report*, vol. 59, no. SS-5, June 4, 2010, http://www.cdc.gov/mmwr/pdf/ss/ss5905.pdf (accessed February 2, 2012)

national effort will be needed to encourage and fund the needed research, raise awareness of the problem among LGBT and suicide prevention leaders, and develop the interventions, prevention strategies, and policy changes through which suicidal behavior and suicide risk in LGBT populations can be reduced."

EUTHANASIA AND PHYSICIAN-ASSISTED SUICIDE

The U.S. Constitution does not guarantee the right to choose to die. However, the U.S. Supreme Court recognizes that Americans have a fundamental right to privacy, or what is sometimes called the "right to be left alone." Even though the right to privacy is not explicitly mentioned in the Constitution, the Supreme Court has interpreted

several amendments as encompassing this right. For example, in *Roe v. Wade* (410 U.S. 113 [1973]), the court ruled that the 14th Amendment protects the right to privacy against state action, specifically a woman's right to abortion. Another example is the landmark Karen Ann Quinlan case, which was based on right-to-privacy rulings by the U.S. Supreme Court. In *In re Quinlan* (70 N.J. 10, 355 A.2d 647 [1976]), the New Jersey Supreme Court held that the right to privacy included the right to refuse unwanted medical treatment and, as a consequence, the right to die (see Chapter 8).

The Acceptability of Euthanasia and Physician-Assisted Suicide

Stéphanie Frileux et al. examine in "When Is Physician Assisted Suicide or Euthanasia Acceptable?" (*Journal of Medical Ethics*, vol. 29, no. 6, December 2003) the opinion of the general public on euthanasia and physician-assisted suicide. The researchers define these terms as follows: "In physician assisted suicide, the physician provides the patient with the means to end his or her own life. In euthanasia, the physician deliberately and directly intervenes to end the patient's life; this is sometimes called 'active euthanasia' to distinguish it from withholding or withdrawing treatment needed to sustain life." Their study posed the questions: "Should a terminally ill patient be allowed to die? Should the medical profession have the option of helping such a patient to die?" Frileux et al. find that acceptability of euthanasia and physician-assisted suicide by the general public appears to depend on four factors: the level of patient suffering, the extent to which the patient requested death, the age of the patient, and the degree of curability of the illness.

According to Lydia Saad of the Gallup Organization, in *Doctor-Assisted Suicide Is Moral Issue Dividing Americans Most* (May 31, 2011, http://www.gallup.com/poll/147842/Doctor-Assisted-Suicide-Moral-Issue-Dividing-Americans.aspx), 45% of Americans supported physician-assisted suicide in 2011, and 48% thought it was morally

TABLE 6.7

Percentage of high school students who seriously considered attempting suicide, and who made a suicide plan, by sex, race/ethnicity, and grade, 2009

Category	Seriously considered attempting suicide			Made a suicide plan		
	Female %	Male %	Total %	Female %	Male %	Total %
Race/ethnicity						
White*	16.1	10.5	13.1	12.3	8.5	10.3
Black*	18.1	7.8	13.0	13.3	6.2	9.8
Hispanic	20.2	10.7	15.4	15.4	9.0	12.2
Grade						
9	20.3	10.0	14.8	14.9	7.3	10.8
10	17.2	10.0	13.4	14.3	9.3	11.7
11	17.8	11.4	14.5	13.4	9.4	11.3
12	13.6	10.5	12.1	9.6	8.8	9.2
Total	**17.4**	**10.5**	**13.8**	**13.2**	**8.6**	**10.9**

Note: Time period is the 12 months before the survey.
*Non-Hispanic.

SOURCE: Adapted from Danice K. Eaton et al., "Table 22. Percentage of High School Students Who Seriously Considered Attempting Suicide and Who Made a Plan about How They Would Attempt Suicide, by Sex, Race/Ethnicity, and Grade—United States, Youth Risk Behavior Survey, 2009," in "Youth Risk Behavior Surveillance—United States, 2009," *Morbidity and Mortality Weekly Report*, vol. 59, no. SS-5, June 4, 2010, http://www.cdc.gov/mmwr/pdf/ss/ss5905.pdf (accessed February 2, 2012)

wrong. (See Table 6.11.) Saad lists physician-assisted suicide as one of three most controversial issues among Americans, the other two being abortion and out-of-wedlock births.

Joris Gielen et al. interviewed 14 physicians and 13 nurses working in palliative care programs to determine what they thought about palliative sedation in end-of-life care and reported their findings in "The Attitudes of Indian Palliative-Care Nurses and Physicians to Pain Control and Palliative Sedation" (*Indian Journal of Palliative Care*, vol. 17, no. 1, January–April 2011). The health care providers all thought that palliative care painkillers were fine to administer, provided that they were titrated (gradually increased to achieve efficacy with the least amount of side effects) to the patient's pain. They thought that such light sedation was useful but disagreed whether deep sedation was acceptable.

Antoine Baumann et al. note in "The Ethical and Legal Aspects of Palliative Sedation in Severely Brain-Injured Patients: A French Perspective" (*Philosophy, Ethics, and Humanities in Medicine*, vol. 6, February 8, 2011) that in patients in which the presence and severity of pain cannot be known, and in lieu of the 2005 French law that provides legal and ethical safeguards against euthanasia, the law "reminds physicians of their duty to respect the patient's right to receive palliative care, including major palliative sedation when considered proportionate to the patient's potential suffering." The researchers also state that "transparency of the decision-making process, collegial decision making, information of the relatives, and documentation of the entire decision-making process in the medical files are legal requirements that constitute safeguards against the

inappropriate use of palliative sedation." Baumann et al. suggest that this approach may be appropriate and beneficial for physicians working in countries in which physician-assisted suicide and euthanasia are illegal.

Patients Requesting Assisted Suicide and Euthanasia

Table 6.12 shows the characteristics of patients at the end of life in Oregon, where assisted suicide is legal. (It is also legal in Washington and Montana.) These results are from patients who died between 1998 and 2010 and in 2011. The patients who died after ingesting a lethal dose of medication were predominantly male (53.7%) between 1998 and 2010 and predominantly female (63.4%) in 2011, 55 to 84 years old (77% between 1998 and 2010 and 80.3% in 2011), and white (97.9% between 1998 and 2010 and 95.6% in 2011). More than 40% were college graduates (44.2% between 1998 and 2010 and 48.5% in 2011), and a majority had a primary diagnosis of cancer (80.8% between 1998 and 2010 and 82.4% in 2011).

Reasons for Assisted Suicide Requests

Linda Ganzini, Elizabeth R. Goy, and Steven K. Dobscha reveal in "Oregonians' Reasons for Requesting Physician Aid in Dying" (*Archives of Internal Medicine*, vol. 169, no. 5, March 9, 2009) patients' reasons for requesting physician-assisted suicide. The primary reasons for wanting physician-assisted suicide were:

- Wanting to control circumstances of death
- Future poor quality of life
- Future pain

TABLE 6.8

Percentage of high school students who felt sad or hopeless, by sex and selected U.S. sites, 2009

Site	Female %	Male %	Total %
State surveys			
Alabama	34.5	22.8	28.6
Alaska	33.5	17.2	25.2
Arizona	41.0	28.9	34.9
Arkansas	35.3	21.0	28.1
Colorado	31.7	19.3	25.4
Connecticut	32.9	17.2	25.0
Delaware	32.8	20.2	26.5
Florida	33.0	19.6	26.3
Georgia	35.9	21.6	28.8
Hawaii	39.0	22.9	30.6
Idaho	36.2	20.9	28.3
Illinois	32.9	22.9	27.8
Indiana	37.0	19.6	28.1
Kansas	28.0	15.4	21.5
Kentucky	32.1	21.7	26.7
Louisiana	35.5	26.1	31.2
Maine	26.9	18.5	22.7
Maryland	30.1	20.2	25.1
Massachusetts	29.1	19.2	24.0
Michigan	34.7	20.3	27.4
Mississippi	36.3	21.8	29.0
Missouri	33.2	21.3	27.1
Montana	33.2	21.7	27.3
Nevada	37.9	23.0	30.3
New Hampshire	32.1	18.4	25.1
New Jersey	—	—	—
New Mexico	37.3	22.3	29.7
New York	28.3	16.5	22.6
North Carolina	32.8	21.6	27.4
North Dakota	30.6	15.6	22.9
Oklahoma	36.8	20.1	28.2
Pennsylvania	31.5	15.8	23.5
Rhode Island	29.5	20.3	25.0
South Carolina	31.3	18.8	25.1
South Dakota	—	—	—
Tennessee	33.9	21.6	27.6
Texas	34.9	20.8	27.7
Utah	32.8	19.4	26.0
Vermont	27.3	15.0	21.1
West Virginia	36.7	22.9	29.7
Wisconsin	25.9	16.1	20.8
Wyoming	35.3	19.2	26.9
Median	33.1	20.2	27.0
Range	25.9–41.0	15.0–28.9	20.8–34.9
Local surveys			
Boston, MA	36.0	21.1	28.8
Broward County, FL	33.0	19.9	26.6
Charlotte-Mecklenburg, NC	34.3	21.5	28.2
Chicago, IL	36.7	24.9	30.5
Clark County, NV	39.0	24.3	31.5
Dallas, TX	35.5	30.6	33.0
Detroit, MI	37.5	20.4	28.8
Duval County, FL	31.5	22.7	27.3
Los Angeles, CA	35.9	24.6	30.1
Memphis, TN	29.0	16.7	23.0
Miami-Dade County, FL	35.7	21.8	28.7
Milwaukee, WI	37.1	23.5	30.3
New York City, NY	34.4	21.5	28.3
Orange County, FL	32.3	20.2	26.2
Palm Beach County, FL	32.3	21.0	26.5
Philadelphia, PA	40.8	26.1	33.8
San Bernardino, CA	38.2	25.7	31.9
San Diego, CA	33.8	18.3	25.9
San Francisco, CA	26.8	21.0	23.9

- Future inability to care for self

- Loss of independence

- Wanting to die at home

Site	Female %	Male %	Total %
Seattle, WA	24.3	17.0	20.6
Median	34.9	21.5	28.5
Range	24.3–40.8	16.7–30.6	20.6–33.8

Notes: Per centage of students who were sad or felt hopeless almost every day for 2 or more weeks in a row so that they stopped doing some usual activities during the 12 months before the survey.
—Not available.

SOURCE: Adapted from Danice K. Eaton et al., "Table 21. Percentage of High School Students Who Felt Sad or Hopeless, by Sex—Selected U.S. Sites, Youth Risk Behavior Survey, 2009," in "Youth Risk Behavior Surveillance—United States, 2009," *Morbidity and Mortality Weekly Report*, vol. 59, no. SS-5, June 4, 2010, http://www.cdc.gov/mmwr/pdf/ss/ss5905.pdf (accessed February 2, 2012)

Other important reasons were:

- Perception of self as burden

- Loss of dignity

- Future mental confusion

- Worry about loss of sense of self

- Future dyspnea (difficulty in breathing)

- Ready to die

- Future fatigue

Ganzini, Goy, and Dobscha indicate that even though patients nearing death have concerns about physical pain and suffering, they are also highly focused on the loss of dignity, the loss of control, and of being a burden or dependent on others.

SUPPORTERS OF ASSISTED SUICIDE

Compassion & Choices and Derek Humphry

In 2003 the Hemlock Society officially became End-of-Life Choices. Two years later, in 2005, End-of-Life Choices merged with Compassion and Dying to form Compassion & Choices. The organization advocates for legislation that allows Americans to live with the freedom of choosing a dignified death and informs and educates the public about the right to die.

Compassion & Choices was founded as the Hemlock Society in 1980 by Derek Humphry (1930–), a British journalist. In 1975 Humphry helped his wife take her own life to end the pain and suffering that was caused by her terminal bone cancer. Humphry recounted this incident in *Jean's Way* (1978). The book launched his career in the voluntary euthanasia movement two years later.

TABLE 6.9

Trends in suicide-related behaviors, selected years, 1991–2009

	1991	1993	1995	1997	1999	2001	2003	2005	2007	2009	Changes from 1991–2009[a]	Change from 2007–2009[b]
Seriously considered attempting suicide (during the 12 months before the survey)	29.0	24.1	24.1	20.5	19.3	19.0	16.9	16.9	14.5	13.8	Decreased, 1991–2009	No change
Made a plan about how they would attempt suicide (during the 12 months before the survey)	18.6	19.0	17.7	15.7	14.5	14.8	16.5	13.0	11.3	10.9	Decreased, 1991–2009	No change
Attempted suicide one or more times (during the 12 months before the survey)	7.3	8.6	8.7	7.7	8.3	8.8	8.5	8.4	6.9	6.3	No change, 1991–2001 Decreased, 2001–2009	No change
Suicide attempt resulted in an injury, poisoning, or an overdose that had to be treated by a doctor or nurse (during the 12 months before the survey)	1.7	2.7	2.8	2.6	2.6	2.6	2.9	2.3	2.0	1.9	No change, 1991–2003 Decreased, 2003–2009	No change

[a]Based on trend analyses using a logistic regression model controlling for sex, race/ethnicity, and grade.
[b]Based on t-test analyses, p < 0.05.

SOURCE: Adapted from "Trends in the Prevalence of Suicide-Related Behaviors, National YRBS: 1991–2009," in *National Youth Risk Behavior Survey, 1991–2009*, Centers for Disease Control and Prevention, http://www.cdc.gov/healthyyouth/yrbs/pdf/us_suicide_trend_yrbs.pdf (accessed February 2, 2012)

TABLE 6.10

Number of suicide deaths, death rates, and age-adjusted death rates, by mechanism of suicide, 2008

Mechanism of suicide	Number of deaths	Rate of death (per 100,000 population)
All mechanisms	36,035	11.9
Firearm	18,223	6.0
Suffocation	8,578	2.8
Poisoning	6,442	2.1
Fall	709	0.2
Cut/pierce	666	0.2
Drowning	407	0.1
Other specified, classifiable	301	0.1
Other specified, not elsewhere classified	222	0.1
Unspecified	188	0.1
Fire/flame	169	0.1
All transport	129	0.0

SOURCE: Adapted from Arialdi M. Miniño et al., "Table 18. Number of Deaths, Death Rates, and Age-Adjusted Death Rates for Injury Deaths, by Mechanism and Intent of Death: United States, 2008," in "Deaths: Final Data for 2008," *National Vital Statistics Reports*, vol. 59, no. 10, December 7, 2011, http://www.cdc.gov/nchs/data/nvsr/nvsr59/nvsr59_10.pdf (accessed February 21, 2012)

TABLE 6.11

Physician-assisted suicide divides Americans most, 2011

Ranked by "difference"

	Morally acceptable %	Morally wrong %	Difference pct. pts.
Doctor-assisted suicide	45	48	3
Abortion	39	51	12
Having a baby outside of marriage	54	41	13
Buying and wearing clothing made of animal fur	56	39	17
Gay or lesbian relations	56	39	17
Medical testing on animals	55	38	17
Sex between an unmarried man and woman	60	36	24
Cloning animals	32	62	30
Medical research using stem cells obtained from human embryos	62	30	32
Gambling	64	31	33
Pornography	30	66	36
The death penalty	65	28	37
Divorce	69	23	46
Suicide	15	80	
Cloning humans	12	84	72
Polygamy, when a married person has more than one spouse at the same time	11	86	75
Married men and women having an affair	7	91	84

SOURCE: Lydia Saad, "U.S. Perceived Moral Acceptability of Behaviors and Social Policies," in *Doctor-Assisted Suicide Is Moral Issue Dividing Americans Most*, The Gallup Organization, May 31, 2011, http://www.gallup.com/poll/147842/Doctor-Assisted-Suicide-Moral-Issue-Dividing-Americans.aspx (accessed February 26, 2012). Copyright © 2011 by The Gallup Organization. Reproduced by permission of The Gallup Organization.

In 1991 Humphry published *Final Exit: The Practicalities of Self-Deliverance and Assisted Suicide for the Dying*. The suicide manual, which was on the *New York Times* best-seller list for 18 weeks, gives explicit instructions on how to commit suicide. Even though Humphry insisted that his how-to book was written only for those who were terminally ill, and not for those suffering from depression, some physicians were concerned about how the book would affect those suffering from depression. In October 1991 Humphry's second wife, Wickett Humphry (1942–1991), whom he had divorced the year before, committed suicide. She had been diagnosed with cancer and was reportedly depressed.

Humphry retired from the Hemlock Society in 1992, but his activities continued to spark controversy. In 1999 he recorded a video that depicted a variety of methods for committing suicide. Even though it had been available from the Hemlock Society USA for several months, the video drew more criticism when it aired on public television in Oregon a number of

TABLE 6.12

Characteristics and end-of-life care of Death with Dignity Act patients who ingested lethal medication, Oregon, 1998–2011

Characteristics	2011 (N = 71)		1998–2010 (N = 525)		Total (N = 596)	
	N	(%)[a]	N	(%)[a]	N	(%)[a]
Sex						
Male (%)	26	(36.6)	282	(53.7)	308	(51.7)
Female (%)	45	(63.4)	243	(46.3)	288	(48.3)
Age						
18–34 (%)	0	(0.0)	6	(1.1)	6	(1.0)
35–44 (%)	1	(1.4)	13	(2.5)	14	(2.3)
45–54 (%)	5	(7.0)	39	(7.4)	44	(7.4)
55–64 (%)	16	(22.5)	107	(20.4)	123	(20.6)
65–74 (%)	23	(32.4)	147	(28.0)	170	(28.5)
75–84 (%)	18	(25.4)	150	(28.6)	168	(28.2)
85+ (%)	8	(11.3)	63	(12.0)	71	(11.9)
Median years (range)	70	(41–96)	71	(25–96)	71	(25–96)
Race						
White (%)	65	(95.6)	514	(97.9)	579	(97.6)
African American (%)	0	(0.0)	1	(0.2)	1	(0.2)
American Indian (%)	0	(0.0)	1	(0.2)	1	(0.2)
Asian (%)	0	(0.0)	7	(1.3)	7	(1.2)
Pacific Islander (%)	1	(1.5)	0	(0.0)	1	(0.2)
Other (%)	0	(0.0)	0	(0.0)	0	(0.0)
Two or more races (%)	0	(0.0)	0	(0.0)	0	(0.0)
Hispanic (%)	2	(2.9)	2	(0.4)	4	(0.7)
Unknown	3		0		3	
Marital status						
Married (%)	26	(38.2)	245	(46.7)	271	(45.7)
Widowed (%)	19	(27.9)	115	(21.9)	134	(22.6)
Never married (%)	7	(10.3)	42	(8.0)	49	(8.3)
Divorced (%)	16	(23.5)	123	(23.4)	139	(23.4)
Unknown	3		0		3	
Education						
Less than high school (%)	3	(4.4)	37	(7.1)	40	(6.8)
High school graduate (%)	9	(13.2)	130	(24.9)	139	(23.5)
Some college (%)	23	(33.8)	125	(23.9)	148	(25.0)
Baccalaureate or higher (%)	33	(48.5)	231	(44.2)	264	(44.7)
Unknown	3		2		5	
Residence						
Metro counties (%)[b]	27	(39.7)	226	(43.0)	253	(42.7)
Coastal counties (%)	6	(8.8)	41	(7.8)	47	(7.9)
Other western counties (%)	31	(45.6)	219	(41.7)	250	(42.2)
East of the Cascades (%)	4	(5.9)	39	(7.4)	43	(7.3)
Unknown	3		0		3	
End of life care						
Hospice						
Enrolled (%)[c]	59	(96.7)	463	(88.9)	522	(89.7)
Not enrolled (%)	2	(3.3)	58	(11.1)	60	(10.3)
Unknown	10		4		14	
Insurance						
Private (%)[d]	31	(50.8)	351	(68.0)	382	(66.2)
Medicare, Medicaid or other governmental (%)	28	(45.9)	157	(30.4)	185	(32.1)
None (%)	2	(3.3)	8	(1.6)	10	(1.7)
Unknown	10		9		19	

times in 2000. Critics asserted that this airing provided dangerous information, particularly to people who were depressed or mentally ill.

In 2004 Humphry published *The Good Euthanasia Guide 2004: Where, What, and Who in Choices in Dying.* Much of the book describes international suicide laws. His memoir *Good Life, Good Death: Memoir of a Writer Who Became a Euthanasia Advocate* was published in 2008. As of April 2012, Humphry was president of the Euthanasia Research and Guidance Organization.

Jack Kevorkian

Jack Kevorkian (1928–2011) first earned the nickname "Dr. Death" when, as a medical resident, he photographed patients at the time of death to gather data that would help him differentiate death from coma, shock, and fainting. During his study and residency, he suggested unconventional ideas, such as the harvesting of organs from death-row inmates. His career as a doctor was also "checkered" (Kevorkian's own word) and notable for controversy.

TABLE 6.12

Characteristics and end-of-life care of Death with Dignity Act patients who ingested lethal medication, Oregon, 1998–2011 [CONTINUED]

Characteristics	2011 (N = 71)		1998–2010 (N = 525)		Total (N = 596)	
	N	(%)[a]	N	(%)[a]	N	(%)[a]
Underlying illness						
Malignant neoplasms (%)	56	(82.4)	424	(80.8)	480	(80.9)
Lung and bronchus (%)	16	(23.5)	96	(18.3)	112	(18.9)
Breast (%)	11	(16.2)	41	(7.8)	52	(8.8)
Colon (%)	2	(2.9)	34	(6.5)	36	(6.1)
Pancreas (%)	4	(5.9)	38	(7.2)	42	(7.1)
Prostate (%)	1	(1.5)	25	(4.8)	26	(4.4)
Ovary (%)	3	(4.4)	22	(4.2)	25	(4.2)
Other (%)	19	(27.9)	168	(32.0)	187	(31.5)
Amyotrophic lateral sclerosis (%)	2	(2.9)	42	(8.0)	44	(7.4)
Chronic lower respiratory disease (%)	5	(7.4)	20	(3.8)	25	(4.2)
Heart disease (%)	1	(1.5)	9	(1.7)	10	(1.7)
HIV/AIDS (%)	0	(0.0)	8	(1.5)	8	(1.3)
Other illnesses (%)[e]	4	(5.9)	22	(4.2)	26	(4.4)
Unknown	3		0		3	
DWDA process						
Referred for psychiatric evaluation (%)	1	(1.4)	39	(7.4)	40	(6.7)
Patient informed family of decision (%)[f]	70	(98.6)	423	(93.8)	493	(94.4)
Patient died at						
Home (patient, family or friend) (%)	64	(94.1)	498	(94.9)	562	(94.8)
Long term care, assisted living or foster care facility (%)	4	(5.9)	21	(4.0)	25	(4.2)
Hospital (%)	0	(0.0)	1	(0.2)	1	(0.2)
Other (%)	0	(0.0)	5	(1.0)	5	(0.8)
Unknown	3		0		3	
Lethal medication						
Secobarbital (%)	56	(78.9)	318	(60.6)	374	(62.8)
Pentobarbital (%)	15	(21.1)	200	(38.1)	215	(36.1)
Other (%)[g]	0	(0.0)	7	(1.3)	7	(1.2)
End of life concerns[h]	(N = 71)		(N = 521)		(N = 592)	
Losing autonomy (%)	63	(88.7)	475	(91.2)	538	(90.9)
Less able to engage in activities making life enjoyable (%)	64	(90.1)	459	(88.1)	523	(88.3)
Loss of dignity (%)[i]	53	(74.6)	333	(84.1)	386	(82.7)
Losing control of bodily functions (%)	24	(33.8)	294	(56.4)	318	(53.7)
Burden on family, friends/caregivers (%)	30	(42.3)	184	(35.3)	214	(36.1)
Inadequate pain control or concern about it (%)	23	(32.4)	111	(21.3)	134	(22.6)
Financial implications of treatment (%)	2	(2.8)	13	(2.5)	15	(2.5)
Health-care provider present[j]	(N = 71)		(N = 455)		(N = 526)	
When medication was ingested[k]						
Prescribing physician	6		94		100	
Other provider, prescribing physician not present	3		228		231	
No provider	5		67		72	
Unknown	57		66		123	
At time of death						
Prescribing physician (%)	6	(8.5)	83	(18.7)	89	(17.3)
Other provider, prescribing physician not present (%)	2	(2.8)	252	(56.9)	254	(49.4)
No provider (%)	63	(88.7)	108	(24.4)	171	(33.3)
Unknown	0		12		12	
Complications[k]	(N = 71)		(N = 525)		(N = 596)	
Regurgitated	1		21		22	
Seizures	0		0		0	
None	11		456		467	
Unknown	59		48		107	
Other outcomes						
Regained consciousness after ingesting DWDA medications[l]	2		3		5	

During the late 1980s Kevorkian retired from pathology work and pursued an interest in the concept of physician-assisted suicide, becoming one of its best-known and most passionate advocates. He constructed the Mercitron, a machine that allowed a patient to press a red button and self-administer a lethal dose of poisonous potassium chloride, along with thiopental, a painkiller.

The first patient to commit suicide with Kevorkian's assistance and his Mercitron was Janet Adkins. Adkins, a Hemlock Society member, sought Kevorkian's aid because she did not want to wait until she lost her cognitive abilities to Alzheimer's disease. In June 1990 Adkins committed suicide in Kevorkian's van in a public campground.

In 1991 Kevorkian assisted in the deaths of two Michigan women on the same day. Sherry Miller, aged 43, had multiple sclerosis, and Marjorie Wantz, aged 58, complained of a painful pelvic disease. Neither one was terminally ill, but court findings showed that they both suffered from

TABLE 6.12

Characteristics and end-of-life care of Death with Dignity Act patients who ingested lethal medication, Oregon, 1998–2011 [CONTINUED]

Characteristics	2011 (N = 71)		1998–2010 (N = 525)		Total (N = 596)	
	N	(%)[a]	N	(%)[a]	N	(%)[a]
Timing of DWDA event						
Duration (weeks) of patient-physician relationship[m]						
Median	12		12		12	
Range	1–1,379		0–1,905		0–1,905	
Number of patients with information available	71		523		594	
Number of patients with information unknown	0		2		2	
Duration (days) between 1st request and death						
Median	47		46		46	
Range	15–872		15–1,009		15–1,009	
Number of patients with information available	71		525		596	
Number of patients with information unknown	0		0		0	
Minutes between ingestion and unconsciousness[k]						
Median	5		5		5	
Range	2–10		1–38		1–38	
Number of patients with information available	8		454		462	
Number of patients with information unknown	63		71		134	
Minutes between ingestion and death[k]						
Median	27		25		25	
Range (minutes–hours)	15 min–1.5 hrs		1 min–104 hrs		1 min–104 hrs	
Number of patients with information available	8		459		467	
Number of patients with information unknown	63		66		129	

[a]Unknowns are excluded when calculating percentages.
[b]Clackamas, Multnomah, and Washington counties.
[c]Includes patients that were enrolled in hospice at the time the prescription was written or at time of death.
[d]Private insurance category includes those with private insurance alone or in combination with other insurance.
[e]Includes deaths due to benign and uncertain neoplasms, other respiratory diseases, diseases of the nervous system (including multiple sclerosis, Parkinson's disease and Huntington's disease), musculoskeletal and connective tissue diseases, viral hepatitis, diabetes mellitus, cerebrovascular disease, and alcoholic liver disease.
[f]First recorded beginning in 2001. Since then, 21 patients (4.0%) have chosen not to inform their families, and 8 patients (1.5%) have had no family to inform. There was one unknown case in 2002, two in 2005, and one in 2009.
[g]Other includes combinations of secobarbital, pentobarbital, and/or morphine.
[h]Affirmative answers only ("Don't know" included in negative answers). Categories are not mutually exclusive. Data unavailable for four patients in 2001.
[i]First asked in 2003. Data available for 71 patients in 2011, 396 patients between 1998–2010, and 467 patients for all years.
[j]The data shown are for 2001–2011 since information about the presence of a health care provider/volunteer, in the absence of the prescribing physician, was first collected in 2001.
[k]A procedure revision was made mid-year in 2010 to standardize reporting on the follow-up questionnaire. The new procedure accepts information about time of death and circumstances surrounding death only when the physician or another health care provider is present at the time of death. This resulted in a larger number of unknowns beginning in 2010.
[l]Patients who regained consciousness after ingesting prescribed medications are not included in the total number of DWDA deaths. In 2005, one patient regained consciousness 65 hours after ingesting the medication, subsequently dying from underlying illness 14 days after awakening. In 2010, two patients regained consciousness after ingesting medications. One patient regained consciousness 88 hours after ingesting the medication, subsequently dying from underlying illness three months later. The other patient regained consciousness within 24 hours, subsequently dying from underlying illness five days following ingestion. In 2011, two patients regained consciousness after ingesting the medication. One of the patients very briefly regained consciousness after ingesting the prescribed medication and died from underlying illness about 30 hours later. The other patient regained consciousness approximately 14 hours after ingesting the medication and died from underlying illness about 38 hours later.
[m]Previous reports listed 20 records missing the date care began with the attending physician. Further research with these cases has reduced the number of unknowns.

SOURCE: "Table 1. Characteristics and End-of-Life Care of 596 DWDA Patients Who Died after Ingesting a Lethal Dose of Medication as of February 29, 2012, by Year, Oregon, 1998–2011," in *Death with Dignity Act 2011 Annual Report*, Oregon Department of Human Services, February 29, 2012, http://public.health .oregon.gov/ProviderPartnerResources/EvaluationResearch/DeathwithDignityAct/Documents/year14-tbl-1.pdf (accessed April 30, 2012)

depression. In 1996 Kevorkian was tried for the assisted deaths of Miller and Wantz under the common law that considers assisted suicide illegal. Common law against assisted suicide means there is a precedent of customs, usage, and court decisions that support prosecution of an individual assisting in a suicide. Kevorkian was acquitted.

He continued to draw media attention with increasingly controversial actions. In February 1998, 21-year-old Roosevelt Dawson, a paralyzed university student, became the youngest person to commit suicide with Kevorkian's help. In June 1998 Kevorkian announced that he was donating kidneys from Joseph Tushkowski, a quadriplegic whose death he had assisted. His actions were denounced by transplant program leaders, medical ethicists, and most of the public. The organs were refused by all medical centers and transplant teams.

In October 1998 Kevorkian euthanized 52-year-old Thomas Youk, a man afflicted with ALS, at the patient's request. Kevorkian videotaped the death and gave the video to the CBS television show *60 Minutes* for broadcast. The death was televised nationwide in November 1998 during primetime and included an interview with Kevorkian. He taunted Oakland County, Michigan, prosecutors to file charges against him. They did, and Kevorkian was convicted of second-degree murder in March 1999. In April 1999 the 70-year-old retired pathologist was sentenced to 10 to 25 years in prison. While in prison, Kevorkian staged three hunger strikes and was subjected to force-feeding by prison officials. Kevorkian was released from prison in June 2007 due to good behavior.

In March 2008 Kevorkian announced plans to run for Congress as an independent in Michigan's ninth congressional district. Espousing a platform of freedoms based on the Ninth Amendment, Kevorkian held that the amendment meant that the government had no right to ban actions such as smoking, abortion, homosexual marriage, or assisted suicide. (The Ninth Amendment is part of the U.S. Constitution's Bill of Rights and addresses rights that are not specifically enumerated elsewhere in the Constitution.) Ken Thomas reports in "Democrat Defeats GOP Rep. Knollenberg" (Associated Press, November 5, 2008) that during the November 2008 election Kevorkian garnered only 2.6% of the vote in his Oakland County congressional district, losing to Democrat Gary Peters.

During the last two years of his life, Kevorkian lectured, was on television, and had a movie made about him titled *You Don't Know Jack* (2010). He walked the red carpet with Al Pacino (1940–), who played him and won an Emmy for his portrayal. In May 2011 Kevorkian was hospitalized with kidney problems and pneumonia. His situation worsened, and he died in June 2011.

ASSISTED SUICIDE'S DETRACTORS

In general, physician-assisted suicide is seen as being at odds with the work of doctors and nurses. In 2012 the American College of Physicians again officially opposed physician-assisted suicide, reaffirming its opposition from 2001 and 2005. The organization's formal position statement on this topic was published within the sixth edition of *Ethics Manual* (2012, http://www.acponline.org/running _practice/ethics/manual/). The statement reads:

> The College does not support legalization of physician-assisted suicide or euthanasia. After much consideration, the College concluded that making physician-assisted suicide legal raised serious ethical, clinical, and social concerns and that the practice might undermine patient trust; distract from reform in end-of-life care; and be used in vulnerable patients, including those who are poor, are disabled, or are unable to speak for themselves or minority groups who have experienced discrimination. The major emphasis of the College and its members, including those who lawfully participate in the practice, should be ensuring that all persons can count on good care through to the end of life, with prevention or relief of suffering insofar as possible, an unwavering commitment to human dignity and relief of pain and other symptoms, and support for family and friends. Physicians and patients must continue to search together for answers to the problems posed by the difficulties of living with serious illness before death, neither violating the physician's personal and professional values, nor abandoning the patient to struggle alone.

In 1994 the American Nurses Association's (ANA; 2012, http://www.nursingworld.org/MainMenuCategories/ Policy-Advocacy/Positions-and-Resolutions/ANAPosition Statements/Position-Statements-Alphabetically/prtetsuic

14456.html) position statements on assisted suicide and active euthanasia were adopted by its board of directors. According to the ANA, "the nurse should not participate in assisted suicide. Such an act is in violation of the Code for Nurses with Interpretive Statements (Code for Nurses) and the ethical traditions of the profession. Nurses, individually and collectively, have an obligation to provide comprehensive and compassionate end-of-life care which includes the promotion of comfort and the relief of pain, and at times, foregoing life-sustaining treatments." Concerning active euthanasia, the ANA indicates its stance in a similarly worded statement.

The American Medical Association (AMA) updated its position statement on physician-assisted suicide in 1996. Its position statement is incorporated into the AMA's *Code of Medical Ethics: Principles, Opinions, and Reports* (2012, http://www.ama-assn.org/ama/pub/physician-resources/ medical-ethics/code-medical-ethics/opinion2211.page?). The AMA states that "allowing physicians to participate in assisted suicide would cause more harm than good. Physician-assisted suicide is fundamentally incompatible with the physician's role as healer, would be difficult or impossible to control, and would pose serious societal risks."

THE BATTLE OVER LEGALIZING PHYSICIAN-ASSISTED SUICIDE

As of April 2012, Oregon, Washington, and Montana were the only states that allowed physician-assisted suicide and then only in limited circumstances. Oregon was the first state to allow the practice by passing the Oregon Death with Dignity Act in November 1994. The law took effect in 1998. In November 2008 Washington voters passed the Washington Death with Dignity Act and the law went into effect the following year, and in December 2009 the Montana Supreme Court ruled that state law protects the right of terminally ill patients to choose physician-assisted suicide.

The Oregon Death with Dignity Act

In November 1994 Oregon voters approved Measure 16 by a vote of 51% to 49%, making Oregon the first state in the nation to legalize physician-assisted suicide. Under the Oregon Death with Dignity Act (DWDA), a mentally competent adult resident of Oregon who is terminally ill (likely to die within six months) may request a prescription for a lethal dose of medication to end his or her life. At least two physicians must concur on the terminal diagnosis, and the patient must request the medication in writing, witnessed by two individuals who are not related to or caregivers of the patient. Furthermore, the patient must take the medication him- or herself.

Between 1994 and 1997 the DWDA was kept on hold due to legal challenges. In November 1997 Oregonians voted to defeat a measure to repeal the 1994 law. Immediately after this voter reaffirmation of the DWDA, the U.S. Drug Enforcement Administration (DEA) warned Oregon doctors that they could be arrested or have their medical licenses revoked for prescribing lethal doses of drugs. The DEA administrator Thomas A. Constantine (1938–), who was under pressure from some members of Congress, stated that prescribing a drug for suicide would be a violation of the Controlled Substances Act (CSA) of 1970 because assisted suicide was not a "legitimate medical purpose." Janet Reno (1938–), the U.S. attorney general, overruled Constantine in 1998 and decided that that portion of the CSA would not apply to states that legalize assisted suicide. Those opposed to the practice observed that Reno's ruling was inconsistent with other rulings, citing the government's opposite ruling in states that have legalized marijuana for medical use. (Reno maintained that the prescription of marijuana was still illegal, regardless of its medicinal value.)

In response to the DEA decision, Congress moved toward the passage of the Pain Relief Promotion Act. This law would promote the use of federally controlled drugs for the purpose of palliative care but would prevent their use for euthanasia and assisted suicide. In 2000 the U.S. House of Representatives passed the bill, but the U.S. Senate did not. The act never became law.

On November 6, 2001, John D. Ashcroft (1942–), who succeeded Reno as the U.S. attorney general, over-turned Reno's 1998 ruling that prohibited the DEA from acting against physicians who administer drugs under the DWDA. Ashcroft said that taking the life of terminally ill patients was not a "legitimate medical purpose" for federally controlled drugs. The Oregon Medical Association and the Washington State Medical Association opposed Ashcroft's ruling. Even physicians who were opposed to assisted suicide expressed concern that the ruling might compromise patient care and that any DEA investigation might discourage physicians from prescribing pain medication to patients in need.

The state of Oregon disagreed so vehemently with Ashcroft's interpretation of the CSA that on November 7, 2001, the attorney general of Oregon filed suit, claiming that Ashcroft was acting unconstitutionally. A November 8, 2001, restraining order allowed the DWDA to remain in effect while the case was tried.

On April 17, 2002, in *State of Oregon and Peter A. Rasmussen et al. v. John Ashcroft* (Civil No. 01-1647-JO), Judge Robert E. Jones (1927–) of the U.S. District Court for the District of Oregon ruled in favor of the DWDA. His decision read, in part:

> State statutes, state medical boards, and state regulations control the practice of medicine. The CSA was never intended, and the [U.S. Department of Justice] and DEA were never authorized, to establish a national medical practice or act as a national medical board. To

allow an attorney general—an appointed executive whose tenure depends entirely on whatever administration occupies the White House—to determine the legitimacy of a particular medical practice without a specific congressional grant of such authority would be unprecedented and extraordinary.... Without doubt there is tremendous disagreement among highly respected medical practitioners as to whether assisted suicide or hastened death is a legitimate medical practice, but opponents have been heard and, absent a specific prohibitive federal statute, the Oregon voters have made the legal, albeit controversial, decision that such a practice is legitimate in this sovereign state.

The U.S. Department of Justice appealed the ruling to the U.S. Court of Appeals for the Ninth Circuit in San Francisco. On May 26, 2004, the court stopped Ash-croft's attempts to override the Oregon law. The divided three-judge panel ruled that Ashcroft overstepped his authority when he declared that physicians who prescribe lethal drug doses are in violation of the CSA and when he instructed the DEA to prosecute the physicians. In addition, the court noted that Ashcroft's interpretation of the CSA violated Congress's intent.

The administration of George W. Bush (1946–) appealed the case to the U.S. Supreme Court, and in February 2005 the High Court agreed to hear the DWDA challenge. On January 17, 2006, the court ruled in the favor of Oregon in *Gonzales v. Oregon* (546 U.S. 243), holding that the CSA "does not allow the Attorney General to prohibit doctors from prescribing regulated drugs for use in physician-assisted suicide under state law permitting the procedure." Justice Anthony M. Kennedy (1936–), writing for the majority, stated that the U.S. attorney general did not have the power to override the Oregon physician-assisted suicide law. Kennedy also added that it should not be the attorney general who determines what is a "legitimate medical purpose" for the administration of drugs, because the job description for the attorney general does not include making health and medical policy.

ANALYSIS OF THE EFFECTS OF THE DWDA. In March 1998 an Oregon woman in her mid-80s who had terminal breast cancer ended her life with a lethal dose of barbiturates. Hers was the first known death under the DWDA. According to the Oregon Department of Human Services, in *Death with Dignity Act 2011 Annual Report* (February 29, 2012, http://public.health.oregon.gov/ProviderPartner Resources/EvaluationResearch/DeathwithDignityAct/ Documents/year14-tbl-1.pdf), between 1998 and 2010 a total of 525 people had reportedly committed suicide with a doctor's assistance under the DWDA. (See Table 6.12.) Seventy-one Oregon patients requested and received lethal medications in 2011. (See Figure 6.1.) Prescriptions for lethal medications increased every year between 1998 and 2003, leveled off between 2004 and 2006, and increased again beginning in 2007 through 2011.

FIGURE 6.1

Number of DWDA (Death with Dignity Act) prescription recipients and deaths, Oregon, 1998–2011

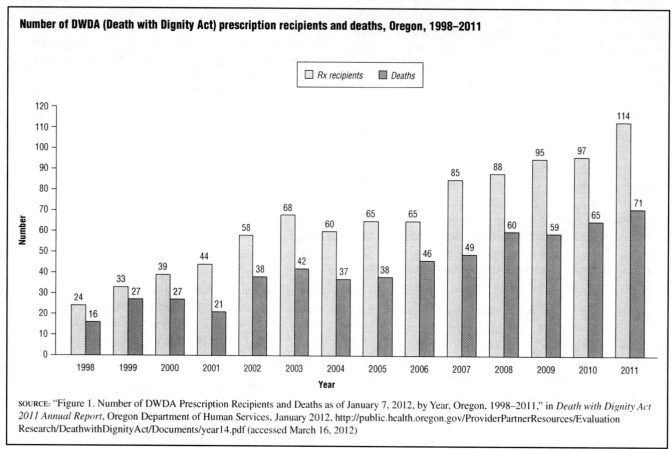

SOURCE: "Figure 1. Number of DWDA Prescription Recipients and Deaths as of January 7, 2012, by Year, Oregon, 1998–2011," in *Death with Dignity Act 2011 Annual Report*, Oregon Department of Human Services, January 2012, http://public.health.oregon.gov/ProviderPartnerResources/Evaluation Research/DeathwithDignityAct/Documents/year14.pdf (accessed March 16, 2012)

Table 6.12 shows (under the physician-suicide process) that of the patients who died under the DWDA, 94.9% between 1998 and 2010 and 94.1% in 2011 did so at home. The remainder died in long-term care or in other similar facilities. Other than a few instances in which the lethal medication was regurgitated, medical complications have been few.

The Washington Death with Dignity Act

On November 4, 2008, voters chose 58% to 42% to make Washington the second state in the nation to allow physician-assisted suicide. Like the Oregon law, the Washington Death with Dignity Act allows terminally ill patients over the age of 18 years to self-administer lethal medication that is prescribed by a physician to end their life. William Yardley notes in "First Death for Washington Assisted-Suicide Law" (*New York Times*, May 22, 2009) that Linda Fleming, a terminal patient with pancreatic cancer, became the first person in Washington to die under the new law on May 21, 2009. The Washington State Department of Health reveals in *2010 Death with Dignity Act Report* (March 2011, http://www.doh.wa.gov/dwda/forms/DWDA2010 .pdf) that 87 patients received medication and 72 died under the law in 2010. Most (78%) of the patients who died had terminal cancer, 12% had heart disease or other diseases, and 10% had neurodegenerative disease (including ALS).

Montana's Right-to-Die Ruling

In Montana it was not the voters but the Montana Supreme Court that allowed physician-assisted suicide in the state. Kirk Johnson explains in "Montana Ruling Bolsters Doctor-Assisted Suicide" (*New York Times*, December 31, 2009) that the court ruling protects physicians from prosecution in physician-assisted suicide but does not declare that physician-assisted suicide is a right allowed Montana residents. The court left this issue to be debated by the state legislature. The court case was originally initiated at the district level by Robert Baxter, a 76-year-old Montana truck driver with terminal cancer, who won the case.

In "Montana Lawmakers Punt on Physician-Assisted Suicide" (Associated Press, February 20, 2011), Matt Volz notes that Montana legislators had been asked in 2010 and 2011 to choose between banning assisted suicide or creating regulations for physicians to follow. Thus, the state of Montana was still in "legal limbo" since the court ruled in 2009. Physician-assisted suicide is legal, but there are no rules to follow and "no way to track how many people have ended their lives this way." According to Volz, it will be likely be at least 2013 before such bills are considered again. As of April 2012, the state of Montana had not decided one way or the other regarding physician-assisted suicide.

EUTHANASIA AND PHYSICIAN-ASSISTED SUICIDE AROUND THE WORLD

According to the article "The Legality of Assisted Suicide around the World" (Associated Press, June 3, 2011), euthanasia and/or physician-assisted suicide are legal in the Netherlands, Belgium, and Luxembourg. Recently, Switzerland's Supreme Court ruled that "deciding on one's own death is a human right, regardless of whether a person is terminally ill." In Germany, assisted suicide is legal but cannot involve a physician. The article states that in 1997 Colombia's Supreme Court "ruled that penalties for mercy killing should be removed. However, the ruling does not go into effect until guidelines are approved by the Colombian Congress, which has never happened." Euthanasia and physician-assisted suicide are not legal elsewhere in the world.

The Netherlands

Euthanasia became legal in the Netherlands on April 10, 2001. Before that date, active euthanasia was a criminal offense under article 293 of the Dutch Penal Code, which read, "He who takes the life of another person on this person's explicit and serious request will be punished with imprisonment of up to twelve years or a fine of the fifth category." At the same time, however, section 40 of the same penal code stated that an individual was not punishable if he or she was driven by "an irresistible force" (legally known as force majeure) to put another person's welfare above the law. This might include a circumstance in which a physician is confronted with the conflict between the legal duty of not taking a life and the humane duty to end a patient's intolerable suffering.

ORIGIN OF OPEN PRACTICE. In 1971 Geertruida Postma granted an elderly nursing home patient's request to die by injecting the patient with morphine and ending her life. The patient was her 78-year-old mother, who was partially paralyzed and was tied to a chair to keep her from falling. Postma was found guilty of murder, but her penalty consisted of a one-week suspended jail sentence and one-year probation. This light sentence encouraged other physicians to come forward, admitting that they had also assisted in patients' suicides.

Two years later the Royal Dutch Medical Association announced that, should a physician assist in the death of a terminally ill patient, it was up to the court to decide if the physician's action could be justified by "a conflict of duties." In Alkmaar, Netherlands, Piet Schoonheim helped 95-year-old Marie Barendregt to die in 1982 by using a lethal injection. Barendregt, who was severely disabled, had initially signed an advance directive refusing artificial (life-prolonging) treatment. Schoonheim assisted in Barendregt's death with the knowledge of the patient's son and after consultation with two independent physicians. In 1984 the Dutch Supreme Court, ruling on this well-known Alkmaar case (in the Netherlands the court case is referred to by the name of the city where the trial takes place), found Schoonheim not guilty of murder.

Thereafter, and until euthanasia was legalized, each euthanasia case brought under prosecution was judged on its individual circumstances. The force majeure defense ensured acquittal, and compliance with certain guidelines for performing euthanasia laid down by the Royal Dutch Medical Association and the Dutch courts in 1984 protected physicians from prosecution.

On April 10, 2001, the Dutch Parliament voted 46–28 to legalize physician-assisted suicide by passing the Termination of Life on Request and Assisted Suicide (Review Procedures) Act. Arguments in favor of the bill included public approval ratings of 90%. In May 2001 the results of a Dutch public opinion poll revealed that nearly half of respondents favored making lethal drugs available to older adults who no longer wanted to live.

Euthanasia in Belgium

The Belgian Act on Euthanasia passed in 2002 after the Dutch law, making Belgium the second country to legalize euthanasia. The law applies to competent adults who have an incurable illness causing unbearable, constant suffering and to patients in a persistent vegetative state who made their wishes known within the previous five years in front of two witnesses. It allows someone to terminate the life of another at his or her "voluntary, well-considered, and repeated" request, but does not allow physician-assisted suicide. All acts of euthanasia must be reported.

Euthanasia in Luxembourg

In February 2008 the Parliament of the Grand Duchy of Luxembourg passed a bill that decriminalized euthanasia. However, Henri Guillaume (1955–), the grand duke of Luxembourg, refused to sign the bill into law. In 2009 his power was curtailed by the parliament, and his signature is no longer required for bills to become law. In April of that year the bill that decriminalized euthanasia officially went into force, making Luxembourg the third country to legalize euthanasia.

Switzerland and Germany Allow Assisted Suicide but Not Euthanasia

Euthanasia is not a legal medical treatment in Switzerland as it is in the Netherlands, Belgium, and Luxembourg, but the country does not punish suicide that is assisted by physicians or people with no medical training if they conduct the act for altruistic reasons. Assisted suicide is a crime if it is motivated by financial gain or by selfish or negative reasons. In Germany, the law on assisted suicide is murky, but the practice is legal.

Assisted suicide is not considered to be an appropriate part of medical practice in both Switzerland and Germany, so physicians generally do not assist in suicides of the terminally ill in Switzerland and cannot assist in Germany. Members of EXIT (the Swiss Society for Humane Dying) are allowed to help the terminally ill commit suicide in their home. In January 2006 the Vaud University Hospital Center in Lausanne began allowing EXIT to help patients already admitted to the hospital and who can no longer go home to take their own life. Many Germans travel to Switzerland to seek help in dying.

CHAPTER 7
ADVANCE DIRECTIVES

The movement toward greater patient participation in health care that began during the 1960s and 1970s focused increasing attention on patients' desire for control over nearly all aspects of medical care, including critical care. Dramatic medical and technological advances further underscored the importance of planning ahead for end-of-life care. Baby boomers (people born between 1946 and 1964), who were on the threshold of aging and faced with caring for elderly parents, became increasingly aware of the need to make provisions for their own future medical treatment. Advance directives filled this need.

ADVANCE DIRECTIVES
What Are Advance Directives?

Advance directives are legal documents that help protect patients' rights of self-determination (the right to make one's own medical decisions, including the right to accept or refuse treatment). These documents are a person's requests concerning health care, should he or she be unable to do so when the need arises due to physical or mental disabilities. There are two main documents in an advance directive: a living will and a durable power of attorney for health care.

A living will is a legal document that states a person's wishes for dealing with life-sustaining medical procedures in case he or she is debilitated and cannot speak for him- or herself. A living will is different from a last will and testament. A last will and testament deals with property and comes into effect after a person is dead. A living will deals with health and personal care and is in effect when a person is alive. A durable power of attorney, the other part of an advance directive, is a legal document in which one person gives another (called the agent or proxy) legal authority to act or speak on his or her behalf should he or she become debilitated and not able to make decisions on his or her own.

A Brief History of Advance Directives

In 1967 the Euthanasia Society of America and the attorney Luis Kutner (1908–1993), the cofounder of Amnesty International, devised the first living will. California was the first state to recognize the legality of living wills (1976) and the durable powers of attorney for health care (1984). The California Natural Death Act of 1976 states that to preserve "dignity and privacy...any adult person may execute a directive directing the withholding or withdrawal of life-sustaining procedures in a terminal condition." As of December 2009, all 50 states and the District of Columbia had laws recognizing the use of living wills and the durable powers of attorney for health care, although the provisions of these laws varied from state to state. (See Table 7.1.)

Charles P. Sabatino of the American Bar Association conducted an extensive literature review of health care advance planning and published his findings in "The Evolution of Health Care Advance Planning Law and Policy" (*Milbank Quarterly*, vol. 88, no. 2, June 2010). He indicates that in the 30 years since advance health care planning has been available, laws from various states evolved in a heterogeneous manner but with important points of convergence. Sabatino notes that one convergent point is the movement from a "legal transactional approach" to a "communications approach." The latter is evolving into Physician Orders for Life-Sustaining Treatment (POLST), and the communications approach and its evolution toward POLST help translate patients' wishes and desires in end-of-life care into "visible and portable medical orders."

LIVING WILLS

As mentioned previously, a living will is one part of an advance directive. It is a document that outlines a patient's preferences about end-of-life medical treatments in the event that he or she is unable to communicate or make his or her own decisions. The laws that regulate living wills vary from state to state, and they change often. In "State

TABLE 7.1

Health care power of attorney and combined advance directive legislation, December 2009

State	Type	Provides form	Limits on agent's powers	Prohibited agents	Formalities of execution	Prohibited witnesses Note: "Provider" includes employees of provider	Registry for advance directives	Out-of-state directives recognized	POLST protocol state wide
1. Alabama Ala. Stat. §22-8A-2 to -14 (West 2007). "Natural Death Act" *See also Durable Power of Attorney Act, §26-1-2* *Separate Living Will Statute: No*	Combined advance directive *[Modeled on UHCDA]*	Yes Must be substantially followed	• Mental health facility admission and treatments • Psycho-surgery • Sterilization • Abortion • Pregnancy limitation • Nutrition & hydration—refusal permitted if expressly authorized	• Individual provider* *Exception for relatives employed by the provider	• 2 or more witnesses age 19 or older	• Minor = 18 • Agent • Proxy signor • Relative/spouse • Heir/beneficiary • Person responsible for care costs		Yes	
2. Alaska Alaska Stat. §13.52.010 to -.395 (West 2007) "Health Care Decisions Act" *Separate Living Will Statute: No*	Combined advance directive *[Modeled on UHCDA]* plus incorporates mental health directive	Yes Optional	• Psycho-surgery* • Sterilization* • Abortion* • Removal of bodily organs* • Temporary admission to mental health facility* • Electro-convulsive therapy* • Psychotropic mediation* • Life-sustaining procedures* • Pregnancy limitation *Consent/refusal permitted only if expressly authorized.	• Facility provider* *Exception for relatives	• 2 witness or notarized	• Agent • Facility provider One may not be: • Relative/spouse • Heir/beneficiary		Yes	
3. Arizona Ariz. Rev. Stat. Ann. §36-3201 to -3262 (West 2007)	Combined advance directive	Yes Optional	None specified	None specified	• 1 witness or notarized	• Agent • Provider If only <u>one</u> witness, person may not be: • Relative/spouse • Heir/beneficiary	Yes §§36-3291 to -3297	Yes	
4. Arkansas Ark. Code. Ann. §20-13-104 (2007) "Durable Power of Attorney for Health Care Act" *See also* Ark. Code Ann. §20-17-201 to -218 (proxy appointment in Living Will Declaration)	Special DPA	No (but proxy appointment in Living Will Declaration does have optional form)	• Life-sustaining treatment—unless the DPA incorporates a proxy authorization from the Living Will Declaration statute, §20-17-202 • Pregnancy limitation	None specified	• 2 witnesses	None specified		Yes, if part of a (living will) declaration	

TABLE 7.1

Health care power of attorney and combined advance directive legislation, December 2009 [CONTINUED]

State	Type	Provides form	Limits on agent's powers	Prohibited agents	Formalities of execution	Prohibited witnesses Note: "Provider" includes employees of provider	Registry for advance directives	Out-of-state directives recognized	POLST protocol state wide
5. California Cal. Probate Code §4600 to -4948 806 (West 2007) *Separate Living Will Statute: No*	Combined advance directive	Yes Optional	• Civil commitment • Electro-convulsive therapy • Psycho-surgery • Sterilization • Abortion	• Supervising individual provider (exception for relatives who are employees of) • Facility provider (exception for relatives who are employees of) • Conservator—unless conditions are met	• 2 witnesses or notarized • Special institutional requirements	• Agent • Individual provider • Facility provider One may not be: • Relative/spouse • Heir/beneficiary	Yes §§4800-4802	Yes	Yes Cal. Probate Code §§4780-4785 (8/4/08) "Physician Order for Life-Sustaining Treatment"
6. Colorado Colo. Rev. Stat §15-14-503 to -509 (West 2007). "Colorado Patient Autonomy Act" See also §15-14-501 to -502 and §15-14-601 to -611 re DPA *Separate Living Will Statute:* Colo. Rev. Stat. §15-18-101 to -113	Special DPA	No	None specified	None specified	None specified	N/A		Yes	
7. Connecticut Conn. Gen. Stat. §19a-570 to -580d (West 2007) See also Conn. Gen. Stat. §1-43 et seq. (2007) (statutory short form DPA) and §1-56r (Designation of person for decision-making) *Separate Living Will Statute: No*	Combined advance directive	Yes Optional	None specified (but authority is described as authority to "convey" principal's wishes, rather than to make decisions for principal.) • Pregnancy limitation	• Facility provider* • Attending physician • Administrator or employee of government agency financially responsible for care* *Exception for relatives	• 2 witnesses • Special institutional requirements	• Agent		Not addressed	
8. Delaware Del. Code Ann. tit. 16, §2501 to 2518 (2007) *Separate Living Will Statute: No*	Combined advance directive [Modeled on UHCDA]	Yes Optional	• Pregnancy limitation	• Residential LTC Facility provider* *Exception for relatives	• 2 witnesses • Special institutional requirements	• Facility provider • Relative/spouse • Heir/beneficiary • Creditor • Person responsible for care costs		Yes	
9. District of Columbia D.C. Code Ann. §21-2201 to -2213 (2007) *Separate Living Will Statute:* D.C. Code Ann. §7-621 to -630 (2007)	Special DPA	Yes Optional	• Decision to medicate defendant to render him/her competent to stand trial	• Individual provider • Facility provider	• 2 witnesses	• Principal • Individual Provider • Facility provider • One may not be Relative/spouse or Heir/beneficiary		Not addressed	

TABLE 7.1

Health care power of attorney and combined advance directive legislation, December 2009 [CONTINUED]

State	Type	Provides form	Limits on agent's powers	Prohibited agents	Formalities of execution	Prohibited witnesses Note: "Provider" includes employees of provider	Registry for advance directives	Out-of-state directives recognized	POLST protocol state wide
10. Florida Fla. Stat. Ann. §765.101 to -.404 (West 2007) *Separate Living Will Statute: No*	Combined advance directive	Yes Optional	• Mental health facility admission* • Electro-convulsive therapy* • Psycho-surgery* • Sterilization* • Abortion* • Experimental treatments not approved by IRB* • Life-sustaining procedures while pregnant* • Pregnancy limitation* *Consent/refusal permissible if expressly authorized	None specified	• 2 witnesses	• Agent • <u>One</u> may not be relative/spouse		Yes	
11. Georgia Ga. Code Ann. §§31-36-1 to -13 (West 2008) *Separate LW Statute: No*	Combined advance directive	Yes Optional	• Mental health facility admission or treatment (incl. mental retardation or addiction) • Psycho-surgery • Sterilization • Pregnancy limitation	• Individual provider directly or indirectly involved	• 2 witnesses • Special institutional requirements	• Agent • Heir/beneficiary • Individual provider <u>One</u> may not be • Institutional provider		Yes	
12. Hawaii Hawaii Rev. Stat. §327E-1 to -16 (2007) *See also Hawaii Rev. Stat. §551D-2.5 re DPA for health care* *Separate LW Statute: No*	Combined advance directive *[Modeled on UHCDA]*	Yes Optional	None specified	• Facility provider* *Exception for relatives	• 2 witnesses <u>or</u> notarized	• Individual provider • Facility provider • Agent <u>One</u> may not be • Relative/spouse • Heir/beneficiary		Yes	
13. Idaho Idaho Code §39-4501 to -4509 (West 2007), specifically §39-4505. *Separate LW Statute: No*	Combined advance directive	Yes Optional	• Pregnancy limitation	• Individual provider* • Community care facility provider* *Exception for relatives who are employees of	• 2 witnesses <u>or</u> notarized	• Agent • Individual provider • Community care facility • <u>One</u> may not be relative/ spouse or heir/ beneficiary	Yes §39-4515	Not addressed	Yes
14. Illinois 755 ILCS 45/4-1 through 4-12 (West 2007) *Separate LW Statute: 755 ILCS 35/1 to 35/10*	Special DPA	Yes Optional	None specified	• Individual provider	None specified	None specified		Yes	
15. Indiana Ind. Code §§30-5-1-1 to 30-5-5-19 (West 2007), specifically §30-5-5-16 and -17, AND Ind. Code §§16-36-1-1 thru -19, specifically §§16-36-1-6 and -7 *Separate LW Statute: Ind. Code Ann. §16-36-4-1 to -21*	General DPA with health powers.	No, but mandatory language for authority re life-sustaining treatment (§30-5-5-17)	None specified	None specified	• Notarized <u>or</u> one witness	• Agent		Yes	

TABLE 7.1

Health care power of attorney and combined advance directive legislation, December 2009 [CONTINUED]

State	Type	Provides form	Limits on agent's powers	Prohibited agents	Formalities of execution	Prohibited witnesses Note: "Provider" includes employees of provider	Registry for advance directives	Out-of-state directives recognized	POLST protocol state wide
Ind. Code Ann. §16-36-1-1 to -14 (West 2007)	Health Care Consent Statute including appointment of health-care representative	No, but mandatory language above is incorporated by reference at §16-36-1-14	None specified	None specified	• 1 witness	• Agent		Not addressed	
16. Iowa Iowa Code Ann. §144B.1 to .12 (West 2007) *Separate LW Statute:* Iowa Code Ann. §144A.1 to .12	Special DPA	Yes Optional	None specified	• Individual provider* *Exception for relatives	• 2 witnesses or notarized	• Agent • Individual provider One may not be relative/spouse		Yes	
17. Kansas Kan. Stat. Ann. §58-625 to -632 (2003) *Separate LW Statute:* Kan. Stat. Ann. §65-28,101 to 28,109	Special DPA	Yes Must be substantially followed	• Cannot revoke previous living will	• Individual provider* • Facility provider* *Exception for relatives & religious community members	• 2 witnesses or notarized	• Agent • Relative/spouse • Heir/beneficiary • Person responsible for care costs		Yes	
18. Kentucky Ky. Rev. Stat. §311.621 to .643 (Baldwin 2007) *Separate LW Statute: No*	Combined advanced directive (but called "Living Will Directive")	Yes Must be substantially followed	• Nutrition & hydration* • Pregnancy limitation *Refusal permissible if specified conditions are met	• Facility provider* *Exception for relatives	• 2 witnesses or notarized	• Relative/spouse • Facility provider • Attending physician • Heir/beneficiary • Person responsible for care costs		Not addressed	
19. Louisiana La. Rev. Stat. Ann 40: 1299.58.1 to .10 (West 2007) See also DPA ("Procuration") statute: La. Civ. Code Ann. Art 2985 to 3034 (West 2007), specifically art. 2997 *Separate LW Statute: No*	Proxy contained in Living Will statute	Yes Optional	• Powers implicitly limited to executing a living will declaration on behalf of principal However, a DPA (a "procuration") may confer health decision powers generally on an agent (a "mandatary")	None specified	• 2 witnesses	• Relative/spouse • Heir/beneficiary	Yes §1299.58.3D	Yes	
20. Maine Me. Rev. Stat. Ann. tit. 18A, §5-801 to §5-817 (West 2007) *Separate LW Statute: No*	Combined advance directive *[Modeled on UHCDA]*	Yes Optional	• Mental health facility admission, consent permissible if expressly authorized	• LTC facility provider* *Exception for relatives	• 2 witnesses	None specified		Yes	
21. Maryland Md. Code Ann. [Health-Gen.] §5-601 to -618 (2007) *Separate LW Statute: No*	Combined advance directive	Yes Optional	None specified	• Facility provider* *Exception for relatives	• 2 witnesses • Also recognizes oral directive to a physician with one witness	• Agent • One must not be: heir, or have any other financial interest in person's death	Yes §§5-619 to -626	Yes	Yes* §5-608.1 *Not technically POLST, but similar: "Instructions on Current Life-Sustaining Treatment Options"

TABLE 7.1

Health care power of attorney and combined advance directive legislation, December 2009 [CONTINUED]

State	Type	Provides form	Limits on agent's powers	Prohibited agents	Formalities of execution	Prohibited witnesses Note: "Provider" includes employees of provider	Registry for advance directives	Out-of-state directives recognized	POLST protocol state wide
22. Massachusetts Mass. Gen. Laws Ann. Ch. 201D (West 2007) *Separate LW Statute: None*	Special DPA	No	None specified	•Facility provider* *Exception for relatives	•2 witnesses	•Agent		Yes	
23. Michigan Mich. Comp. Laws Ann. §700.5506 to 5512 (West 2007) *Separate LW Statute: None*	Special DPA	Only for agent's acceptance	•Pregnancy limitation •Life-sustaining procedures* *Refusal permissible if expressly authorized	None specified	•2 witnesses Agent must accept in writing before acting as agent ("patient advocate")	•Agent •Relative/spouse •Heir/beneficiary •Individual provider •Facility provider •Employee of life/health insurance provider for patient		Not addressed	
24. Minnesota Minn. Stat. Ann. §145C.01 to .16 (West 2007) *Separate LW Statute: Minn. Stat. §145B.01 to .17 (West 2007)*	Combined advance directive	Yes Optional	None specified	•Individual provider* •Facility provider* *Exception for relatives	•2 witnesses or notarized	•Agent •One may not be provider		Yes	
25. Mississippi Miss. Code Ann. §41-41-201 to -229 (West 2007) *Separate LW Statute: No*	Combined advance directive [Modeled on UHCDA]	Yes Optional	•Mental health facility admission, consent permissible if expressly authorized	•LTC Facility* *Exception for relatives	•2 witnesses or notarized	•Agent •Individual provider •Facility provider •One may not be relative/spouse or heir/beneficiary		Yes, but only if directive complies with this Act	
26. Missouri Mo. Ann. Stat. §404.800 -.872 (West 2007) and cross-referenced parts of §404.700 to .735 (DPA statute) *Separate LW Statute: Mo. Ann. Stat. §459.010 to 459.055 (West 2007)*	Special DPA	No	•Nutrition & hydration* *Refusal permissible if expressly authorized	•Attending physician* •Facility provider* *Exception for relatives and members of same religious community	•Must contain language of durability and be acknowledged as conveyance of real estate (i.e., must be notarized)	None specified		Yes	
27. Montana Mont. Code Ann. §50-9-101 to -206 (2007). Also incorporates by reference §72-5-501 and -502 (DPA statute) *Separate LW Statute: No*	Proxy contained in Living Will statute	Yes Optional	•Pregnancy limitation	None specified	•2 witnesses under LW statute •DPA statute: none, although customarily notarized	None specified	Yes §§50-9-501 to 505	Yes	
28. Nebraska Neb. Rev. Stat. §30-3401 to -3432 (2007) *Separate LW Statute: Neb. Rev. Stat. §20-401 to -416 (2007)*	Special DPA	Yes Optional	•Life-sustaining procedures* •Nutrition & hydration* •Pregnancy limitation *Refusal permissible if expressly authorized	•Attending physician* •Facility* •Any agent serving 10 or more principals* *Exception for relatives who are employees of	•2 witnesses or notarized	•Agent •Relative/spouse •Heir/beneficiary •Attending physician •Insurer One may not be facility provider		Yes	

TABLE 7.1

Health care power of attorney and combined advance directive legislation, December 2009 [CONTINUED]

State	Type	Provides form	Limits on agent's powers	Prohibited agents	Formalities of execution	Prohibited witnesses Note: "Provider" includes employees of provider	Registry for advance directives	Out-of-state directives recognized	POLST protocol state wide
29. Nevada Nev. Rev. Stat. §449.800 to .860 (2007) *Separate LW Statute:* Nev. Rev. Stat. 449.535 to 690 (2007) with proxy designation. NB. LW statute recognizes an agent under a regular DPA with authority to w/h or w/d life-sustaining treatment.	Special DPA	Yes Form with disclosure statement must be substantially followed	• Mental health facility admission • Electro-convulsive therapy • Aversive intervention • Psycho-surgery • Sterilization • Abortion	• Individual provider* • Facility provider* *Exception for relatives	• 2 witnesses *or* notarized	• Agent • Individual provider • Facility provider • <u>One</u> may not be relative/spouse or heir/beneficiary	Yes §449.915 to -.965	Not addressed	
30. New Hampshire N.H. Rev. Stat. Ann. §137-J:1 to -J:16 (2007) *LW Statute: Repealed*	Combined advanced directive	Form and disclosure statement must be substantially followed	• Mental health facility admission • Sterilization • Pregnancy limitation • Nutrition & hydration* *Refusal permissible if expressly authorized	• Facility provider* *Exception for relatives who are employees of	• 2 witnesses *or* notarized • Principal must acknowledge receipt of mandatory notice	• Agent • Spouse • Heir/beneficiary • AH Physician • <u>One</u> may not be residential care provider		Yes	
31. New Jersey N.J. Stat. Ann. §26:2H-53 to -81 (West 2007) *Separate LW Statute: No*	Combined advance directive	No	None specified	• Attending physician • Facility provider* *Exception for relatives	• 2 witnesses *or* notarized	• Agent			
32. New Mexico N.M. Stat. Ann. §24-7A-1 to -18 (West 2007) *Separate LW Statute: No*	Combined advance directive *[Modeled on UHCDA]*	Yes Optional	• Mental health facility admission	• LTC facility provider* *Exception for relatives	• 2 witnesses recommended, but not required	None specified		Yes, but only if directive complies with this Act	
33. New York N.Y. Pub. Health Law §2994 (McKinney 2007) *Separate LW Statute: None*	Special DPA	Yes Optional	• Nutrition & hydration* *Principal must make his/her wishes "reasonably known"	• Attending physician* • Facility provider* • Any agent serving 10 or more principals* *Exception for relatives who are employees of	• 2 witnesses • Special institutional requirements	• Agent		Yes	Yes N.Y. Surr. Ct. Pro. §1750-b "Medical Orders for Life-Sustaining Treatment"
34. North Carolina N.C. Gen. Stat. §32A-15 to -27 (2008) *Separate LW Statute:* N.C. Gen. Stat. §§90-320 to -323 (2008)	Special DPA	Yes Optional	None specified	None specified	• 2 witnesses *and* notarized	• Relative/spouse • Heir/beneficiary • Individual provider • Facility provider • Creditor	Yes §§130A-465 to -471	Yes	Yes §90-21.17 "Medical Orders for Scope of Treatment"

TABLE 7.1

Health care power of attorney and combined advance directive legislation, December 2009 [CONTINUED]

State	Type	Provides form	Limits on agent's powers	Prohibited agents	Formalities of execution	Prohibited witnesses Note: "Provider" includes employees of provider	Registry for advance directives	Out-of-state directives recognized	POLST protocol state wide
35. North Dakota N.D. Cent. Code §23-06.5-01 to -18 (2007)	Special DPA	Yes Optional	• Mental health facility admission >45 days • Psycho-surgery • Abortion • Sterilization	• Individual provider* • Facility provider* *Exception for relatives who are employees of	• 2 witnesses or notarized • Agent must accept in writing	• Agent* • Relative/spouse* • Heir/beneficiary* • Creditor* One may not be: • Individual provider • Facility provider *Also disqualifies notary	Yes §23-06. 5-19	Yes	
36. Ohio Ohio Rev. Code §1337.11 to .17 (West 2007) *Separate LW Statute:* Ohio Rev. Code §2133.01 to .15 (West 2007)	Special DPA	Only for mandatory disclosure statement	• Life-sustaining procedures* • Nutrition & hydration* • Pregnancy limitation *Refusal permissible if specified conditions are met	• Attending physician* • Nursing home administrator* *Exception for relatives who are employees of	• 2 witnesses or notarized	• Agent • Relative/spouse • Attending physician • Nursing home administrator		Yes	
37. Oklahoma Okla. Stat. Ann. tit. 63, §3101.1 to .16 (West 2007) *Separate LW Statute: No*	Combined advance directive	Yes Must be substantially followed	• Nutrition & hydration* • Pregnancy limitation *Refusal permissible if expressly authorized	None specified	• 2 witnesses	• Heir/beneficiary	Yes §3102.1 to .3	Yes	
38. Oregon Or. Rev. Stat. §127.505 to .660 and 127.995 (2007) *Separate LW Statute: No*	Combined advance directive	Yes Must be followed (but recognizes that any other form "constitutes evidence of the patient's desires and interests")	• Mental health facility admission • Electro-convulsive therapy • Psycho-surgery • Sterilization • Abortion • Life-sustaining procedures* • Nutrition & hydration* *Refusal permissible if expressly authorized or if specified conditions are met	• Attending physician* • Facility provider* *Exception for relatives	• 2 witnesses • Agent must accept in writing • Special institutional requirements	• Agent • Att. physician • One may not be relative/spouse heir/beneficiary, or facility provider	Yes 2007 Or. Law Ch. 697 (S.B. 329) [not codified]	Yes	Yes No statute "Physician Order for Life-Sustaining Treatment"
39. Pennsylvania Pa. Stat. Ann. tit. 20, §5401 to 5416 (West 2007). *And* 20 Pa. Cons. Stat. Ann. §5601 to 5611 (DPA)	Living Will Statute Statutory Form DPA includes health decisions powers	Yes Optional	LW: Unclear whether agent is permitted to act only if principal is in a • terminal condition, or • state of permanent unconsciousness • nutrition & hydration* • pregnancy limitation *Refusal permissible if expressly authorized Statutory Form DPA defines powers specifically.	None specified	• LW: 2 witnesses • Statutory Form DPA: None required	• LW: Person who signs declaration on declarant's behalf • Statutory Form DPA: None specified		• LW: Not addressed • Statutory Form DPA: Yes	

TABLE 7.1

Health care power of attorney and combined advance directive legislation, December 2009 [CONTINUED]

State	Type	Provides form	Limits on agent's powers	Prohibited agents	Formalities of execution	Prohibited witnesses Note: "Provider" includes employees of provider	Registry for advance directives	Out-of-state directives recognized	POLST protocol state wide
40. Rhode Island R.I. Gen. Laws §23-4.10-1 to -12 (2007) *Separate LW Statute:* R.I. Gen Laws §23-4.11-1 to -15 (2007)	Special DPA	Yes Not clear whether optional or mandatory	None specified	• Individual provider* • Community care facility* *Exception for relatives who are employees of	• 2 witnesses • Principal must be Rhode Island resident	• Agent • Individual provider • Community care facility • <u>One</u> may not be relative/spouse or heir/beneficiary		Yes	
41. South Carolina S.C. Code §62-5-501 to -505 (2007), particularly §62-5-504. *Separate LW Statute:* S. C. Code §44-77-10 to -160 (also permits appointment of agent)	Special DPA (within general DPA statute)	Yes Must be substantially followed (but conventional DPAs may also contain health powers)	• Nutrition & hydration necessary for comfort care or alleviation of pain* • Pregnancy limitation *Refusal permissible if expressly authorized	• Individual provider* • Facility provider* • Spouse of a provider* *Exception for relatives	• 2 witnesses	• Agent • Relative/spouse • Heir/beneficiary • Attending physician • Creditor • Life insurance beneficiary • Person responsible for care costs • <u>One</u> may not be facility provider		Yes	
42. South Dakota S.D. Codified Laws §59-7-1 to -9 (2007) See also §34-12C-1 to -8 (Health care consent procedures) *Separate LW Statute:* S.D. Codified Laws §34-12D-1 to -22 (2007)	General DPA that permits health decisions authority	No	• Pregnancy limitation • Nutrition & hydration* *Refusal permissible if expressly authorized or other conditions are met	None specified	None specified	None specified		Yes	
43. Tennessee Tenn. Code Ann §68-11-1801 to -1815 (2007) *Separate LW Statute: No*	Combined advance directive	No	None specified	None specified	• 2 witnesses <u>or</u> notarized	• Agent • Provider • Facility • <u>One</u> may not be relative/spouse or heir/beneficiary		Yes	
44. Texas Tex. [Health & Safety] Code Ann. §166.001 to -.166 (Vernon 2007) *Separate LW Statute: No*	(1) Special DPA (2) Proxy contained in LW	(1) Special DPA: (Medical PoA): Yes. Must be substantially followed plus mandatory disclosure statement. (2) LW: Yes Optional	• Mental health facility admission • Electro-convulsive therapy • Psycho-surgery • Abortion • Comfort care	• Individual provider* • Facility provider* *Exception for relatives who are employees of	• 2 witnesses	<u>One</u> may not be: • Agent • Attending physician • Relative/spouse • Facility • Heir/beneficiary • Creditor		Yes	

TABLE 7.1

Health care power of attorney and combined advance directive legislation, December 2009 [CONTINUED]

State	Type	Provides form	Limits on agent's powers	Prohibited agents	Formalities of execution	Prohibited witnesses Note: "Provider" includes employees of provider	Registry for advance directives	Out-of-state directives recognized	POLST protocol state wide
45. Utah Utah Code Ann. §75-2A-101 to -125 (2008) New Law. Eff. 1/1/08 *Separate LW Statute: No*	Combined advance directive	No	• Pregnancy limitation • Long-term custodial placement in licensed facility other than for assessment, rehabilitative, or respite care.	• Individual provider* • Facility provider* *Exception for relatives who are employees of	• One witness	• Agent • Relative/spouse • Provider • Facility • Heir • Beneficiary under any instrument/plan/ account • Person responsible for care costs		Yes	Yes 75-2a-106 "Life with Dignity Order"
46. Vermont Vt. Stat. Ann. tit. 18, §9700 to 9720 (2009)	Combined advance directive	No	None specified (may make certain decisions over the protest of the principal if certain conditions met)	• Individual provider • Facility provider* • Funeral/crematory/ cemetery/organ procurement representative (when authorized to dispose of remains or donate organs)* *Exception for relatives who are employees of	• 2 witnesses • Special institutional requirements	• Agent • Spouse or reciprocal beneficiary • Relative	Yes §§9701, 9704, 9709, 9712, 9714, 9719	Yes	Yes 2009 Vt. Laws No. 25 (H. 435) §97-1(6)
47. Virginia Va. Code §54.1-2981 to -2993 (West 2007) *Separate LW Statute: No*	Combined advance directive	Yes Optional	• Mental health facility admission • Psycho-surgery • Sterilization • Abortion • Decisions about "visitation" unless expressly authorized (may make certain decisions over the protest of the principal if certain conditions met.)	None specified	• 2 witnesses	• Relative/spouse	Yes §54.1-2983, -2985, and -2994 to -2996	Yes	
48. Washington Wash. Rev. Code Ann. §11.94.010 to .900 (West 2007) *Separate LW Statute:* Wash. Rev. Code Ann. §70.l22.010 to -.920 (West 2007)	General DPA	No	Cross reference to guardianship law [RCWA 11.92.043(5)]: • Electro-convulsive therapy • Psycho-surgery • Other psychiatric • Amputation	• Individual provider* • Facility provider* *Exception for relatives	None specified	N/A	Yes §70.122.130	Yes	Yes Wash. Rev. Code Ann. §43.70.480 "Physician Order for Life-Sustaining Treatment"

TABLE 7.1

Health care power of attorney and combined advance directive legislation, December 2009 [CONTINUED]

State	Type	Provides form	Limits on agent's powers	Prohibited agents	Formalities of execution	Prohibited witnesses Note: "Provider" includes employees of provider	Registry for advance directives	Out-of-state directives recognized	POLST protocol state wide
49. West Virginia W. VA. Code Ann. §16-30-1 to -25 (West 2007) *Separate LW Statute: No*	Combined advance directive (but maintains separate Living Will and Medical Power of Attorney documents)	Yes Optional	• Limit on agent's authority to revoke a pre-need funeral contract	• Individual provider* • Facility provider* *Exception for relatives who are employees of	• 2 witnesses and notarized	• Agent • Att. Physician • Principal's signatory • Relative/spouse • Heir/beneficiary • Person responsible for care costs		Yes	Yes §16-30-25 and others "Physician Order for Scope of Treatment"
50. Wisconsin Wis. Stat. Ann. §155.01 to .80 (West 2007) See DPA cross reference §243.07 (6m) (West 2007) *Separate LW Statute:* Wisc. Stat. Ann. §§ l54.01 to -l5 (West 2007)	Special DPA	Yes Optional (but disclosure statement is mandatory)	• Admission to facility for mental health/retardation or other listed conditions • Electro-convulsive therapy • Mental health research • Drastic mental health treatment • Admission to nursing home or residential facility—very limited unless expressly authorized in the document • Nutrition & hydration* • Pregnancy limitation *Refusal permissible only if specified conditions are met	• Individual provider* • Facility provider* *Exception for relatives	• 2 witnesses	• Agent • Individual provider • Facility provider* • Relative/spouse • Heir/beneficiary • Person responsible for care costs *Exception for chaplains & social workers		Yes	
51. Wyoming Wyo. Stat. §35-22-401 to -416 (2004) *Separate LW Statute:* Wyo. Stat §§ 35-22-101 to -109 (2004)	Combined advance directive	Yes Optional	None specified	• Residential or community care provider* *Exception for relatives who are employees of	• 2 witnesses or notarized	• Agent • Individual provider • Facility provider		Not addressed	
Uniform Health-Care Decisions Act *Separate LW Statute: No*	Combined advance directive	Yes Optional	• Mental health facility admission, consent permissible if expressly authorized	• LTC Facility provider	• 2 witnesses recommended, but not required	None		Yes, but only if directive complies with this Act	

LW = Living Will. DPA = Durable Power of Attorney. UHCDA = Uniform Health Care Decisions Act. POLST = Physician Order for Life-sustaining Treatment, or similar protocol.
Notes: The descriptors in the chart are generalizations of statutory language and not quotations, so the statutes must be consulted for precise meaning. All states limit appointed agent's from acting over the objection of the principal, unless otherwise noted in the column under Limits on Agent's Powers.
Caution: The descriptions and limitations listed in this chart are broad characterizations for comparison purposes and not as precise quotations from legislative language.

SOURCE: "Health Care Power of Attorney and Combined Advance Directive Legislation: Selected Features Compared—December 2009," published by the American Bar Association, Commission on Law and Aging, 2009, http://www.americanbar.org/content/dam/aba/migrated/aging/PublicDocuments/hcpa_cht09.authcheckdam.pdf (accessed February 7, 2012). Copyright © 2009 by the American Bar Association. Reprinted with permission. This information or any portion thereof may not be copied or disseminated in any form or by any means or stored in an electronic database or retrieval system without the express written consent of the American Bar Association.

Living Wills Laws" (2012, http://law.findlaw.com/state-laws/living-wills/), FindLaw offers an up-to-date compendium of living will laws for each state.

Living wills enable people to list the types of medical treatments they want or do not want. It is therefore important for an individual contemplating a living will to know what these treatments involve. Some examples of life-prolonging treatments patients should consider when preparing a living will include cardiopulmonary resuscitation, mechanical ventilation, artificial nutrition and hydration, and kidney dialysis.

An advance directive form is included in the model Uniform Health-Care Decisions Act (UHCDA; February 7, 1994, http://www.law.upenn.edu/bll/archives/ulc/fnact99/1990s/uhcda93.pdf). The UHCDA consolidates various state laws that deal with all decisions about adult health care and health care powers of attorney. This model law was approved by the National Conference of Commissioners on Uniform State Laws in 1993 to provide some consistency among state advance directives and remained a model law as of April 2012. Its advance directive form offers several options that include treatments to prolong life. (See Table 7.2.) The states whose advance directives were modeled on the UHCDA are noted in Table 7.1.

Another form, called "Five Wishes," was developed in Florida by the nonprofit organization Aging with Dignity and is now distributed nationwide. The document probes legal and medical issues as well as spiritual and emotional ones. It even outlines small details, such as requests for favorite music to be played and poems to be read, and provides space for individuals to record their wishes for funeral arrangements. The document is relatively easy to complete because it uses simplified language rather than legal or medical jargon.

In February 2012 "Five Wishes" met living will or advance directive criteria in 42 states and the District of Columbia. (See Figure 7.1.) It did not meet advance directive criteria in eight states: Alabama, Indiana, Kansas, New Hampshire, Ohio, Oregon, Texas, and Utah. Other forms were necessary in these states, although the "Five Wishes" document could still serve as a guide for family and physicians and could be attached to the state's required form.

Pro-Life Alternative to Living Wills

The National Right to Life Committee opposes active and passive euthanasia (active euthanasia is the administration of lethal drugs to hasten death; passive euthanasia is the withdrawal of life-sustaining treatment with the intention of hastening death) and offers an alternative to the standard living will. Called the "Will to Live" (2012, http://www.nrlc.org/euthanasia/willtolive/index.html), it does not consider artificial nutrition and hydration as forms of medical treatment, but as basic necessities for the preservation of life.

DURABLE POWER OF ATTORNEY FOR HEALTH CARE

Even though living wills provide specific directions about medical treatment, most apply only to limited circumstances, such as terminal illness or permanent coma. Living wills cannot address every possible future medical situation. Many medical treatments, such as surgical procedures, diagnostic tests, blood transfusions, antibiotics, radiation therapy, and chemotherapy, require decision making.

A durable power of attorney for health care, also called a medical power of attorney, addresses this need. It is the other part of an advance directive and is generally more flexible than a living will. It allows individuals to appoint agents (proxies) who will use their judgment to respond to unforeseen situations based on their knowledge of the patient and the patient's values and beliefs. (See Table 7.2.) The role of this agent or proxy begins as soon as the physician certifies that a patient is incompetent to make his or her own decisions.

Because there is no uniform advance directive statute nationally, the rights of health care agents vary across states. Limits on agents' powers in each state and the District of Columbia as of December 2009 are shown in Table 7.1.

In the Absence of a Durable Power of Attorney for Health Care

Physicians usually involve family members in medical decisions when the patient has not designated a health care proxy in advance. This person is called a surrogate. Many states have surrogate consent laws for this purpose. Some have laws that designate the order in which family members may assume the role of surrogate decision maker. For example, the spouse may be the prime surrogate, followed by an adult child, then the patient's parent, and so on.

Most states specify a decision-making standard for surrogates: either a substituted judgment standard, a best interests standard, or a combination of the two. A substituted judgment standard requires the surrogate to do what the patient would do in the situation were the patient competent. A best interests standard requires the surrogate to weigh health care options for the patient and then decide what is in the patient's best interest.

ADDITIONAL INSTRUCTIONS IN ADVANCE DIRECTIVES
Artificial Nutrition and Hydration

Some living wills contain a provision for the withdrawal of artificial nutrition and hydration (ANH). (See Table 7.2.) ANH is legally considered to be a medical treatment and may, therefore, be refused. However, this form of treatment remains controversial in regards to the

TABLE 7.2

Advance health-care directive

Optional Form

The following form may, but need not, be used to create an advance health-care directive. The other sections of this [Act] govern the effect of this or any other writing used to create an advance health-care directive. An individual may complete or modify all or any part of the following form:

ADVANCE HEALTH-CARE DIRECTIVE

Explanation

You have the right to give instructions about your own health care. You also have the right to name someone else to make health-care decisions for you. This form lets you do either or both of these things. It also lets you express your wishes regarding donation of organs and the designation of your primary physician. If you use this form, you may complete or modify all or any part of it. You are free to use a different form.

Part 1 of this form is a power of attorney for health care. Part 1 lets you name another individual as agent to make health-care decisions for you if you become incapable of making your own decisions or if you want someone else to make those decisions for you now even though you are still capable. You may also name an alternate agent to act for you if your first choice is not willing, able, or reasonably available to make decisions for you. Unless related to you, your agent may not be an owner, operator, or employee of [a residential long-term health-care institution] at which you are receiving care.

Unless the form you sign limits the authority of your agent, your agent may make all health-care decisions for you. This form has a place for you to limit the authority of your agent. You need not limit the authority of your agent if you wish to rely on your agent for all health-care decisions that may have to be made. If you choose not to limit the authority of your agent, your agent will have the right to:

(a) consent or refuse consent to any care, treatment, service, or procedure to maintain, diagnose, or otherwise affect a physical or mental condition;
(b) select or discharge health-care providers and institution;
(c) approve or disapprove diagnostic tests, surgical procedures, programs of medication, and orders not to resuscitate; and
(d) direct the provision, withholding, or withdrawal of artificial nutrition and hydration and all other forms of health care.

Part 2 of this form lets you give specific instructions about any aspect of your health care. Choices are provided for you to express your wishes regarding the provision, withholding, or withdrawal of treatment to keep you alive, including the provision of artificial nutrition and hydration, as well as the provision of pain relief. Space is also provided for you to add to the choices you have made or for you to write out any additional wishes.

Part 3 of this form lets you express an intention to donate your bodily organs and tissues following your death.

Part 4 of this form lets you designate a physician to have primary responsibility for your health care.

After completing this form, sign and date the form at the end. It is recommended but not required that you request two other individuals to sign as witnesses. Give a copy of the signed and completed form to your physician, to any other health-care providers you may have, to any health-care institution at which you are receiving care, and to any health-care agents you have named. You should talk to the person you have named as agent to make sure that he or she understands your wishes and is willing to take the responsibility.

You have the right to revoke this advance health-care directive or replace this form at any time.

* * * * * * * * *

PART 1
POWER OF ATTORNEY FOR HEALTH CARE

1. DESIGNATION OF AGENT: I designate the following individual as my agent to make health-care decisions for me:

_____
(name of individual you choose as agent)

_____
(address)   (city)   (state)   (zip code)

_____
(home phone)   (work phone)

OPTIONAL: If I revoke my agent's authority or if my agent is not willing, able, or reasonably available to make a health-care decision for me, I designate as my first alternate agent:

_____
(name of individual you choose as first alternate agent)

_____
(address)   (city)   (state)   (zip code)

_____
(home phone)   (work phone)

OPTIONAL: If I revoke the authority of my agent and first alternate agent or if neither is willing, able, or reasonably available to make a health-care decision for me, I designate as my second alternate agent:

_____
(name of individual you choose as first alternate agent)

_____
(address)   (city)   (state)   (zip code)

_____
(home phone)   (work phone)

(Add additional sheets if needed.)

right-to-die issue because food and liquid are the most basic forms of life sustenance, yet they are not usually needed by dying people and may even make them less comfortable.

The unresolved problem is mirrored by the fact that not all states' advance directive statutes (laws) address this issue, and the ones that do show no consensus.

TABLE 7.2

Advance health-care directive [CONTINUED]

2. AGENT'S AUTHORITY: My agent is authorized to make all health-care decisions for me, including decisions to provide, withhold, or withdraw artificial nutrition and hydration and other forms of health care to keep me alive, except as I state here:

_____

_____

_____

3. WHEN AGENT'S AUTHORITY BECOMES EFFECTIVE: My agent's authority becomes effective when my primary physician determines that I am unable to make my own health-care decisions unless I mark the following box. If I mark this box [ ], my agent's authority to make health-care decisions for me takes effect immediately.

4. AGENT'S OBLIGATION: My agent shall make health-care decisions for me in accordance with this power of attorney for health care, any instructions I give in Part 2 of this form, and my other wishes to the extent known to my agent. To the extent my wishes are unknown, my agent shall make health-care decisions for me in accordance with what my agent determines to be in my best interest. In determining my best interest, my agent shall consider my personal values to the extent known to my agent.

NOMINATION OF GUARDIAN: If a guardian of my person needs to be appointed for me by a court, I nominate the agent designated in this form. If that agent is not willing, able, or reasonably available to act as guardian, I nominate the alternate agents whom I have named, in the order designated.

PART 2

INSTRUCTIONS FOR HEALTH CARE

If you are satisfied to allow your agent to determine what is best for you in making end-of-life decisions, you need not fill out this part of the form. If you do fill out this part of the form, you may strike any wording you do not want.

6. END-OF-LIFE DECISIONS: I direct that my health-care providers and others involved in my care provide, withhold, or withdraw treatment in accordance with the choice I have marked below:

[　] (a) Choice Not To Prolong Life
   I do not want my life to be prolonged if (i) I have an incurable and irreversible condition that will result in my death within a relatively short time, (ii) I become unconscious and, to a reasonable degree of medical certainty, I will not regain consciousness, or (iii) the likely risks and burdens of treatment would outweigh the expected benefits, OR

[　] (b) Choice To Prolong Life
   I want my life to be prolonged as long as possible within the limits of generally accepted health-care standards.

7. ARTIFICIAL NUTRITION AND HYDRATION: Artificial nutrition and hydration must be provided, withheld, or withdrawn in accordance with the choice I have made in paragraph (6) unless I mark the following box. If I mark this box [　], artificial nutrition and hydration must be provided regardless of my condition and regardless of the choice I have made in paragraph (6).

8. RELIEF FROM PAIN: Except as I state in the following space, I direct that treatment for alleviation of pain or discomfort be provided at all times, even if it hastens my death:

_____

_____

_____

9. OTHER WISHES: (If you do not agree with any of the optional choices above and wish to write your own, or if you wish to add to the instructions you have given above, you may do so here.) I direct that:

_____

_____

_____

(Add additional sheets if needed.)

PART 3

DONATION OF ORGANS AT DEATH (OPTIONAL)

10. Upon my death (mark applicable box)

[　] (a) I give any needed organs, tissues, or parts, OR
[　] (b) I give the following organs, tissues, or parts only

_____

[　] (c) My gift is for the following purposes (strike any of the following you do not want)
   (i) Transplant
   (ii) Therapy
   (iii) Research
   (iv) Education

One crux of the ANH controversy is the comfort care–pain relief mandate. If ANH is seen as a procedure that comforts the dying patient or helps relieve pain, then a state may require it be given regardless of what a health care proxy or surrogate wants. A state may, however, prohibit ANH if it is expected to cause pain. Again, the

TABLE 7.2

Advance health-care directive [CONTINUED]

PART 4
PRIMARY PHYSICIAN (OPTIONAL)

11. I designate the following physician as my primary physician:

_____
(name of physician)

_____
(address)   (city)   (state)   (zip code)

_____
(phone)

OPTIONAL: If the physician I have designated above is not willing, able, or reasonably available to act as my primary physician, I designate the following physician as my primary physician:

_____
(name of physician)

_____
(address)   (city)   (state)   (zip code)

_____
(phone)

* * * * * * * * * *

EFFECT OF COPY: A copy of this form has the same effect as the original.

12. SIGNATURES: Sign and date the form here:

_____   _____
(date)   (sign your name)

_____   _____
(address)   (print name)

_____
(city)   (state)

Optional SIGNATURES OF WITNESSES:

_____   _____
(First witness)   (Second witness)

_____   _____
(print name)   (print name)

_____   _____
(address)   (address)

_____   _____
(city)   (state)   (city)   (state)

_____   _____
(signature of witness)   (signature of witness)

_____   _____
(date)   (date)

SOURCE: "Advance Health-Care Directive," in *Patient Self-Determination Act: Providers Offer Information on Advance Directives but Effectiveness Uncertain,* U.S. General Accounting Office, August 1995, http://www.gao.gov/archive/1995/he95135.pdf (accessed February 3, 2012).

proxy or surrogate would have no say. Complicating the matter even further, a state may require that ANH be deemed to have no impact on the patient's illness or to potentially harm the patient before the agent or surrogate would be allowed to forgo ANH.

Relief from Pain

Some living wills also enable an individual to give instructions about the management of pain. Even though a number of studies show that pain is not the primary motivation for assisted suicide requests, many people have seen family and friends suffer painful deaths, and they fear the same fate. Experts advise that advance directives should expressly indicate desires for pain control and comfort care, even when individuals have chosen to forgo life-sustaining treatments.

In the past, patient pain may not have been adequately treated because medical professionals lacked training or feared overprescribing pain medications. A variety of legislative and education initiatives by states and medical professional societies have dramatically improved pain management. The Federation of State

FIGURE 7.1

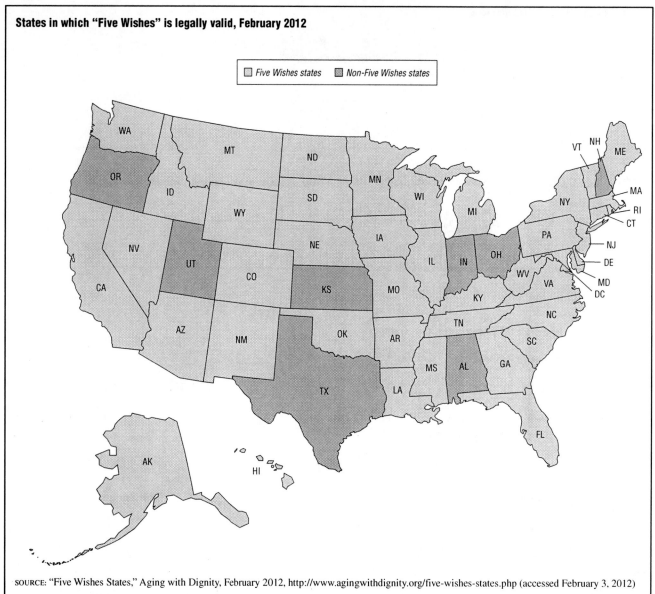

States in which "Five Wishes" is legally valid, February 2012

Five Wishes states   Non-Five Wishes states

SOURCE: "Five Wishes States," Aging with Dignity, February 2012, http://www.agingwithdignity.org/five-wishes-states.php (accessed February 3, 2012)

Medical Boards has developed guidelines to help physicians use medication to manage pain safely and effectively. Special instruction in pain management for patients with life-limiting illnesses is now offered in many medical and nursing schools.

COMBINED ADVANCE DIRECTIVE LAWS

Some states have separate laws that govern living wills and durable powers of attorney for health care. The National Conference of State Legislatures (NCSL) and the Center to Improve Care of the Dying (CICD) believe that rather than having separate laws for these two documents, states should combine right-to-die laws into a single statute. As of December 2009, 26 states had done just that. (See Table 7.1.) Of these states, Alabama, Alaska, Delaware, Hawaii, Maine, Mississippi, and New Mexico had also adopted the UHCDA as a model.

The UHCDA has been recommended by the NCSL and the CICD as a model law because it is simple and comprehensive. It contains provisions governing living wills and durable powers of attorney, as well as limits on an agent's powers. The law permits instructions regarding one's future health care to be either written or oral. States using the law as a model may adopt the optional combined directive, which does not require witnesses to the document. It further enables individuals to express their preferences about organ donation and to designate a primary physician. (See Table 7.2.)

Along with showing the type of health care power of attorney and combined advance directive legislation in each state, Table 7.1 provides other related information, including the comity provision. If a state has a comity provision, that means it has legislation specifically requiring that another state's living will, health care power of attorney, or both, be honored within its borders.

IMPORTANCE OF COMMUNICATION FOR END-OF-LIFE CARE

The consideration of an advance directive should be the start of an ongoing discussion among the individual, family members, and the family doctor about end-of-life health care. Discussions about one's advance directive do not have to be limited to treatment preferences and medical circumstances. Sometimes knowing things such as the patient's religious beliefs and values can be important for the proxy when speaking for the patient's interests. The Institute for Ethics at the University of New Mexico has devised a values history form (http://hsc.unm.edu/ethics/docs/Values_History.pdf) to help people examine their attitudes about issues related to illness, health care, and dying. It may serve as a valuable tool to guide discussions between the patient and the proxy, as well as among family members.

When preparing an advance directive, it is vitally important for the family and proxy to fully understand the care and measures that are wanted. Even when a patient has a living will calling for no "heroic measures," if the family demands such medical intervention, it is likely that the hospital or doctor will comply with the family's wishes rather than risk a lawsuit.

THE PATIENT SELF-DETERMINATION ACT

In 1990 Congress enacted the Patient Self-Determination Act (PSDA) as part of the Omnibus Budget Reconciliation Act of 1990. This legislation was intended to "reinforce individuals' constitutional right to determine their final health care."

The PSDA took effect on December 1, 1991, and was still in force as of April 2012. It requires most health care institutions to provide patients, on admission, with a summary of their health care decision-making rights and to ask them if they have an advance directive. Health care institutions must also inform the patient of their facility's policies with respect to honoring advance directives. The PSDA requires health care providers to educate their staff and the community about advance directives. It also prohibits hospital personnel from discriminating against patients based on whether they have an advance directive, and patients are informed that having an advance directive is not a prerequisite to receiving medical care.

ADVANCE DIRECTIVES AND THE COST FOR END-OF-LIFE CARE

In "Regional Variation in the Association between Advance Directives and End-of-Life Medicare Expenditures" (*Journal of the American Medical Association*, vol. 306, no. 13, October 5, 2011), Lauren Hersch Nicholas et al. seek to determine if there is a connection between advance directives and Medicare costs for end-of-life care. The researchers find that there is a variability of Medicare costs nationally in end-of-life care and that there are some regions of the country in which end-of-life care costs much more than in other regions. These are the regions in which there appears to be a connection between end-of-life care costs and advance directives.

By using a variety of statistical methods, Nicholas et al. note that "advance directives are associated with important differences in treatment during the last 6 months of life for patients who live in areas of high medical expenditures but not in other regions." The researchers also indicate, "This suggests that the clinical effect of advance directives is critically dependent on the context in which a patient receives care. Advance directives may be especially important for ensuring treatment consistent with patients' preferences for those who prefer less aggressive treatment at the end of life but are patients in systems characterized by high intensity of treatment." What Nicholas et al. mean is that Medicare payments might go down in areas of the country in which high-intensity care is given at the end of life. Many people in their advance directives indicate whether they want certain high-intensity care.

CHAPTER 8
COURTS AND THE END OF LIFE

Traditionally, death was said to have occurred when circulation and respiration stopped. However, in 1968 the Ad Hoc Committee of the Harvard Medical School defined irreversible coma, or brain death, as the new criterion for death. As medical technology has become increasingly able to maintain patients who would otherwise die from severe injuries or illnesses, the debate about defining death, and about whether patients have the right to choose to die, has intensified.

THE RIGHT TO PRIVACY: KAREN ANN QUINLAN

The landmark case of Karen Ann Quinlan was the first to deal with the dilemma of withdrawing life-sustaining treatment from a patient who was not terminally ill but who was not really "alive." The decision to terminate life support, which was once a private matter between the patient's family and doctor, became an issue to be decided by the courts. The New Jersey Supreme Court ruling on this case became the precedent for nearly all right-to-die cases nationwide.

In 1975, 21-year-old Karen Ann Quinlan suffered cardiopulmonary arrest after ingesting a combination of alcohol and drugs. She subsequently went into a persistent vegetative state (PVS). Fred Plum (1924–2010), a world-renowned neurologist who had coined the term *persistent vegetative state*, described her as no longer having any cognitive function but retaining the capacity to maintain the vegetative parts of neurological function. She grimaced, made chewing movements, uttered sounds, and maintained a normal blood pressure, but she was entirely unaware of anyone or anything. The medical opinion was that Quinlan had some brain stem function, but that it could not support breathing. She had been on a respirator since her admission to the hospital.

Quinlan's parents asked that her respirator be removed and that she be allowed to die. Quinlan's doctor refused, claiming that his patient did not meet the Harvard Criteria for brain death. Joseph Quinlan, Quinlan's father, went to court to seek appointment as his daughter's guardian (because she was of legal age) and to gain the power to authorize "the discontinuance of all extraordinary medical procedures now allegedly sustaining Karen's vital processes." The court refused to grant him guardianship over his daughter and denied his petition to have Quinlan's respirator turned off.

First and Eighth Amendments
Are Irrelevant to the Case

Joseph Quinlan subsequently appealed to the New Jersey Supreme Court. He requested, as a parent, to have Quinlan's life support removed based on the U.S. Constitution's First Amendment (the right to religious freedom). In *In re Quinlan* (70 N.J. 10, 355 A.2d 647 [1976]), the court rejected his request. It also indicated that the Eighth Amendment (protection against cruel and unusual punishment) did not apply to Quinlan's case, explaining that this amendment applied to protection from excessive criminal punishment. The court considered Quinlan's cruel and unusual circumstances not punishment inflicted by the law or state, but as the result of "an accident of fate and nature."

The Right to Privacy

However, the New Jersey Supreme Court stated that an individual's right to privacy was most relevant to the case. Even though the Constitution does not expressly indicate a right to privacy, U.S. Supreme Court rulings in past cases had not only recognized this right but had also determined that some areas of the right to privacy are guaranteed by the Constitution. The New Jersey Supreme Court ruled that "Karen's right of privacy may be asserted in her behalf, in this respect, by her guardian and family under the particular circumstances presented by this record," and further noted, "We have no doubt...that if Karen were herself miraculously lucid for an interval (not altering the existing prognosis of the condition to which she would soon return) and perceptive of her irreversible condition, she could effectively decide upon discontinuance of the life-support apparatus, even if it meant the prospect of natural death."

The State's Interest

Balanced against Quinlan's constitutional right to privacy was the state's interest in preserving life. Judge Richard J. Hughes (1909–1992) of the New Jersey Supreme Court noted that in many cases the court had ordered medical treatment continued because the minimal bodily invasion (usually blood transfusion) resulted in recovery. He indicated that in Quinlan's case bodily invasion was far greater than minimal, consisting of 24-hour nursing care, antibiotics, respirator, catheter, and feeding tube. Judge Hughes further noted, "We think that the State's interest ... weakens and the individual's right to privacy grows as the degree of bodily invasion increases and the prognosis dims. Ultimately there comes a point at which the individual's rights overcome the State's interest."

Prevailing Medical Standards and Practices

Quinlan's physicians had refused to remove the respirator because they did not want to violate the prevailing medical standards and practices. Even though Quinlan's physicians assured the court that the possibility of lawsuits and criminal sanctions did not influence their decision in this specific case, the court believed that the threat of legal ramifications strongly influenced the existing medical standards and practices of health care providers.

The court also observed that life-prolongation advances had rendered the existing medical standards ambiguous (unclear), leaving doctors in a quandary. Moreover, modern devices used for prolonging life, such as respirators, had confused the issue of "ordinary" and "extraordinary" measures. Therefore, the court suggested that respirators could be considered "ordinary" care for a curable patient, but "extraordinary" care for irreversibly unconscious patients.

The court also suggested that hospitals should form ethics committees to assist physicians with difficult cases such as Quinlan's. These committees would be similar to a multijudge panel exploring different solutions to an appeal. The committees would not only diffuse professional responsibility but would also eliminate any possibly unscrupulous motives of physicians or families. The justices considered the court's intervention on medical decisions an infringement on the physicians' field of competence.

The state had promised to prosecute anyone who terminated Quinlan's life support because such an act would constitute homicide. However, the New Jersey Supreme Court rejected this consequence because the resulting death would be from natural causes.

After the Respirator Was Removed

In March 1976 the New Jersey Supreme Court ruled that, if the hospital ethics committee agreed that Quinlan would not recover from irreversible coma, her respirator could be removed. Furthermore, all parties involved would be legally immune from criminal and civil prosecution. However, after Quinlan's respirator was removed, she continued to breathe on her own and remained in a PVS until she died of multiple infections in 1985.

Some people wondered why the Quinlans did not request permission to discontinue Karen's artificial nutrition and hydration. In *Karen Ann: The Quinlans Tell Their Story* (1977), the Quinlans state that they had moral problems with depriving their daughter of food and antibiotics.

SUBSTITUTED JUDGMENT

Superintendent of Belchertown State School et al. v. Joseph Saikewicz

Joseph Saikewicz was a mentally incompetent resident of the Belchertown State School of the Massachusetts Department of Mental Health. In April 1976 Saikewicz was diagnosed with acute myeloblastic monocytic leukemia (cancer of the blood). He was 67 years old but had the mental age of about two years and eight months. The superintendent of the mental institution petitioned the court for a guardian ad litem (a temporary guardian for the duration of the trial). The court-appointed guardian recommended that it would be in the patient's best interests that he not undergo chemotherapy.

In May 1976 the probate judge ordered nontreatment of the disease based in part on findings of medical experts, who indicated that chemotherapy might produce remission of leukemia in 30% to 50% of the cases. If remission occurred, it would last between two and 13 months. Chemotherapy, however, would make Saikewicz suffer adverse side effects that he would not understand. Without chemotherapy, the patient might live for several weeks or months, but would die without the pain or discomfort associated with chemotherapy.

Saikewicz died on September 4, 1976, from pneumonia, a complication of the leukemia. Nevertheless, his case, *Superintendent of Belchertown State School et al. v. Joseph Saikewicz* (Mass., 370 N.E.2d 417 [1977]), was heard by the Massachusetts Supreme Court to establish a precedent on the question of substituted judgment—letting another entity, such as a court, ethics committee, surrogate, or guardian, determine what the patient would do in the situation were the patient competent.

The court agreed that extraordinary measures should not be used if the patient will not recover from the disease. The court also ruled that a person has a right to the preservation of his or her bodily integrity and can refuse medical invasion. The Massachusetts Supreme Court turned to *In re Quinlan* for support of its right of privacy argument.

THE RIGHTS OF AN INCOMPETENT PATIENT. Once the right to refuse treatment had been established, the court declared that everyone, including an incompetent person, has the right of choice. Referring to *Quinlan*, the court recommended that the patient not receive the treatment most people with leukemia would choose. (Unlike some later courts, the *Quinlan* court accepted the premise that a vegetative patient would not want to remain "alive.") The *Saikewicz* court believed that the "substituted judgment" standard would best preserve respect for the integrity and autonomy of the patient. In other words, the decision maker—in this case, the court—would put itself in Saikewicz's position and make the treatment decision the patient most likely would make were he competent. The court believed Saikewicz would have refused treatment.

In evaluating the role of the hospital and the guardian in the decision-making process, the *Saikewicz* court rejected the *Quinlan* court's recommendation that an ethics committee should be the source of the decision. The court instead concluded that the judicial branch of government was the proper venue.

Charles S. Soper, as Director of Newark Developmental Center et al. v. Dorothy Storar

John Storar, a 52-year-old mentally retarded man with a mental age of about 18 months, was diagnosed with terminal cancer. His mother, Dorothy Storar, petitioned the court to discontinue blood transfusions that were delaying her son's death, which would probably occur within three to six months.

At the time of the hearing, Storar required two units of blood about every one to two weeks. He found the transfusions disagreeable and had to be given a sedative before the procedure. He also had to be restrained during the transfusions. Storar's physician reported that after the transfusions, however, Storar had more energy and was able to resume most of his normal activities. Without the blood transfusions there would be insufficient oxygen in his blood, causing his heart to beat faster and his respiratory rate to increase, impeding normal activities.

The probate court granted Dorothy Storar the right to terminate the treatments, but the order was stayed and treatment continued pending an appeal to the New York Appellate Division (or appellate court). Storar died before the case, *Charles S. Soper, as Director of Newark Developmental Center et al. v. Dorothy Storar* (N.Y., 420 N.E.2d 64 [1981]), could be heard, rendering the decision moot, but because the issue was considered to be of public importance, the appellate court proceeded to hear the case.

The appellate court agreed with the probate court that a guardian can make medical decisions for an incompetent patient. However, the parent/guardian "may not deprive a child of life-saving treatment." In this case there were two threats to Storar's life: the incurable cancer and the loss of blood that could be remedied with transfusions. Because the transfusions did not, in the eyes of the majority opinion written by Judge Sol Wachtler (1930–), cause much pain, the appellate court overturned the probate court's ruling.

Dissenting from this determination, Judge Hugh R. Jones (1914–2001) believed the treatments did not serve Storar's best interests. They did not relieve his pain and, in fact, caused him additional pain. Because the blood transfusions would not cure his cancer, they could be considered extraordinary treatments. Finally, Judge Jones reasoned that Storar's mother had cared for him for a long time and knew best how he felt, and therefore the court should respect her decision.

COMPETENT PATIENTS' WISHES

Michael J. Satz etc. v. Abe Perlmutter

Not all the cases of patients seeking to terminate life support concern incompetent people. Abe Perlmutter, aged 73, was suffering from amyotrophic lateral sclerosis (ALS; a degenerative neurologic condition commonly known as Lou Gehrig's disease). ALS is always fatal after prolonged physical degeneration, but it does not affect mental function.

Perlmutter's 1978 request to have his respirator removed was approved by the Circuit Court of Broward County, Florida. At a bedside hearing, the court questioned whether the patient truly understood the consequences of his request. Perlmutter told the judge that if the respirator were removed, "It can't be worse than what I'm going through now."

The state appealed the case before the Florida District Court of Appeals (appellate court), citing the state's duty to preserve life and to prevent the unlawful killing of a human being. The state also noted the hospital's and the doctors' fear of criminal prosecution and civil liability. In *Michael J. Satz, State Attorney for Broward County, Florida v. Abe Perlmutter* (Fla. App., 362 So.2d, 160 [1978]), the appellate court concluded that Perlmutter's right to refuse treatment overrode the state's interests and found in Perlmutter's favor.

THE STATE'S INTERESTS. An individual's right to refuse medical treatment is generally honored as long as it is consistent with the state's interests, which include:

- Interest in the preservation of life

- Need to protect innocent third parties

- Duty to prevent suicide

- Requirement that it help maintain the ethical integrity of medical practice

In the *Perlmutter* case, the Florida District Court of Appeals found that the preservation of life is an important goal, but not when the disease is incurable and causes the patient to suffer. The need to protect innocent third parties refers to cases in which a parent refuses treatment for him- or herself and a third party suffers, such as the abandonment of a minor child when the parent dies. Perlmutter's children were all adults and Perlmutter was not committing suicide. Were it not for the respirator, he would be dead; therefore, disconnecting it would not cause his death but would result in the disease running its natural course. Finally, the court turned to *Quinlan* and *Saikewicz* to support its finding that there are times when medical ethics dictates that a dying person needs comfort more than treatment. The court concluded:

> Abe Perlmutter should be allowed to make his choice to die with dignity.... It is all very convenient to insist on continuing Mr. Perlmutter's life so that there can be no question of foul play, no resulting civil liability and no possible trespass on medical ethics. However, it is quite another matter to do so at the patient's sole expense and against his competent will, thus inflicting never-ending physical torture on his body until the inevitable, but artificially suspended, moment of death. Such a course of conduct invades the patient's constitutional right of privacy, removes his freedom of choice and invades his right to self-determine.

The state again appealed the case, this time to the Supreme Court of Florida, which, in *Michael J. Satz etc. v. Abe Perlmutter* (Fla., 379 So.2d 359 [1980]), supported the decision by the Florida District Court of Appeals. Shortly after this ruling, Perlmutter's respirator was disconnected, and he died of his disease on October 6, 1980.

THE SUBJECTIVE, LIMITED-OBJECTIVE, AND PURE-OBJECTIVE TESTS

In the Matter of Claire C. Conroy

Claire Conroy was an 84-year-old nursing-home patient suffering from "serious and irreversible mental and physical impairments with a limited life expectancy." In March 1984 her nephew (her guardian and only living relative) petitioned the Superior Court of Essex County, New Jersey, to remove her nasogastric feeding tube. Conroy's court-appointed guardian ad litem opposed the petition. The superior court approved the nephew's request, and the guardian ad litem appealed. Conroy died with the nasogastric tube in place while the appeal was pending. Nonetheless, the appellate court chose to hear the case *In the Matter of Claire C. Conroy* (486 A.2d 1209 [N.J. 1985]). The court reasoned that this was an important case and that its ruling could influence future cases with comparable circumstances.

Conroy suffered from heart disease, hypertension, and diabetes. She also had a gangrenous leg, bedsores, and an eye problem that required irrigation. She lacked bowel control, could not speak, and had a limited swallowing ability. In the appeals trial one medical expert testified that

Conroy, although awake, was seriously demented. Another doctor testified that "although she was confused and unaware, 'she responds somehow.'"

Both experts were not sure if Conroy could feel pain, although she had moaned when subjected to painful stimuli. However, they agreed that if the nasogastric tube were removed, Conroy would die a painful death.

Conroy's nephew testified that his aunt would never have wanted to be maintained in this manner. She feared doctors and had avoided them all her life. Because she was Roman Catholic, a priest was brought in to testify. In his judgment the removal of the tube would be ethical and moral even though her death might be painful.

The appeals court held that "the right to terminate life-sustaining treatment based on a guardian's judgment was limited to incurable and terminally ill patients who are brain dead, irreversibly comatose, or vegetative, and who would gain no medical benefit from continued treatment."

Furthermore, a guardian's decision did not apply to food withdrawal, which hastens death. The court deemed this active euthanasia, which it did not consider ethically permissible.

THE THREE TESTS. The court proposed three tests to determine if Conroy's feeding tube should have been removed. The subjective test served to clarify what Conroy would have decided about her tube feeding if she were able to do so. The court listed acceptable expressions of intent that should be considered by surrogates or by the court: spoken expressions, living wills, durable power of attorney, oral directives, prior behavior, and religious beliefs.

If the court determines that patients in Conroy's circumstance have not explicitly expressed their wishes, two other "best interests" tests may be used: the limited-objective and the pure-objective tests. The limited-objective test permits discontinuing life-sustaining treatment if medical evidence shows that the patient would reject treatment that would only prolong suffering and that medication would not alleviate pain. Under this test, the court requires the additional evidence from the subjective test. The pure-objective test applies when there is no trustworthy evidence, or any evidence at all, to help guide a decision. The burden imposed on the patient's life by the treatment should outweigh whatever benefit would result from the treatment.

In January 1985 the court concluded that Conroy failed the tests. Her intentions, while perhaps clear enough to help support a limited-objective test (she had shown some evidence of a desire to reject treatment), were not strong enough for the subjective test (clear expressions of her intent). In addition, the information on her possible pain versus benefits of remaining alive was not sufficient for either the limited-objective test (her pain might outweigh her pleasure in life) or the pure-objective test (her pain would be so great it would be inhumane to continue treatment). Had Conroy survived the appellate court's decision, the court would have required her guardian to investigate these matters further before reaching a decision.

Justice Alan B. Handler (1931–), dissenting in part, disagreed with the majority's decision to measure Conroy's "best interests" in terms of the possible pain she could have been experiencing. First, in many cases pain can be controlled through medication. Second, pain levels cannot always be determined, as was shown in Conroy's case. Finally, not all patients decide based on pain. Some fear being dependent on others, especially when their bodily functions deteriorate; others value personal privacy and dignity.

CAN DOCTORS BE HELD LIABLE?
Barber v. Superior Court of the State of California

Historically, physicians have been free from prosecution for terminating life support. However, a precedent was set in 1983, when two doctors (Neil Barber and Robert Nejdl) were charged with murder and conspiracy to commit murder after agreeing to requests from a patient's family to discontinue life support.

Clarence Herbert suffered cardiorespiratory arrest following surgery. He was revived and placed on a respirator. Three days later his doctors diagnosed him as deeply comatose. The prognosis was that he would likely never recover. The family requested in writing that Herbert's respirator and other life-sustaining equipment be removed. The doctors complied, but Herbert continued to breathe on his own. After two days the family asked the doctors to remove the intravenous tubes that provided nutrition and hydration. The request was honored. From that point until his death, Herbert received care that provided a clean and hygienic environment and allowed for the preservation of his dignity.

A superior court judge ruled that because the doctors' behavior intentionally shortened the patient's life, they had committed murder. However, the court of appeals found in *Barber v. Superior Court of the State of California* (195 Cal.Rptr. 484 [Cal.App. 2 Dist. 1983]) that a patient's right to refuse treatment, and a surrogate's right to refuse treatment for an incompetent, superseded any liability that could be attributed to the physicians.

In ruling that the physicians' compliance with the request of Herbert's family did not constitute murder, the court of appeals stated that "cessation of 'heroic' life support measures is not an affirmative act but rather a withdrawal or omission of further treatment." In addition, artificial nutrition and hydration also constituted a medical treatment.

WHAT ARE THE HOSPITAL'S RIGHTS?
Patricia E. Brophy v. New England Sinai Hospital

In 1983 Paul E. Brophy Sr. suffered the rupture of an aneurysm (a part of an artery wall that weakens, causing it to balloon outward with blood) that left him in a PVS. He was neither brain dead nor terminal. He had been a fireman and an emergency medical technician and often expressed the opinion that he never wanted to be kept alive artificially.

Patricia Brophy brought suit when physicians refused to remove or clamp a gastrostomy tube (g-tube) that supplied nutrition and hydration to her husband. The Massachusetts Appeals Court ruled against Brophy, but in *Patricia E. Brophy v. New England Sinai Hospital* (497 N.E.2d 626 [Mass. 1986]) the Massachusetts Supreme Court allowed substituted judgment for a comatose patient who had previously made his intentions clear.

However, the Massachusetts Supreme Court did agree with the Massachusetts Appeals Court ruling that the hospital could not be forced to withhold food and water, which went against the hospital's ethical beliefs. Consequently, the Massachusetts Supreme Court ordered New England Sinai Hospital to facilitate Brophy's transfer to another facility or to his home, where his wife could carry out his wishes.

In October 1986 Brophy was moved to Emerson Hospital in Concord, Massachusetts. He died there on October 23 after eight days with no food. The official cause of death was pneumonia.

VITALIST DISSENSIONS. In *Brophy*, Justices Joseph Richard Nolan (1925–) and Neil L. Lynch (1930–) of the Massachusetts Supreme Court strongly disagreed with the majority opinion to allow withdrawal of nutrition and hydration. Justice Nolan argued that food and water were not medical treatments that could be refused. In his view, food and water are basic human needs, and by permitting the removal of the g-tube, the court gave its stamp of approval to euthanasia and suicide.

Justice Lynch believed the Massachusetts Supreme Court majority had ignored what he considered to be valid findings by the Massachusetts Appeals Court, which found that Brophy's wishes, as expressed in his wife's substituted-judgment decision of withholding food and water, did not concern intrusive medical treatment. Rather, Brophy's decision, if he were competent to make it, was to knowingly terminate his life by declining food and water. This was suicide and the state was, therefore, condoning suicide.

In the Matter of Beverly Requena

Beverly Requena was a competent 55-year-old woman with ALS. She informed St. Clare's/Riverside Medical Center—a Roman Catholic hospital—that when she lost the ability to swallow, she would refuse artificial feeding. The hospital filed a suit to force Requena to leave the hospital, citing its policy against withholding food or fluids from a patient.

Requena was paralyzed from the neck down and was unable to make sounds, although she could form words with her lips. At the time of the hearing, she could not eat but could suck some nutrient liquids through a straw. Her abilities were quickly deteriorating, however.

The court did not question Requena's right to refuse nutrition, nor did the hospital question that right. That was a right that had been upheld in many previous cases. However, reasserting its policy of refusing to participate in the withholding or withdrawal of artificial nutrition and hydration, the hospital offered to help transfer Requena to another facility that was willing to fulfill her wishes.

Requena did not want to transfer to another hospital. In the last 17 months, she had formed a relationship of trust in, and affection for, the staff. She also liked the familiar surroundings. The court found that being forced to leave would upset her emotionally and psychologically. The hospital staff was feeling stress as well. It was fond of Requena and did not want to see her die a presumably painful death from dehydration.

Judge Reginald Stanton ruled in *In the Matter of Beverly Requena* (517 A.2d 869 [N.J.Super.A.D. 1986]) that Requena could not be removed from the hospital without her consent and that the hospital would have to comply with her wishes. He stressed the importance of preserving the personal worth, dignity, and integrity of the patient. The hospital may provide her information about her prognosis and treatment options, but Requena alone had the right to decide what was best for her. Following the ruling, the hospital honored Requena's request and stopped giving her artificial nutrition. She died in December 1987.

WHAT ARE THE NURSING HOME'S RIGHTS?
In the Matter of Nancy Ellen Jobes

In 1980, 24-year-old Nancy Ellen Jobes was in a car accident. At the time, she was four-and-a-half months pregnant. Doctors who treated her determined that her fetus was dead. During the surgery to remove the fetus, Jobes suffered a loss of oxygen and blood flow to the brain. Never regaining consciousness, she was moved to the Lincoln Park Nursing Home several months later.

The nursing home provided nourishment to Jobes through a jejunostomy tube (j-tube) that was inserted into the jejunum (midsection) of her small intestine. Five years later Jobes's husband, John Jobes, asked the nursing home to stop his wife's artificial feeding. The nursing home refused, citing moral considerations.

The trial court appointed a guardian ad litem, who, after reviewing the case, filed in favor of John Jobes. The nursing home moved to appoint a life advocate (a person who would support retaining the feeding tube), which was turned down by the trial court. The New Jersey Supreme Court heard the case *In the Matter of Nancy Ellen Jobes* (529 A.2d 434 [N.J. 1987]).

DIFFERING INTERPRETATIONS OF PVS. Whether Jobes was in a PVS was hotly debated, which revealed how different medical interpretations of the same patient's condition can produce different conclusions. After John Jobes initiated the suit, his wife was transferred to Cornell Medical Center for four days of observation and testing. The neurologist Fred Plum and his associate David Levy concluded, after extensive examination and testing, that Jobes was indeed in a PVS and would never recover.

On the contrary, Maurice Victor and Allan Ropper testified for the nursing home. Having examined Jobes for about one-and-a-half hours, Victor reported that even though the patient was severely brain damaged, he did not believe she was in a PVS. She had responded to his commands, such as to pick up her head or to stick out her tongue. However, he could not back up his testimony with any written record of his examination.

Ropper had also examined Jobes for about an hour and a half. He testified that some of the patient's motions, such as lifting an arm off the bed, excluded her from his definition of PVS. (His definition of PVS differed from Plum's in that it excluded patients who made reflexive responses to outside stimuli—a definition that would have also excluded Quinlan.) Testimony from the nurses who had cared for Jobes over the past years was also contradictory, with some asserting she smiled or responded to their care and others saying they saw no cognitive responses.

The New Jersey Supreme Court concluded that the neurological experts, especially Plum and Levy, "offered sufficiently clear and convincing evidence to support the trial court's finding that Jobes is in an irreversibly vegetative state." However, the court could find no "clear and convincing" evidence that Jobes, if she were competent, would want the j-tube removed. Jobes's family and friends, including her minister, had testified that in general conversation she had mentioned that she would not want to be kept alive with artificial life support measures. The court did not accept these past remarks as clear evidence of the patient's intent.

With no clear and convincing evidence of Jobes's beliefs about artificial feeding, the New Jersey Supreme Court turned to *In re Quinlan* for guidance. The court stated, "Our review of these cases and medical authorities confirms our conclusion that we should continue to defer, as we did in *Quinlan*, to family members' substituted judgments about medical treatment for irreversibly vegetative patients who did not clearly express their medical preferences while they were competent. Those decisions are best made because the family is best able to decide what the patient would want."

THE NURSING HOME'S RESPONSIBILITY. The New Jersey Supreme Court reversed the trial court decision that had allowed the nursing home to refuse to participate in the withdrawal of the feeding tube. The court noted, "Mrs. Jobes's family had no reason to believe that they were surrendering the right to choose among medical alternatives when they placed her in the nursing home." The court pointed out that it was not until 1985, five years after Jobes's admission to the Lincoln Park Nursing Home, and only after her family requested the removal of her feeding tube, that her family learned of the nursing home's policy. The court ordered the nursing home to comply with the family's request. Jobs died in August 1987 after the court ruling allowed her husband to have the feeding tube removed.

Justice Daniel J. O'Hern (1930–2009) dissented on both issues. He claimed that not all families may be as loving as Jobes's. He was concerned for other individuals whose family might not be so caring, but who would still have the authority to order the withdrawal of life-sustaining treatments. He also disagreed with the order given the nursing home to comply with the family's request to discontinue Jobes's feeding. "I believe a proper balance could be obtained by adhering to the procedure adopted [in] *In re Quinlan*, that would have allowed the non-consenting physician not to participate in the life-terminating process."

CLEAR AND CONVINCING EVIDENCE

Throughout the history of right-to-die cases, there has been considerable debate about how to determine a patient's wishes. How clearly must a patient have expressed his or her wishes before becoming incompetent? Does a parent or other family member best represent the patient? Are casual conversations sufficient to reveal intentions, or must there be written instructions?

In the Matter of Philip K. Eichner, on Behalf of Joseph C. Fox v. Denis Dillon, as District Attorney of Nassau County

Eighty-three-year-old Joseph C. Fox went into a PVS after a hernia operation. He was a member of the Society of Mary, a Roman Catholic religious order. The local director of the society, Philip K. Eichner, filed suit, asking for permission to have Fox's respirator removed.

In *In the Matter of Philip K. Eichner, on Behalf of Joseph C. Fox v. Denis Dillon, as District Attorney of Nassau County* (N.Y., 420 N.E.2d 64 [1981]), the court reasoned that "the highest burden of proof beyond a reasonable doubt should be required when granting the relief that may result in the patient's death." The need for high

standards "forbids relief whenever the evidence is loose, equivocal, or contradictory." Fox, however, had discussed his feelings in the context of formal religious conversations. Only two months before his final hospitalization, he had stated that he did not want his life prolonged if his condition became hopeless. The court argued, "These were obviously solemn pronouncements and not casual remarks made at some social gathering, nor can it be said that he was too young to realize or feel the consequences of his statements." Following the ruling, Fox's respirator was removed, and he died from congestive heart failure on January 24, 1980.

Fox's case was the first where the reported attitudes of an incompetent patient were accepted as "clear and convincing."

In the Matter of Westchester County Medical Center, on Behalf of Mary O'Connor

Not all patients express their attitudes about the use of life-sustaining treatments in serious religious discussions as did Fox. Nonetheless, courts have accepted evidence of "best interests" or "substituted judgments" in allowing the termination of life-sustaining treatments.

In 1985 Mary O'Connor had a stroke that rendered her mentally and physically incompetent. More than two years later she suffered a second major stroke, after which she had additional disabilities and difficulty swallowing. O'Connor's two daughters moved her to a long-term geriatric facility that was associated with the Westchester County Medical Center. During her hospital admission, her daughters submitted a signed statement to be added to her medical records. The document stated that O'Connor had indicated in many conversations that "no artificial life support be started or maintained in order to continue to sustain her life."

In June 1988, when O'Connor's condition deteriorated, she was admitted to Westchester County Medical Center. Because she was unable to swallow, her physician prescribed a nasogastric tube. The daughters objected to the procedure, citing their mother's expressed wish. The hospital petitioned the court for permission to provide artificial feeding, without which O'Connor would starve to death within seven to 10 days. The lower court found in favor of O'Connor's daughters. The hospital subsequently brought the case *In the Matter of Westchester County Medical Center, on Behalf of Mary O'Connor* (531 N.E.2d 607 [N.Y. 1988]) before the New York Court of Appeals.

O'Connor's physician testified that she was not in a coma. Even though he anticipated that O'Connor's awareness might improve in the future, he believed she would never regain the mental ability to understand complex matters. This included the issue of her medical condition and treatment. The physician further indicated that, if his patient were allowed to starve to death, she would experience pain and "extreme, intense discomfort."

A neurologist testifying for the daughters reported that O'Connor's brain damage would keep her from experiencing pain. If she did have pain in the process of starving to death, she could be given medication. However, the doctor admitted he could not be "medically certain" because he had never had a patient die under the same circumstances.

The New York Court of Appeals majority concluded that even though family and friends testified that O'Connor "felt that nature should take its course and not use further artificial means" and that it is "monstrous" to keep someone alive by "machinery," these expressions did not constitute clear and convincing evidence of her present desire to die. Also, she had never specifically discussed the issue of artificial nutrition and hydration. Nor had she ever expressed her wish to refuse artificial medical treatment should such refusal result in a painful death.

The court further noted that O'Connor's statements about refusing artificial treatments had generally been made in situations involving terminal illness, specifically cancer: her husband, two of her brothers, her stepmother, and a close friend had all died of cancer. Speaking for the court of appeals majority, Judge Wachtler stressed that O'Connor was not terminally ill, was conscious, and could interact with others, albeit minimally. Her main problem was that she could not eat on her own, and her physician could help her with that. Writing for the majority, Judge Wachtler stated, "Every person has a right to life, and no one should be denied essential medical care unless the evidence clearly and convincingly shows that the patient intended to decline the treatment under some particular circumstances. This is a demanding standard, the most rigorous burden of proof in civil cases. It is appropriate here because if an error occurs it should be made on the side of life."

THIS IS TOO RESTRICTIVE. Judge Richard D. Simons (1927–) of the New York Court of Appeals differed from the majority in his opinion of O'Connor's condition. O'Connor's "conversations" were actually limited to saying her name and words such as "okay," "all right," and "yes." Neither the hospital doctor nor the neurologist who testified for her daughters could say for sure that she understood their questions. The court majority mentioned the patient squeezing her doctor's hand in response to some questions, but failed to add that she did not respond to most questions.

Even though O'Connor was not terminally ill, her severe mental and physical injuries—should nature take its course—would result in her death. Judge Simons believed the artificial feeding would not cure or improve her deteriorating condition.

Judge Wachtler noted that O'Connor had talked about refusing artificial treatment in the aftermath of the deaths of loved ones from cancer. He claimed this had no bearing on her present condition, which was not terminal. Judge Simons pointed out that O'Connor had worked for 20 years in a hospital emergency room and pathology laboratory. She was no casual observer of death, and her "remarks" about not wanting artificial treatment for herself carried a lot of weight. Her expressed wishes to her daughters, who were nurses and coworkers in the same hospital, could not be considered "casual," as the majority observed. Judge Simons stated that "Judges, the persons least qualified by training, experience or affinity to reject the patient's instructions, have overridden Mrs. O'Connor's wishes, negated her long held values on life and death, and imposed on her and her family their ideas of what her best interests require." O'Connor died 10 months later with the feeding tube still in place.

Daniel Gindes suggests in "Judicial Postponement of Death Recognition: The Tragic Case of Mary O'Connor" (*American Journal of Law and Medicine*, vol. 15, nos. 2–3, 1989) that the court made an error in its judgment. He concludes by stating that "artificial hydration and nutrition is not 'food.' It is a desperate treatment best used as a transition from acute crisis to normal functioning. This miraculous technology, misused, harms the very patients medicine purports to help. One can argue that the 'sanctity of life' is more offended by warehousing bodies, than by cessation of treatment. Incompetent patients, who have suffered structural damage to necessary nerve centers, do not get better. Feeding tubes cannot regenerate this fragile tissue. Perhaps one day doctors will be able to make people like Mary O'Connor well. Until then, they should leave them alone."

THE CASE OF NANCY BETH CRUZAN

Even though *O'Connor* set a rigorous standard of proof for the state of New York, *Cruzan* was the first right-to-die case to be heard by the U.S. Supreme Court. It confirmed the legality of such strict standards for the entire country.

Nancy Beth Cruzan, by Co-guardians, Lester L. Cruzan Jr. and Joyce Cruzan v. Robert Harmon

In January 1983, 25-year-old Nancy Beth Cruzan lost control of her car. A state trooper found her lying facedown in a ditch. She was in cardiac and respiratory arrest. Paramedics were able to revive her, but a neurosurgeon indicated that she had "a probable cerebral contusion compounded by significant anoxia." The final diagnosis estimated that she had suffered anoxia (deprivation of oxygen) for 12 to 14 minutes. After six minutes of oxygen deprivation, the brain generally suffers permanent damage.

Doctors surgically implanted a feeding tube about a month after the accident, following the consent of her husband. However, within a year of the accident, Cruzan's husband had their marriage dissolved. In January 1986 Cruzan became a ward of the state of Missouri.

Medical experts diagnosed Cruzan to be in a PVS and indicated that she was capable of living another 30 years. Cruzan's parents, Joyce and Lester Cruzan Jr., believed that their daughter would not want to live in a PVS sustained by a feeding tube and asked the hospital to remove the tube; hospital employees refused to do so. Because Cruzan was an adult, her parents had no legal standing in the courts, so they became the legal guardians of their daughter. They petitioned a Missouri trial court to have the feeding tube removed. The court gave Cruzan's parents the right to terminate artificial nutrition and hydration. However, the state and the court-appointed guardian ad litem appealed to the Missouri Supreme Court. Even though the guardian ad litem believed it was in Cruzan's best interests to have the artificial feeding tube removed, he felt it was his duty as her attorney to take the case to the state supreme court because it was a case of first impression (without a precedent) in the state of Missouri.

THE RIGHT TO PRIVACY. In *Nancy Beth Cruzan, by Co-guardians, Lester L. Cruzan Jr. and Joyce Cruzan v. Robert Harmon* (760 S.W.2d 408 [Mo.banc 1988]), the Missouri Supreme Court stressed that the state constitution did not expressly provide for the right of privacy, which would support an individual's right to refuse medical treatment. Even though the U.S. Supreme Court had recognized the right of privacy in cases such as *Griswold v. Connecticut* (381 U.S. 479 [1965]) and *Roe v. Wade* (410 U.S. 113 [1973]), this right did not extend to the withdrawal of food and water. In fact, the U.S. Supreme Court, in *Roe v. Wade*, stressed that it "has refused to recognize an unlimited right of this kind in the past."

THE STATE'S INTEREST IN LIFE. In Cruzan's case the Missouri Supreme Court majority confirmed that the state's interest in life encompassed the sanctity of life and the prolongation of life. The state's interest in the prolongation of life was especially valid in Cruzan's case. She was not terminally ill and, based on medical evidence, would "continue a life of relatively normal duration if allowed basic sustenance." Furthermore, the state was not interested in the quality of life. The court was mindful that its decision would apply not only to Cruzan but also to others and feared treading a slippery slope. "Were the quality of life at issue, persons with all manner of handicaps might find the state seeking to terminate their lives. Instead, the state's interest is in life; that interest is unqualified."

THE GUARDIANS' RIGHTS. The Missouri Supreme Court ruled that Cruzan had no constitutional right to die and that there was no clear and convincing evidence that she would not wish to continue her vegetative existence. The majority further found that her parents, or guardians, had no right to exercise substituted judgment on their daughter's behalf. The court concluded, "We find no principled legal basis which permits the co-guardians in this case to choose the death of their ward. In the absence of such a legal basis for that decision and in the face of this State's strongly stated policy in favor of life, we choose to err on the side of life, respecting the rights of incompetent persons who may wish to live despite a severely diminished quality of life."

Therefore, the Missouri Supreme Court reversed the judgment of the Missouri trial court that had allowed discontinuance of Cruzan's artificial feeding.

THE STATE DOES NOT HAVE AN OVERRIDING INTEREST. In his dissent, Judge Charles B. Blackmar (1922–2007) indicated that the state should not be involved in cases such as Cruzan's. He was not convinced that the state had spoken better for Cruzan's interests than did her parents. He also questioned the state's interest in life in the context of espousing capital punishment, which clearly establishes "the proposition that some lives are not worth preserving."

Judge Blackmar did not share the majority's opinion that yielding to the guardians' request would lead to the mass euthanasia of handicapped people whose conditions did not come close to Cruzan's. He stressed that a court ruling is precedent only for the facts of that specific case. Besides, one of the purposes of courts is to protect incompetent people against abuse. He claimed, "The principal opinion attempts to establish absolutes, but does so at the expense of human factors. In so doing it unnecessarily subjects Nancy and those close to her to continuous torture which no family should be forced to endure."

"ERRONEOUS DECLARATION OF LAW." Judge Andrew J. Higgins (1921–2011), also dissenting, mainly disagreed with the majority's basic premise that the more than 50 precedent-setting cases from 16 other states were based on an "erroneous declaration of law." Yet, he noted that all the cases cited by the majority upheld an individual's right to refuse life-sustaining treatment, either personally or through the substituted judgment of a guardian. He could not understand the majority's contradiction of its own argument.

Cruzan v. Director, Missouri Department of Health

Cruzan's father appealed the Missouri Supreme Court's decision, and in December 1989 the U.S. Supreme Court heard arguments in *Cruzan v. Director, Missouri Department of Health* (497 U.S. 261 [1990]). This was the first time the right-to-die issue had been brought before the U.S. Supreme Court, which chose not to rule on whether Cruzan's parents could have her feeding tube removed. Instead, it considered whether the U.S. Constitution prohibited the state of Missouri from requiring clear and convincing evidence that an incompetent person desires withdrawal of life-sustaining treatment. In a 5–4 decision the court held that the Constitution did not prohibit the state of Missouri from requiring convincing evidence that an incompetent person wants life-sustaining treatment withdrawn.

Chief Justice William H. Rehnquist (1924–2005) wrote the opinion, with Justices Byron R. White (1917–2002), Sandra Day O'Connor (1930–), Antonin Scalia (1936–), and Anthony M. Kennedy (1936–) joining. The court majority believed that the Missouri Supreme Court's rigorous requirement of clear and convincing evidence that Cruzan had refused termination of life-sustaining treatment was justified. An erroneous decision not to withdraw the patient's feeding tube meant that the patient would continue to be sustained artificially. Possible medical advances or new evidence of the patient's intent could correct the error. An erroneous decision to terminate the artificial feeding could not be corrected, because the result of that decision—death—is irrevocable. The chief justice concluded, "No doubt is engendered by anything in this record but that Nancy Cruzan's mother and father are loving and caring parents. If the State were required by the United States Constitution to repose a right of 'substituted judgment' with anyone, the Cruzans would surely qualify. But we do not think the Due Process Clause requires the State to repose judgment on these matters with anyone but the patient herself." The Due Process Clause of the 14th Amendment provides that no state shall "deprive any person of life, liberty, or property, without due process of law."

STATE INTEREST SHOULD NOT OUTWEIGH THE FREEDOM OF CHOICE. Dissenting, Justice William J. Brennan Jr. (1906–1997) pointed out that the state of Missouri's general interest in the preservation of Cruzan's life in no way outweighed her freedom of choice—in this case the choice to refuse medical treatment. He stated, "The regulation of constitutionally protected decisions... must be predicated on legitimate state concerns other than disagreement with the choice the individual has made.... Otherwise, the interest in liberty protected by the Due Process Clause would be a nullity."

Justice Brennan believed the state of Missouri had imposed an uneven burden of proof. The state would only accept clear and convincing evidence that the patient had made explicit statements refusing artificial nutrition and hydration. However, it did not require any proof that she had made specific statements desiring continuance of such treatment. Hence, it could not be said that the state had accurately determined Cruzan's wishes.

Justice Brennan disagreed that it is better to err on the side of life than death. He argued that, to the patient, erring from either side is "irrevocable." He explained, "An erroneous decision to terminate artificial nutrition and hydration, to be sure, will lead to failure of that last remnant of physiological life, the brain stem, and result in complete brain death. An erroneous decision not to terminate life-support, however, robs a patient of the very qualities protected by the right to avoid unwanted medical treatment. His own degraded existence is perpetuated; his family's suffering is protracted; the memory he leaves behind becomes more and more distorted."

STATE USES NANCY CRUZAN FOR "SYMBOLIC EFFECT." In a separate dissenting opinion, Justice John Paul Stevens (1920–) believed the state of Missouri was using Cruzan for the "symbolic effect" of defining life. The state sought to equate Cruzan's physical existence with life. However, Justice Stevens pointed out that life is more than physiological functions. In fact, life connotes a person's experiences that make up his or her whole history, as well as "the practical manifestation of the human spirit."

Justice Stevens viewed the state's refusal to let Cruzan's guardians terminate her artificial feeding as ignoring their daughter's interests, and therefore, was "unconscionable":

> Insofar as Nancy Cruzan has an interest in being remembered for how she lived rather than how she died, the damage done to those memories by the prolongation of her death is irreversible. Insofar as Nancy Cruzan has an interest in the cessation of any pain, the continuation of her pain is irreversible. Insofar as Nancy Cruzan has an interest in a closure to her life consistent with her own beliefs rather than those of the Missouri legislature, the State's imposition of its contrary view is irreversible. To deny the importance of these consequences is in effect to deny that Nancy Cruzan has interests at all, and thereby to deny her personhood in the name of preserving the sanctity of her life.

CRUZAN CASE FINALLY RESOLVED. On December 14, 1990, nearly eight years after Cruzan's car accident, a Missouri circuit court ruled that new evidence presented by three more friends constituted clear and convincing evidence that she would not want to continue existing in a PVS. The court allowed the removal of her artificial feeding. Within two hours of the ruling, Cruzan's doctor removed the tube. Cruzan's family kept a 24-hour vigil with her, until she died on December 26, 1990. Cruzan's family, however, believed she had left them many years earlier.

THE TERRI SCHIAVO CASE

Like Cruzan, the case of Terri Schiavo involved a young woman in a PVS and the question of whether her nutrition and hydration could be discontinued.

In 1990 Schiavo suffered a loss of potassium in her body due to an eating disorder. This physiological imbalance caused her heart to stop beating, which deprived her brain of oxygen and resulted in a coma. She underwent surgery to implant a stimulator in her brain, an experimental treatment. The brain stimulator implant appeared to be a success, and the young woman appeared to be slowly emerging from her coma.

Nonetheless, even though Schiavo was continually provided with appropriate stimulation to recover, she remained in a PVS years later. Her husband, Michael Schiavo, believing that she would never recover and saying that his wife did not want to be kept alive by artificial means, petitioned a Florida court to remove her feeding tube. Her parents, however, believed that she could feel, understand, and respond. They opposed the idea of removing the feeding tube.

In 2000 a Florida trial court determined that Schiavo did not wish to be kept alive by artificial means based on her clear and direct statement to that effect to her husband. However, Schiavo's parents appealed the ruling, based on their belief that their daughter responded to their voices and could improve with therapy. They also contested the assertion that their daughter did not want to be kept alive by artificial means. Schiavo had left no living will to clarify her position, but under Florida's Health Care Advance Directives Law, a patient's spouse was second in line to decide about whether life support should be suspended (after a previously appointed guardian), adult children were third, and parents were fourth.

Constitutional Breach?

By October 2003 Schiavo's parents had exhausted their appeals, and the Florida appellate courts upheld the ruling of the trial court. At that time, a Florida judge ruled that removal of the tube take place. However, Schiavo's parents requested that the Florida governor Jeb Bush (1953–) intervene. In response, the Florida legislature developed House Bill 35-E (Terri's Law) and passed this bill on October 21, 2003. The law gave Governor Bush the authority to order Schiavo's feeding tube reinserted, and he did that by issuing Executive Order No. 03-201 that same day, six days after the feeding tube had been removed.

Legal experts noted that the Florida legislature, in passing Terri's Law, appeared to have taken judicial powers away from the judicial branch of the Florida government and had given them to the executive branch. If this were the case, then the law was unconstitutional under article 2, section 3 of the Florida constitution, which states, "No person belonging to one branch shall exercise any powers appertaining to either of the other branches unless expressly provided herein." Thus, Michael Schiavo challenged the law's constitutionality in Pinellas County Circuit Court. Governor Bush requested that the Pinellas County Circuit Court judge dismiss Schiavo's lawsuit arguing against Terri's Law. On April 30, 2004, Judge Charles A. Davis Jr. (1948–) rejected the governor's technical challenges, thereby denying the governor's motion to dismiss. In May 2004 the law that allowed Governor Bush to intervene in the case was ruled unconstitutional by a Florida appeals court.

Continued Appeals

Schiavo's parents then appealed the case to the Florida Supreme Court, which heard the case in September 2004. The court upheld the ruling of the lower court, with the seven justices ruling unanimously and writing that Terri's Law was "an unconstitutional encroachment on the power that has been reserved for the independent judiciary." Nonetheless, Schiavo's parents continued their legal fight to keep her alive, so a stay on the tube's removal was put in place while their appeals were pending. In October 2004 Governor Bush asked the Florida Supreme Court to reconsider its decision. The court refused the request.

Attorneys for the Florida governor then asked the U.S. Supreme Court to hear the Schiavo case. The Supreme Court rejected the request, which essentially affirmed the lower court rulings that the governor had no legal right to intervene in the matter. In February 2005 a Florida judge ruled that Michael Schiavo could remove his wife's feeding tube in March of that year. On March 18, 2005, the tube was removed. Days later, in an unprecedented action, the U.S. House of Representatives and the U.S. Senate approved legislation, which was quickly signed by President George W. Bush (1946–), that granted Terri Schiavo's parents the right to sue in federal court. In effect, this legislation allowed the court to intervene in the case and restore Terri's feeding tube. However, when Schiavo's parents appealed to the court, a federal judge refused to order the feeding tube reinserted. They then filed an appeal with the U.S. Supreme Court. Once again, the High Court refused to hear the case.

The Effect of the Schiavo Situation on End-of-Life Decision Making

Terri Schiavo died on March 31, 2005. Her death and the events leading up to her death resulted in an intense debate among Americans over end-of-life decisions and brought new attention to the question of who should make the decision to stop life support.

Timothy Williams reports in "Schiavo's Brain Was Severely Deteriorated, Autopsy Says" (*New York Times*, June 15, 2005) that the medical examiners who conducted Schiavo's autopsy found her brain "severely 'atrophied,'" weighed half the normal size, and noted that "no amount of therapy or treatment would have regenerated the massive loss of neurons." An autopsy cannot definitively establish a PVS, but the Schiavo findings were seen as "consistent" with a PVS.

THE CONSTITUTIONALITY OF ASSISTED SUICIDE

Washington v. Glucksberg

In January 1994 four state of Washington doctors, three terminally ill patients, and the organization Compassion in Dying filed a suit in the U.S. District Court. The plaintiffs sought to have the Washington Revised Code 9A.36.060(1) (1994) declared unconstitutional. This law states, "A person is guilty of promoting a suicide attempt when he knowingly causes or aids another person to attempt suicide."

The plaintiffs argued that under the Equal Protection Clause of the 14th Amendment mentally competent terminally ill adults have the right to a physician's assistance in determining the time and manner of their death. In *Compassion in Dying v. Washington* (850 F. Supp. 1454, 1456 n.2 [WD Wash. 1994]), the U.S. District Court agreed, stating that the Washington Revised Code violated the Equal Protection Clause's provision that "all persons similarly situated...be treated alike."

In its decision, the district court relied on *Planned Parenthood of Southeastern Pennsylvania v. Casey* (505 U.S. 833 [1992]; a reaffirmation of *Roe v. Wade*'s holding of the right to abortion) and *Cruzan v. Director, Missouri Department of Health* (the right to refuse unwanted life-sustaining treatment). The court found Washington's statute against assisted suicide "unconstitutional because it places an undue burden on the exercise of that constitutionally protected liberty interest."

In *Compassion in Dying v. State of Washington* (49 F. 3d 586, 591 [1995]), a panel (three or more judges but not the full court) of the Court of Appeals for the Ninth Circuit Court reversed the district court's decision, stressing that in over 200 years of U.S. history no court had ever recognized the right to assisted suicide. However, in *Compassion in Dying v. State of Washington* (79 F. 3d 790, 798 [1996]), the Ninth Circuit Court reheard the case en banc (by the full court), reversed the panel's decision, and affirmed the district court's ruling.

The en banc Court of Appeals for the Ninth Circuit Court did not mention the Equal Protection Clause violation as indicated by the district court. However, it referred to *Casey* and *Cruzan*, adding that the U.S. Constitution recognizes the right to die. Quoting from *Casey*, Judge Stephen R. Reinhardt (1931–) wrote, "Like the decision of whether or not to have an abortion, the decision how and when to die is one of 'the most intimate and personal choices a person may make in a lifetime,... central to personal dignity and autonomy.'"

THE U.S. SUPREME COURT DECIDES. The state of Washington and its attorney general appealed the case *Washington v. Glucksberg* (521 U.S. 702 [1997]) to the U.S. Supreme Court. Instead of addressing the plaintiffs' initial question of whether mentally competent terminally ill adults have the right to physician-assisted suicide, Chief Justice Rehnquist reframed the issue by focusing on "whether Washington's prohibition against 'caus[ing]' or 'aid[ing]' a suicide offends the Fourteenth Amendment to the United States Constitution."

Chief Justice Rehnquist recalled the more than 700 years of Anglo-American common-law tradition disapproving of suicide and assisted suicide. He added that assisted suicide is considered to be a crime in almost every state, with no exceptions granted to mentally competent terminally ill adults.

PREVIOUS SUBSTANTIVE DUE-PROCESS CASES. The plaintiffs argued that in previous substantive due-process cases, such as *Cruzan*, the U.S. Supreme Court had acknowledged the principle of self-autonomy by ruling "that competent, dying persons have the right to direct the removal of life sustaining medical treatment and thus hasten death." Chief Justice Rehnquist claimed that, even though committing suicide with another's help is just as personal as refusing life-sustaining treatment, it is not similar to refusing unwanted medical treatment. In fact, according to the chief justice, the *Cruzan* court specifically stressed that most states ban assisted suicide.

STATE'S INTEREST. The court pointed out that the state of Washington's interest in preserving human life includes the entire spectrum of that life, from birth to death, regardless of a person's physical or mental condition. The court agreed with the state that allowing assisted suicide might imperil the lives of vulnerable populations such as the poor, the elderly, and the disabled. The state included the terminally ill in this group.

Furthermore, the court agreed with the state of Washington that legalizing physician-assisted suicide would eventually lead to voluntary and involuntary euthanasia. Because a health care proxy's decision is legally accepted as an incompetent patient's decision, what if the patient cannot self-administer the lethal medication? In such a case a physician or a family member would have to administer the drug, thus committing euthanasia.

The court unanimously ruled that:

[The Washington Revised] Code...does not violate the Fourteenth Amendment, either on its face or "as applied to competent, terminally ill adults who wish to hasten their deaths by obtaining medication prescribed by their doctors."

Throughout the Nation, Americans are engaged in an earnest and profound debate about the morality, legality, and practicality of physician assisted suicide. Our holding permits this debate to continue, as it should in a democratic society. The decision of the en banc Court of Appeals is reversed, and the case is remanded [sent back] for further proceedings consistent with this opinion.

PROVISION OF PALLIATIVE CARE. Concurring, Justices O'Connor and Stephen G. Breyer (1938–) wrote that "dying patients in Washington and New York can obtain palliative care [care that relieves pain, but does not cure the illness], even when doing so would hasten their deaths." Hence, the justices did not see the need to address a dying person's constitutional right to obtain relief from pain.

Justice O'Connor believed the court was justified in banning assisted suicide for two reasons, "The difficulty in defining terminal illness and the risk that a dying patient's request for assistance in ending his or her life might not be truly voluntary."

Vacco, Attorney General of New York et al. v. Quill et al.

REFUSING LIFE-SUSTAINING TREATMENT IS ESSENTIALLY THE SAME AS ASSISTED SUICIDE. In 1994 three New York physicians and three terminally ill patients sued the New York attorney general. In *Quill v. Koppell* (870 F. Supp. 78, 84 [SDNY 1994]), they claimed before the U.S. District Court that New York violated the Equal Protection Clause by prohibiting physician-assisted suicide. The state permits a competent patient to refuse life-sustaining treatment, but not to obtain physician-assisted suicide. The plaintiffs claimed that these are "essentially the same thing." The court disagreed, stating that withdrawing life support to let nature run its course differs from intentionally using lethal drugs to cause death.

The plaintiffs brought their case *Quill v. Vacco* (80 F. 3d 716 [1996]) to the Court of Appeals for the Second Circuit (appellate court), which reversed the district court's ruling. The appellate court found that the New York statute does not treat equally all competent terminally ill patients wishing to hasten their death. The court stated, "The ending of life by [the withdrawal of life-support systems] is nothing more nor less than assisted suicide."

REFUSING LIFE-SUSTAINING TREATMENT DIFFERS FROM ASSISTED SUICIDE. New York's attorney general appealed the case to the U.S. Supreme Court. In *Vacco, Attorney General of New York et al. v. Quill et al.* (521 U.S. 793 [1997]), the court distinguished between withdrawing life-sustaining medical treatment and assisted suicide. The court contended that when a patient refuses life support, he or she dies because the disease has run its natural course. By contrast, if a patient self-administers lethal drugs, death results from that medication.

The court also distinguished between the physician's role in both scenarios. A physician who complies with a patient's request to withdraw life support does so to honor a patient's wish because the treatment no longer benefits the patient. Likewise, when a physician prescribes painkilling drugs, the needed drug dosage might hasten death, although the physician's only intent is to ease pain. However, when a physician assists in suicide, his or her prime intention is to hasten death. Therefore, the court reversed the ruling made by the Court of Appeals for the Second Circuit.

MOST STATE LEGISLATURES REJECT PHYSICIAN-ASSISTED SUICIDE

Justices Stevens and David H. Souter (1939–) issued opinions encouraging individual states to enact legislation

to permit physician-assisted suicide in selected cases. In most states ballot initiatives have failed to garner enough votes to legalize physician-assisted suicide. As of April 2012, Oregon, Washington, and Montana were the only states that allowed the practice. The Oregon Death with Dignity Act was approved in 1994 and reaffirmed by voters in 1997. It became effective in 1998. The Washington Death with Dignity Act was approved in 2008; Washington residents began taking advantage of the legislation in 2009. In Montana, no legislation was passed legalizing physician-assisted suicide; instead, the Montana Supreme Court ruled that physicians would not be prosecuted for providing mentally competent terminally ill Montana residents medication to hasten their deaths.

The Montana court case was originally initiated at the district level by Robert Baxter, a 76-year-old Montana truck driver with terminal cancer. Four physicians and the organization Compassion & Choices joined Baxter in the case *Baxter v. State of Montana* (Case No. ADV-2007-787). Baxter had been battling leukemia for over a decade and wished to end his life with prescribed medication. On December 5, 2008, Judge Dorothy McCarter ruled that the Montana constitution protected a mentally competent terminally ill patient's right to die with the help of medication prescribed by a physician. The ruling, which Baxter never heard, came the same day he died of natural causes.

The state of Montana appealed the ruling to the Montana Supreme Court in *Baxter v. State of Montana* (DA 09-0051 [2009 MT 449]). On December 31, 2009, the high court ruled 5–2 that physician-assisted suicide was not criminalized by either the Montana constitution or public policy. Even though the court ruling protected physicians from prosecution in physician-assisted suicide, it did not declare that physician-assisted suicide is a right allowed Montana residents. The high court left that debate to be settled in the state legislature.

THE SUPREME COURT RULING ON PHYSICIAN-ASSISTED SUICIDE IN OREGON

In late 2001 the U.S. attorney general John D. Ashcroft (1942–) reversed a decision made by his predecessor, Janet Reno (1938–), by asserting that the Controlled Substances Act of 1970 could be used against Oregon physicians who helped patients commit suicide by prescribing lethal drugs. If that were the case, then the U.S. Drug Enforcement Administration could disallow the prescription-writing privileges of any Oregon physician who prescribed drugs commonly used for assisted suicide. The possibility would also exist for those physicians to be criminally prosecuted as well. In response, the state of Oregon filed in November 2001 a lawsuit against Ashcroft's decision, claiming that he was acting unconstitutionally.

In April 2002, in *State of Oregon and Peter A. Rasmussen et al. v. John Ashcroft* (Civil No. 01-1647-JO),

Judge Robert E. Jones (1927–) of the U.S. District Court for the District of Oregon ruled in favor of the Oregon Death with Dignity Act. The U.S. Department of Justice appealed the ruling to the U.S. Court of Appeals for the Ninth Circuit in San Francisco. In May 2004 the court upheld the Oregon Death with Dignity Act. The decision, by a divided three-judge panel, said the Department of Justice did not have the power to punish physicians for prescribing medication for the purpose of assisted suicide. The majority opinion stated that Ashcroft overstepped his authority in trying to block enforcement of Oregon's law.

In February 2005 the U.S. Supreme Court agreed to hear the Bush administration's challenge of Oregon's physician-assisted suicide law. On January 17, 2006, the court let stand in *Gonzales v. Oregon* (546 U.S. 243) Oregon's physician-assisted suicide law. The High Court held that the Controlled Substances Act "does not allow the Attorney General to prohibit doctors from prescribing regulated drugs for use in physician-assisted suicide under state law permitting the procedure." Writing for the majority, Justice Kennedy explained that both Ashcroft and Alberto Gonzales (1955–), who succeeded Ashcroft as the U.S. attorney general, did not have the power to override the Oregon physician-assisted suicide law. Furthermore, Justice Kennedy added that the attorney general does not have the authority to make health and medical policy.

CHAPTER 9
THE COST OF HEALTH CARE

Americans want a quality health care system despite its increasingly high cost. Over the decades health care reform has been a topic of recurring debate among Americans and within the U.S. government. On March 23, 2010, health care reform became a reality when the Patient Protection and Affordable Care Act was signed into law by President Barack Obama (1961–). In addition, the Health Care and Education Reconciliation Act, which amended the Patient Protection and Affordable Care Act, was signed into law on March 30, 2010. Together, the two address health care reform.

Will this legislation lower the costs of health care in the United States? The U.S. Senate Democratic Policy Committee states in "Summary of Health Care and Revenue Provisions" (September 17, 2010, http://dpc.senate.gov/healthreformbill/healthbill62.pdf) that "the non-partisan Congressional Budget Office (CBO) has determined that these bills will provide coverage to 32 million Americans while lowering health care costs over the long term. This historic legislation will reduce the deficit by $143 billion over the next ten years, with $1.2 trillion in additional deficit reduction in the following decade." The U.S. Senate Republican Policy Committee (RPC) disagrees, stating in *H.R. 4872—Health Care and Education Reconciliation Act of 2010* (March 22, 2010, http://rpc.senate.gov/public/_files/L35HR4872HealthCareReconciliation032210cj.pdf) that the bill will cost $1.2 trillion "in the bill's first 10 years." The RPC adds that "the Republican staff of the Senate Budget Committee estimates that the total spending in the Senate bill's first 10 years of full implementation (fiscal years 2014–2023) would be $2.4 trillion." Thus, each party has opposing views on the economic costs or savings of the 2010 health care reform legislation.

INCREASING COSTS

Table 9.1 shows the progression of medical costs in the United States between 1960 and 2010. The table compares the growth in national health care expenditures and in gross domestic product (GDP; the total value of all the goods and services that are produced by a nation in a given year) over these years and presents the national health expenditures as a percentage of the GDP.

In 1960 the United States spent 5.2% of its GDP on health care. (See Table 9.1.) In 1970 this percentage rose to 7.2%, and by 1980 it increased to 9.2%. The rise continued, and by 1990 health care consumed 12.5% of the GDP. Growth of the cost of health care continued at a slower pace during the 1990s, so that by 2000 health care was 13.8% of the nation's GDP. However, since 2000 health care costs continued their upward climb at a faster pace. In 2010 health care costs consumed 17.9% of the GDP.

The Consumer Price Index (CPI) is a measure of the average change in prices that are paid by consumers. For most years the medical component of the CPI increased at a greater rate than any other component, even food and housing. Between 1960 and 2009 the average annual percentage change from the previous year shown in the overall CPI was well below the average annual percentage change for medical care. (See Table 9.2.) For example, in 2009 the overall CPI decreased by an annual percentage change of 0.4% from 2008, whereas medical care increased by 3.2%. In 2008 this pattern was opposite: medical care did not increase at a greater rate from 2005 than did the overall CPI. In 2008 the overall CPI increased by 3.8% from 2005, whereas medical care increased by 3.7%. In contrast, the percentage change in the food and energy components of the CPI were 1.8% and −18.4%, respectively, from 2008 to 2009, which were comparatively low from previous years and affected the percentage change of the overall CPI from 2008 to 2009 considerably. In addition, the exceptionally high average annual percentage change in the energy component of the CPI dropped dramatically in 2009, far outdistancing the average annual percentage change in the medical component.

TABLE 9.1

National health expenditures, selected years 1960–2010

Item	1960	1970	1980	1990	2000	2002	2004	2006	2008	2010
					Billions of dollars					
National health expenditures	$27.4	$74.9	$255.8	$724.3	$1,377.2	$1,636.4	$1,900.0	$2,162.4	$2,403.9	$2,593.6
Health consumption expenditure	24.8	67.1	235.7	675.6	1,289.6	1,534.4	1,782.6	2,031.5	2,250.1	2,444.6
Personal health care	23.4	63.1	217.2	616.8	1,165.4	1,372.0	1,589.3	1,804.9	2,010.2	2,186.0
Government administration and net cost of health insurance	1.1	2.6	12.0	38.8	81.2	110.6	139.3	164.0	167.2	176.1
Government public health activities	0.4	1.4	6.4	20.0	43.0	51.9	54.0	62.5	72.7	82.5
Investment	2.6	7.8	20.1	48.7	87.5	102.0	117.4	130.9	153.8	149.0
					Millions					
U.S. population[a]	186	210	230	254	282	288	293	298	304	309
					Billions of dollars					
Gross domestic product[b]	$526	$1,038	$2,788	$5,801	$9,952	$10,642	$11,853	$13,377	$14,292	$14,527
					Per capita amount in dollars					
National health expenditures	$147	$356	$1,110	$2,854	$4,878	$5,687	$6,488	$7,251	$7,911	$8,402
Health consumption expenditure	133	319	1,023	2,662	4,568	5,332	6,087	6,812	7,405	7,919
Personal health care	125	300	943	2,430	4,128	4,768	5,427	6,052	6,615	7,082
Government administration and net cost of health insurance	6	12	52	153	288	384	476	550	550	570
Government public health activities	2	6	28	79	152	180	184	210	239	267
Investment	14	37	87	192	310	355	401	439	506	483
					Percent distribution					
National health expenditures	100.0	100.0	100.0	100.0	100.0	100.0	100.0	100.0	100.0	100.0
Health consumption expenditure	90.6	89.6	92.1	93.3	93.6	93.6	93.8	93.9	93.6	94.3
Personal health care	85.4	84.3	84.9	85.2	84.6	83.8	83.6	83.5	83.6	84.3
Government administration and net cost of health insurance	3.9	3.5	4.7	5.4	5.9	6.8	7.3	7.6	7.0	6.8
Government public health activities	1.4	1.8	2.5	2.8	3.1	3.2	2.8	2.9	3.0	3.2
Investment	9.4	10.4	7.9	6.7	6.4	6.2	6.2	6.1	6.4	5.7
					Percent of gross domestic product					
National health expenditures	5.2	7.2	9.2	12.5	13.8	15.4	16.0	16.2	16.8	17.9
					Average annual percent change from previous year shown					
National health expenditures		10.6	13.1	11.0	7.0	9.5	7.0	6.6	4.7	3.9
Health consumption expenditure		10.5	13.4	11.1	7.4	9.4	7.1	6.8	4.5	4.0
Personal health care		10.4	13.2	11.0	6.9	8.4	7.4	6.3	5.0	3.7
Government administration and net cost of health insurance		9.4	16.4	12.4	15.1	22.8	7.0	9.9	−1.6	7.2
Government public health activities		13.8	16.9	12.0	5.5	9.2	0.4	11.3	5.3	8.2
Investment		11.7	10.0	9.2	2.4	11.8	6.8	3.5	7.1	1.9
U.S. population[a]		1.2	0.9	1.0	1.0	0.9	0.9	0.9	0.9	0.8
Gross domestic product[b]		7.0	10.4	7.6	6.4	3.5	6.4	6.0	1.9	4.2

[a]Census resident-based population less armed forces overseas and population of outlying areas.
[b]U.S. Department of Commerce, Bureau of Economic Analysis.
Note: Numbers and percents may not add to totals because of rounding. Dollar amounts shown are in current dollars.

SOURCE: Adapted from "Table 1. National Health Expenditures Aggregate, per Capita Amounts, Percent Distribution, and Average Annual Percent Change: Selected Calendar Years 1960–2010," in *National Health Expenditure Data: Historical—NHE Web Tables*, Centers for Medicare and Medicaid Services, Office of the Actuary, National Health Statistics Group, January 2012, http://www.cms.gov/NationalHealthExpendData/downloads/tables.pdf (accessed February 3, 2012)

TABLE 9.2

Consumer price index and average annual percentage change for general items and medical care components, selected years 1960–2009

[Data are based on reporting by samples of providers and other retail outlets]

Items and medical care components	1960	1970	1980	1990	1995	2000	2005	2008	2009
					Consumer Price Index (CPI)				
All items	29.6	38.8	82.4	130.7	152.4	172.2	195.3	215.3	214.5
All items less medical care	30.2	39.2	82.8	128.8	148.6	167.3	188.7	207.8	206.6
Services	24.1	35.0	77.9	139.2	168.7	195.3	230.1	255.5	259.2
Food	30.0	39.2	86.8	132.4	148.4	167.8	190.7	214.1	218.0
Apparel	45.7	59.2	90.9	124.1	132.0	129.6	119.5	118.9	120.1
Housing	—	36.4	81.1	128.5	148.5	169.6	195.7	216.3	217.1
Energy	22.4	25.5	86.0	102.1	105.2	124.6	177.1	236.7	193.1
Medical care	22.3	34.0	74.9	162.8	220.5	260.8	323.2	364.1	375.6
Components of medical care									
Medical care services	19.5	32.3	74.8	162.7	224.2	266.0	336.7	384.9	397.3
Professional services	—	37.0	77.9	156.1	201.0	237.7	281.7	311.0	319.4
Physicians' services	21.9	34.5	76.5	160.8	208.8	244.7	287.5	311.3	320.8
Dental services	27.0	39.2	78.9	155.8	206.8	258.5	324.0	376.9	388.1
Eyeglasses and eye care[a]	—	—	—	117.3	137.0	149.7	163.2	174.1	175.5
Services by other medical professionals[a]	—	—	—	120.2	143.9	161.9	186.8	205.5	209.8
Hospital and related services	—	—	69.2	178.0	257.8	317.3	439.9	534.0	567.9
Hospital services[b]	—	—	—	—	—	115.9	161.6	197.2	210.7
Inpatient hospital services[b, c]	—	—	—	—	—	113.8	156.6	190.8	203.6
Outpatient hospital services[a, c]	—	—	—	138.7	204.6	263.8	373.0	456.8	490.6
Hospital rooms	9.3	23.6	68.0	175.4	251.2	—	—	—	—
Other inpatient services[a]	—	—	—	142.7	206.8	—	—	—	—
Nursing homes and adult day care[b]	—	—	—	—	—	117.0	145.0	165.3	171.6
Health insurance[d]	—	—	—	—	—	—	—	114.2	110.5
Medical care commodities	46.9	46.5	75.4	163.4	204.5	238.1	276.0	296.0	305.1
Prescription drugs[e]	54.0	47.4	72.5	181.7	235.0	285.4	349.0	378.3	391.1
Nonprescription drugs and medical supplies[a]	—	—	—	120.6	140.5	149.5	151.7	158.3	161.4
Internal and respiratory over-the-counter drugs	—	42.3	74.9	145.9	167.0	176.9	179.7	188.7	193.0
Nonprescription medical equipment and supplies	—	—	79.2	138.0	166.3	178.1	180.6	185.6	188.2
				Average annual percent change from previous year shown					
All items	. . .	2.7	7.8	9.7	3.1	2.5	6.5	3.8	−0.4
All items excluding medical care	. . .	2.6	7.8	9.2	2.9	2.4	6.2	3.8	−0.6
All services	. . .	3.8	8.3	12.3	3.9	3.0	8.5	3.5	1.4
Food	. . .	2.7	8.3	8.8	2.3	2.5	6.6	5.5	1.8
Apparel	. . .	2.6	4.4	6.4	1.2	−0.4	−4.0	−0.1	1.0
Housing	. . .	—	8.3	9.6	2.9	2.7	7.4	3.2	0.4
Energy	. . .	1.3	12.9	3.5	0.6	3.4	19.2	13.9	−18.4
Medical care	. . .	4.3	8.2	16.8	6.3	3.4	11.3	3.7	3.2
Components of medical care									
Medical care services	. . .	5.2	8.8	16.8	6.6	3.5	12.5	4.2	3.2
Professional services	. . .	—	7.7	14.9	5.2	3.4	8.9	3.4	2.7
Physicians' services	. . .	4.6	8.3	16.0	5.4	3.2	8.4	2.7	3.0
Dental services	. . .	3.8	7.2	14.6	5.8	4.6	12	5.1	3.0
Eyeglasses and eye care[a]	. . .	—	—	—	3.2	1.8	4.4	1.4	0.8
Services by other medical professionals[a]	. . .	—	—	—	3.7	2.4	7.4	4.1	2.1
Hospital and related services	. . .	—	—	20.8	7.7	4.2	17.7	7.0	6.4
Hospital services[b]	. . .	—	—	—	—	—	18.1	7.4	6.9
Inpatient hospital services[b, c]	. . .	—	—	—	—	—	17.3	7.1	6.7
Outpatient hospital services[a, c]	. . .	—	—	—	8.1	5.2	18.9	7.7	7.4
Hospital rooms	. . .	9.8	11.2	20.9	7.4	—	—	—	—
Other inpatient services[a]	. . .	—	—	—	7.7	—	—	—	—
Nursing homes and adult day care[b]	. . .	—	—	—	—	—	11.3	3.6	3.8
Health insurance[d]	. . .	—	—	—	—	—	—	0.6	−3.2
Medical care commodities	. . .	−0.1	5.0	16.7	4.6	3.1	7.7	2.1	3.1
Prescription drugs[e]	. . .	−1.3	4.3	20.2	5.3	4.0	10.6	2.5	3.4
Nonprescription drugs and medical supplies[a]	. . .	—	—	—	3.1	1.2	0.7	0.9	2.0
Internal and respiratory over-the-counter drugs	. . .	—	5.9	14.3	2.7	1.2	0.8	1.2	2.3
Nonprescription medical equipment and supplies	. . .	—	—	11.7	3.8	1.4	0.7	0.3	1.3

The upper portion of Table 9.2 shows the change in prices in a different way—it provides the CPI figure (price level) for each year shown rather than the average annual percent of change from previous years given in the table. The CPI figure is computed by the U.S. Bureau of Labor Statistics (BLS). It is based on the average price of goods and services for the 36-month period covering 1982, 1983, and 1984, which the BLS sets to equal 100.

TABLE 9.2

Consumer price index and average annual percentage change for general items and medical care components, selected years 1960–2009

[CONTINUED]

[Data are based on reporting by samples of providers and other retail outlets]

—Data not available.
. . .Category not applicable.
^aDecember 1986 = 100.
^bDecember 1996 = 100.
^cSpecial index based on a substantially smaller sample.
^dDecember 2005 = 100.
^ePrior to 2006, this category included medical supplies.
Notes: CPI for all urban consumers (CPI-U) U.S. city average, detailed expenditure categories. 1982–1984 = 100, except where noted. Data are not seasonally adjusted.

SOURCE: "Table 123. Consumer Price Index and Average Annual Percent Change for All Items, Selected Items, and Medical Care Components: United States, Selected Years 1960–2009," in *Health, United States, 2010: With Special Feature on Death and Dying*, Centers for Disease Control and Prevention, National Center for Health Statistics, 2011, http://www.cdc.gov/nchs/data/hus/hus10.pdf (accessed February 1, 2012)

(These years are not shown in the top portion of Table 9.2.) Each year, the BLS measures changes in prices in relation to that figure of 100. The resultant figures show the change in relation to the reference years of 1982 to 1984. Thus, the years before the 1982–84 period have price levels below 100, and the years after this period have price levels above 100. For example, an index of 110 means there has been a 10% increase in price since the start of the reference period. "All items" cost slightly more than twice as much in 2009 than they did during the 1982–84 period (214.5 versus 100), whereas medical care cost over three and half times as much (375.6 versus 100).

So where did all the money spent on health care in 2010 come from? Fifty-one percent came from private funds, including private health insurance (33%), out-of-pocket expenses (12%), and other private investment (6%). (See Figure 9.1.) The remaining 49% came from federal or state government sources.

Where did all the money spent on health care in 2010 go? Hospital care and physicians and clinics, which traditionally account for the greatest part of health care expenses, were 31% and 20%, respectively, whereas prescription drugs were 10% of all health care expenses. (See Figure 9.2.) The remaining expenses were nursing care facilities and continuing care retirement communities (6%), government administration and net cost of health insurance (7%), dental services and other professionals (7%), and a composite spending category called "other" (14%). This category includes expenses such as home health care and other medical products (equipment prescribed by physicians for therapeutic home use).

HOW MANY AMERICANS HAVE HEALTH CARE COVERAGE?

One important aspect of the 2010 health care reform legislation was universal health care. Universal health care means health insurance coverage for all residents of a country except those who are not eligible, such as people from foreign countries who have no legal status in the country or those who have not yet met residency requirements (lived in the country long enough to be eligible). Universal health care is typical in all industrialized countries except the United States and exists in many developing countries. However, starting in 2014 the United States will begin operating a universal health care insurance system. As with some countries with universal health care, the U.S. plan will operate with both public and private insurance and medical providers and will be driven by an insurance mandate.

Prior to universal health care in the United States, how many Americans had health insurance coverage? Frank Newport of the Gallup Organization reports in *Health Insurance Coverage Varies Widely by Age and Income* (February 22, 2010, http://www.gallup.com/poll/126143/Health-Insurance-Coverage-Varies-Widely-Age-Income.aspx) that coverage varied widely by age and income in 2009. Many individuals in their late teens to early 20s were covered by their families' health insurance policies, so 75% to 90% of those individuals were covered. Aside from that, health care coverage generally rose with income and with age, rising sharply when Medicare provided medical coverage, generally at age 65.

Only about 50% of individuals in their 20s and 30s who made less than $24,000 per year had health insurance in 2009. (See Figure 9.3.) Approximately 65% to 75% of individuals in that age group who had annual incomes of $24,000 to less than $48,000 had health insurance, and 80% to 95% of individuals in that age group who had annual incomes of $48,000 or more had health insurance. Individuals in their 40s and 50s had higher rates of insurance coverage but showed a similar pattern by income, with approximately 55% to 65% of individuals in that age group in the lowest salary range having health care insurance. Approximately 75% to 85% of individuals in that same age group but in the middle income range ($24,000 to just under $48,000 per year) had health insurance, and about 95% of those in the upper income range ($48,000 per year or more) had health insurance.

FIGURE 9.1

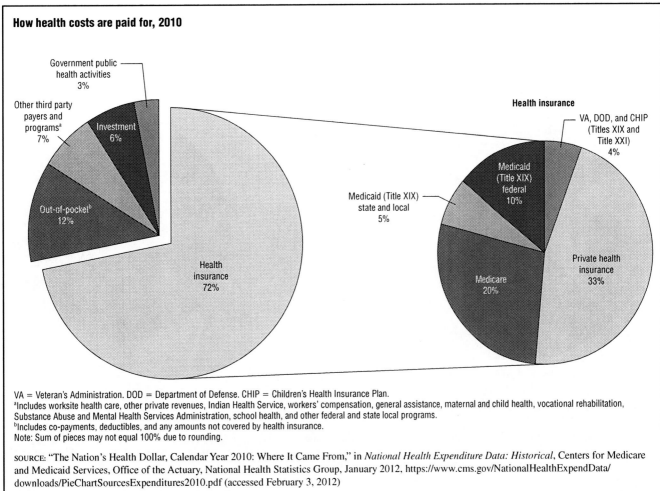

How health costs are paid for, 2010

Government public health activities 3%

Other third party payers and programs[a] 7%

Investment 6%

Out-of-pocket[b] 12%

Health insurance 72%

Health insurance

VA, DOD, and CHIP (Titles XIX and Title XXI) 4%

Medicaid (Title XIX) federal 10%

Medicaid (Title XIX) state and local 5%

Private health insurance 33%

Medicare 20%

VA = Veteran's Administration. DOD = Department of Defense. CHIP = Children's Health Insurance Plan.
[a]Includes worksite health care, other private revenues, Indian Health Service, workers' compensation, general assistance, maternal and child health, vocational rehabilitation, Substance Abuse and Mental Health Services Administration, school health, and other federal and state local programs.
[b]Includes co-payments, deductibles, and any amounts not covered by health insurance.
Note: Sum of pieces may not equal 100% due to rounding.

SOURCE: "The Nation's Health Dollar, Calendar Year 2010: Where It Came From," in *National Health Expenditure Data: Historical*, Centers for Medicare and Medicaid Services, Office of the Actuary, National Health Statistics Group, January 2012, https://www.cms.gov/NationalHealthExpendData/downloads/PieChartSourcesExpenditures2010.pdf (accessed February 3, 2012)

GOVERNMENT HEALTH CARE PROGRAMS

Two government entitlement programs that provide health care coverage for older adults (people aged 65 years and older), the poor, and the disabled are Medicare and Medicaid. Enacted in 1965 as amendments to the Social Security Act of 1935, these programs went into effect in 1966. In 1972 amendments to Medicare extended medical insurance coverage to those disabled long term and to those with chronic kidney disease or end-stage renal disease. In 2008, 45.2 million older adults were enrolled in Medicare, with total expenditures of $468.1 billion. (See Table 9.3.) That same year 58.2 million poor and disabled people were beneficiaries of Medicaid, with total payments of $294.2 billion. (See Table 9.4.)

Medicare

THE ORIGINAL MEDICARE PLAN. The Original Medicare Plan, which was enacted under Title XVIII of the Social Security Act, consists of two health-related insurance plans for adults aged 65 years and older, those under the age of 65 years with certain disabilities, and people of any age with end-stage renal disease:

- Part A (hospital insurance) is funded by Social Security payroll taxes. It pays for inpatient hospital care, which includes physicians' fees, nursing services, meals, a semiprivate room, special care units, operating room costs, laboratory tests, and some prescription drugs and supplies. It also pays for skilled nursing facility care after hospitalization, home health care visits by nurses or medical technicians, and hospice care for the terminally ill. (Skilled nursing facilities are those in which registered nurses provide care for residents 24 hours per day. These facilities are nursing homes that are certified to participate in and be reimbursed by Medicare.) Table 9.3 shows that in 2008, 44.9 million Americans were enrolled in Part A, hospital insurance. Of the $468.1 billion in total Medicare expenditures, $235.6 billion (50.3%) was spent on Medicare hospital insurance-covered expenses.

- Part B (medical insurance) is an elective medical insurance. Because Part A does not pay all health care costs and other expenses that are associated with hospitalization, many beneficiaries enroll in the Part B plan. Most people pay a monthly premium for this coverage. These monthly premiums and general

FIGURE 9.2

Health care expenses, 2010

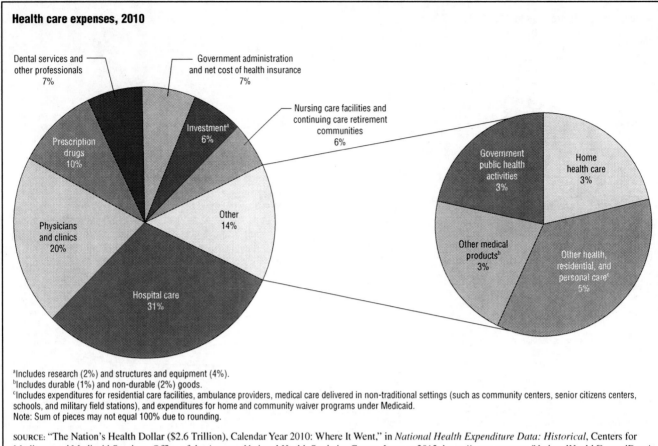

Dental services and
other professionals
7%

Government administration
and net cost of health insurance
7%

Nursing care facilities and
continuing care retirement
communities
6%

Investmentᵃ
6%

Prescription
drugs
10%

Physicians
and clinics
20%

Other
14%

Hospital care
31%

Government
public health
activities
3%

Home
health care
3%

Other medical
productsᵇ
3%

Other health,
residential, and
personal careᶜ
5%

ᵃIncludes research (2%) and structures and equipment (4%).
ᵇIncludes durable (1%) and non-durable (2%) goods.
ᶜIncludes expenditures for residential care facilities, ambulance providers, medical care delivered in non-traditional settings (such as community centers, senior citizens centers, schools, and military field stations), and expenditures for home and community waiver programs under Medicaid.
Note: Sum of pieces may not equal 100% due to rounding.

SOURCE: "The Nation's Health Dollar ($2.6 Trillion), Calendar Year 2010: Where It Went," in *National Health Expenditure Data: Historical*, Centers for Medicare and Medicaid Services, Office of the Actuary, National Health Statistics Group, January 2012, https://www.cms.gov/NationalHealthExpendData/downloads/PieChartSourcesExpenditures2010.pdf (accessed February 3, 2012)

FIGURE 9.3

Health insurance coverage, by age and income, 2009

DO YOU HAVE HEALTH INSURANCE? PERCENTAGE WHO RESPONDED "YES."

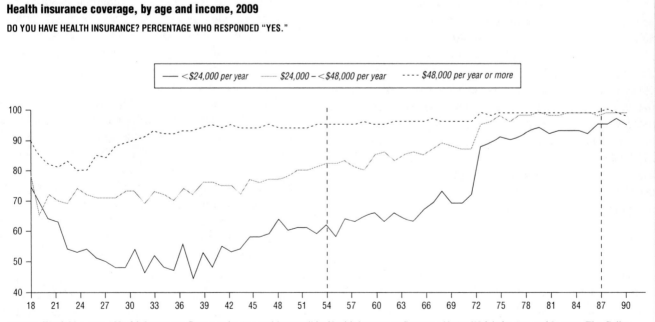

—— <$24,000 per year ········· $24,000 – <$48,000 per year ----- $48,000 per year or more

SOURCE: Frank Newport, "Health Insurance Coverage by Age and Income," in *Health Insurance Coverage Varies Widely by Age and Income*, The Gallup Organization, February 22, 2010, http://www.gallup.com/poll/126143/Health-Insurance-Coverage-Varies-Widely-Age-Income.aspx (accessed February 3, 2012). Copyright © 2010 by The Gallup Organization. Reproduced by permission of The Gallup Organization.

TABLE 9.3

Medicare enrollees and expenditures, by Medicare program and type of service, selected years 1970–2008

[Data are compiled from various sources by the Centers for Medicare & Medicaid Services]

Medicare program and type of service	1970	1980	1990	1995	2000	2003	2004	2005	2006	2007	2008[a]
Enrollees						Number in millions					
Total Medicare[b]	20.4	28.4	34.3	37.6	39.7	41.2	41.9	42.6	43.4	44.3	45.2
Hospital insurance	20.1	28.0	33.7	37.2	39.3	40.7	41.5	42.2	43.1	43.9	44.9
Supplementary medical insurance (SMI)[c]	19.5	27.3	32.6	35.6	37.3	38.6	—	—	—	—	—
Part B	19.5	27.3	32.6	35.6	37.3	38.6	39.1	39.8	40.4	41.1	41.7
Part D[d]	—	—	—	—	—	—	1.2	1.8	27.0	30.8	32.1
Expenditures						Amount in billions					
Total Medicare	$ 7.5	$ 36.8	$ 111.0	$184.2	$221.8	$280.8	$308.9	$336.4	$408.3	$431.7	$468.1
Total hospital insurance (HI)	5.3	25.6	67.0	117.6	131.1	154.6	170.6	182.9	191.9	203.1	235.6
HI payments to managed care organizations[e]	—	0.0	2.7	6.7	21.4	19.5	20.8	24.9	32.9	39.0	50.6
HI payments for fee-for-service utilization	5.1	25.0	63.4	109.5	105.1	134.5	146.5	156.6	159.6	163.4	172.8
Inpatient hospital	4.8	24.1	56.9	82.3	87.1	109.1	117.0	123.2	124.1	124.2	130.5
Skilled nursing facility	0.2	0.4	2.5	9.1	11.1	14.8	17.2	19.4	20.3	22.5	24.2
Home health agency	0.1	0.5	3.7	16.2	4.0	4.9	5.4	6.0	5.9	6.2	6.6
Hospice	—	—	0.3	1.9	2.9	5.7	6.8	8.0	9.3	10.5	11.7
Home health agency transfer[f]	—	—	—	—	1.7	−2.2	—	—	—	—	—
Medicare advantage premiums[g]	—	—	—	—	—	—	—	—	0.0	0.1	0.9
Accounting error (CY 2005–2008)[h]	—	—	—	—	—	—	—	−1.9	−3.9	−2.7	8.5
Administrative expenses[i]	0.2	0.5	0.9	1.4	2.9	2.8	3.3	3.3	3.3	3.2	3.6
Total supplementary medical insurance (SMI)[c]	2.2	11.2	44.0	66.6	90.7	126.1	138.3	153.5	216.4	228.6	232.6
Total part B	2.2	11.2	44.0	66.6	90.7	126.1	137.9	152.4	169.0	178.9	183.3
Part B payments to managed care organizations[e]	0.0	0.2	2.8	6.6	18.4	17.3	18.7	22.0	31.5	38.9	47.6
Part B payments for fee-for-service utilization[j]	1.9	10.4	39.6	58.4	72.2	104.3	116.2	125.0	130.2	134.6	141.0
Physician/supplies[k]	1.8	8.2	29.6	—	—	—	—	—	—	—	—
Outpatient hospital[l]	0.1	1.9	8.5	—	—	—	—	—	—	—	—
Independent laboratory[m]	0.0	0.1	1.5	—	—	—	—	—	—	—	—
Physician fee schedule	—	—	—	31.7	37.0	48.3	54.1	57.7	58.2	58.9	60.8
Durable medical equipment	—	—	—	3.7	4.7	7.5	7.7	8.0	8.3	8.1	8.9
Laboratory[n]	—	—	—	4.3	4.0	5.5	6.1	6.3	6.7	7.1	7.3
Other[o]	—	—	—	9.9	13.6	22.6	25.0	26.7	28.0	28.9	30.2
Hospital[p]	—	—	—	8.7	8.4	15.3	17.4	19.2	21.3	22.4	23.8
Home health agency	0.0	0.2	0.1	0.2	4.5	5.1	5.9	7.1	7.8	9.2	10.0
Home health agency transfer[f]	—	—	—	—	−1.7	2.2	—	—	—	—	—
Medicare advantage premiums	—	—	—	—	—	—	—	—	0.0	0.1	0.1
Accounting error (CY 2005–2008)[h]	—	—	—	—	—	—	—	1.9	3.9	2.7	−8.5
Administrative expenses[i]	0.2	0.6	1.5	1.6	1.8	2.4	2.8	2.6	2.9	2.5	3.0
Part D start-up costs[q]	—	—	—	—	—	—	0.2	0.7	0.2	0.0	0.0
Total part D[d]	—	—	—	—	—	—	0.4	1.1	47.4	49.7	49.3
						Percent distribution of expenditures					
Total hospital insurance (HI)	100.0	100.0	100.0	100.0	100.0	100.0	100.0	100.0	100.0	100.0	100.0
HI payments to managed care organizations[e]	—	0.0	4.0	5.7	16.3	12.6	12.2	13.6	17.2	19.2	21.5
HI payments for fee-for-service utilization	97.0	97.9	94.6	93.1	80.2	87.0	85.9	85.6	83.2	80.5	73.4
Inpatient hospital	91.4	94.3	85.0	70.0	66.4	70.6	68.6	67.4	64.6	61.2	55.4
Skilled nursing facility	4.7	1.5	3.7	7.8	8.5	9.6	10.1	10.6	10.6	11.1	10.3
Home health agency	1.0	2.1	5.5	13.8	3.1	3.1	3.2	3.3	3.1	3.1	2.8
Hospice	—	—	0.5	1.6	2.2	3.7	4.0	4.4	4.9	5.2	5.0
Home health agency transfer[f]	—	—	—	—	1.3	−1.4	—	—	—	—	—
Medicare advantage premiums[g]	—	—	—	—	—	—	—	—	0.0	0.0	0.4
Accounting error (CY 2005–2008)[h]	—	—	—	—	—	—	—	−1.0	−2.0	−1.3	3.6
Administrative expenses[i]	3.0	2.1	1.4	1.2	2.2	1.8	2.0	1.8	1.7	1.6	1.5
Total supplementary medical insurance (SMI)[c]	100.0	100.0	100.0	100.0	100.0	100.0	100.0	100.0	100.0	100.0	100.0

federal revenues finance Part B. Coverage includes physicians' and surgeons' services, diagnostic and laboratory tests, outpatient hospital services, outpatient physical therapy, speech pathology services, home health care services, and medical equipment and supplies. Table 9.3 shows that in 2008, 41.7 million Americans were enrolled in Part B. Of the $468.1 billion in total Medicare expenditures, $183.3 billion (39.2%) was spent on Medicare medical insurance-covered expenses.

MEDICARE SUPPLEMENT INSURANCE (MEDIGAP). The Original Medicare Plan coverage (Part A and Part B) has gaps, which means that it does not cover all medical costs and services. Medigap insurance is supplemental Medicare insurance that pays these expenses. Medigap is not a way to get Medicare benefits; rather, it is extra insurance sold by private insurance companies to those who have Original Medicare Plan coverage. There are 14 standardized plans labeled Plan A through Plan N. According to the Centers for Medicare and Medicaid Services, in *Choosing a Medigap Policy: A Guide to Health Insurance for People with Medicare* (2012, http://www.medicare.gov/Publications/Pubs/pdf/02110.pdf), as of June 1, 2010, only 10 of the plans could be purchased (Plans

TABLE 9.3

Medicare enrollees and expenditures, by Medicare program and type of service, selected years 1970–2008 [CONTINUED]

[Data are compiled from various sources by the Centers for Medicare & Medicaid Services]

Medicare program and type of service	1970	1980	1990	1995	2000	2003	2004	2005	2006	2007	2008[a]
					Percent distribution of expenditures						
Total part B	100.0	100.0	100.0	100.0	100.0	100.0	99.7	99.3	78.1	78.3	78.8
Part B payments to managed care organizations[e]	1.2	1.8	6.4	9.9	20.2	13.7	13.5	14.3	14.5	17.0	20.5
Part B payments for fee-for-service utilization[j]	88.1	92.8	90.1	87.6	79.6	82.7	84.0	81.5	60.2	58.9	60.6
Physician/supplies[k]	80.9	72.8	67.3	—	—	—	—	—	—	—	—
Outpatient hospital[l]	5.2	16.9	19.3	—	—	—	—	—	—	—	—
Independent laboratory[m]	0.5	1.0	3.4	—	—	—	—	—	—	—	—
Physician fee schedule	—	—	—	47.5	40.8	38.3	39.1	37.6	26.9	25.7	26.1
Durable medical equipment	—	—	—	5.5	5.2	6.0	5.6	5.2	3.8	3.5	3.8
Laboratory[n]	—	—	—	6.4	4.4	4.3	4.4	4.1	3.1	3.1	3.2
Other[o]	—	—	—	14.8	15.0	17.9	18.1	17.4	13.0	12.7	13.0
Hospital[p]	—	—	—	13.0	9.3	12.1	12.6	12.5	9.8	9.8	10.2
Home health agency	1.5	2.1	0.2	0.3	4.9	4.0	4.2	4.6	3.6	4.0	4.3
Home health agency transfer[f]	—	—	—	—	−1.9	1.7	—	—	—	—	—
Medicare advantage premiums[g]	—	—	—	—	—	—	—	—	0.0	0.0	0.0
Accounting error (CY 2005–2008)[h]	—	—	—	—	—	—	—	1.2	1.8	1.2	−3.6
Administrative expenses[i]	10.7	5.4	3.5	2.4	2.0	1.9	2.0	1.7	1.3	1.1	1.3
Part D start-up costs[q]							0.1	0.4	0.1	0.0	0.0
Total part D[d]	—	—	—	—	—	—	0.3	0.7	21.9	21.7	21.2

—Category not applicable or data not available.

CY = Calendar year.

0.0 Quantity greater than 0 but less than 0.05.

[a]Preliminary estimates.

[b]Average number enrolled in the hospital insurance (HI) and/or supplementary medical insurance (SMI) programs for the period.

[c]Starting with 2004 data, the SMI trust fund consists of two separate accounts: Part B (which pays for a portion of the costs of physicians' services, outpatient hospital services, and other related medical and health services for voluntarily enrolled individuals) and Part D (Medicare Prescription Drug Account, which pays private plans to provide prescription drug coverage).

[d]The Medicare Modernization Act, enacted on December 8, 2003, established within SMI two Part D accounts related to prescription drug benefits: the Medicare Prescription Drug Account and the Transitional Assistance Account. The Medicare Prescription Drug Account is used in conjunction with the broad, voluntary prescription drug benefits that began in 2006. The Transitional Assistance Account was used to provide transitional assistance benefits, beginning in 2004 and extending through 2005, for certain low-income beneficiaries prior to the start of the new prescription drug benefit. The amounts shown for Total Part D expenditures—and thus for total SMI expenditures and total Medicare expenditures—for 2006 and later years include estimated amounts for premiums paid directly from Part D beneficiaries to Part D prescription drug plans.

[e]Medicare-approved managed care organizations.

[f]For 1998 to 2003 data, reflects annual home health HI to SMI transfer amounts.

[g]When a beneficiary chooses a Medicare Advantage plan whose monthly premium exceeds the benchmark amount, the additional premiums (that is, amounts beyond those paid by Medicare to the plan) are the responsibility of the beneficiary. Beneficiaries subject to such premiums may choose to either reimburse the plans directly or have the additional premiums deducted from their Social Security checks. The amounts shown here are only those additional premiums deducted from Social Security checks. These amounts are transferred to the HI trust and SMI trust funds and then transferred from the trust funds to the plans.

[h]Represents misallocation of benefit payments between the HI trust fund and the Part B account of the SMI trust fund from May 2005 to September 2007, and the transfer made in June 2008 to correct the misallocation.

[i]Includes expenditures for research, experiments and demonstration projects, peer review activity (performed by Peer Review Organizations from 1983 to 2001 and by Quality Review Organizations from 2002 to present), and to combat and prevent fraud and abuse.

[j]Type-of-service reporting categories for fee-for-service reimbursement differ before and after 1991.

[k]Includes payment for physicians, practitioners, durable medical equipment, and all suppliers other than independent laboratory through 1990. Starting with 1991 data, physician services subject to the physician fee schedule are shown. Payments for laboratory services paid under the laboratory fee schedule and performed in a physician office are included under Laboratory beginning in 1991. Payments for durable medical equipment are shown separately beginning in 1991. The remaining services from the Physician/supplies category are included in Other.

[l]Includes payments for hospital outpatient department services, skilled nursing facility outpatient services, Part B services received as an inpatient in a hospital or skilled nursing facility setting, and other types of outpatient facilities. Starting with 1991 data, payments for hospital outpatient department services, except for laboratory services, are listed under Hospital. Hospital outpatient laboratory services are included in the Laboratory line.

[m]Starting with 1991 data, those independent laboratory services that were paid under the laboratory fee schedule (most of the independent lab category) are included in the Laboratory line; the remaining services are included in the Physician fee schedule and Other lines.

[n]Payments for laboratory services paid under the laboratory fee schedule performed in a physician office, independent lab, or in a hospital outpatient department.

[o]Includes payments for physician-administered drugs; freestanding ambulatory surgical center facility services; ambulance services; supplies; freestanding end-stage renal disease (ESRD) dialysis facility services; rural health clinics; outpatient rehabilitation facilities; psychiatric hospitals; and federally qualified health centers.

[p]Includes the hospital facility costs for Medicare Part B services that are predominantly in the outpatient department, with the exception of hospital outpatient laboratory services, which are included on the Laboratory line. Physician reimbursement is included on the Physician fee schedule line.

[q]Part D start-up costs were funded through the SMI Part B account in 2004–2008.

Notes: All data shown are estimates and are subject to revision. Percents may not sum to totals because of rounding. Estimates for Medicare-covered services furnished to Medicare enrollees residing in the United States, Puerto Rico, Virgin Islands, Guam, other outlying areas, foreign countries, and unknown residence. Estimates in this table have been revised and differ from previous editions of *Health, United States*.

SOURCE: "Table 140. Medicare Enrollees and Expenditures and Percent Distribution, by Medicare Program and Type of Service: United States and Other Areas, Selected Years 1970–2008," in *Health, United States, 2010: With Special Feature on Death and Dying*, Centers for Disease Control and Prevention, National Center for Health Statistics, 2011, http://www.cdc.gov/nchs/data/hus/hus10.pdf (accessed February 1, 2012)

A, B, C, D, F, G, K, L, M, and N). Even though some plans were not available to purchase after June 1, 2010, people already subscribed to those plans were able to keep them. Also, Medigap Plans D and G purchased after June 1, 2010, have different benefits from Plans D and G that were purchased before June 1, 2010. Medigap policies only work with the Original Medicare Plan.

MEDICARE ADVANTAGE PLANS (PART C). Medicare Advantage Plans are offered by private companies that have contracts with Medicare to provide Medicare Part

TABLE 9.4

Medicaid recipients and medical vendor payments, by eligibility, race, and ethnicity, selected fiscal years 1999–2008

[Data are compiled by the Centers for Medicare and Medicaid Services from the Medicaid Data System]

Basis of eligibility and race and Hispanic origin	1999	2000	2002	2003	2004	2005	2006	2007	2008
Beneficiaries[a]					Number in millions				
All beneficiaries	40.1	42.8	49.3	52.0	55.6	57.3	57.8	56.8	58.2
					Percent of beneficiaries				
Basis of eligibility:									
Aged (65 years and over)	9.4	8.7	7.9	7.8	7.8	7.6	7.6	7.1	7.1
Blind and disabled	16.7	16.1	15.0	14.8	14.6	14.2	14.4	14.8	14.8
Adults in families with dependent children[b]	18.7	20.5	22.8	22.5	22.5	21.7	21.9	21.8	22.0
Children under age 21[c]	46.9	46.1	47.1	47.8	47.8	47.2	48.0	48.4	47.8
Other Title XIX[d]	8.4	8.6	7.2	7.2	7.3	9.2	8.1	7.8	8.4
Race and Hispanic origin:[e]									
White	—	—	40.9	41.2	41.1	39.1	39.1	38.6	38.0
Black or African American	—	—	22.8	22.4	22.1	21.6	21.8	21.6	21.3
American Indian or Alaska Native	—	—	1.3	1.4	1.3	1.2	1.2	1.2	1.3
Asian or Pacific Islander	—	—	3.4	3.3	3.3	3.5	3.5	3.5	3.3
Hispanic or Latino	—	—	19.0	19.3	19.4	20.7	21.0	21.6	21.8
Multiple race or unknown	—	—	12.6	12.5	12.7	13.9	13.3	13.5	14.4
Payments[f]					Amount in billions				
All payments	$153.5	$168.3	$213.5	$233.2	$257.7	$273.2	$269.0	$276.2	$294.2
					Percent distribution				
Total	**100.0**	**100.0**	**100.0**	**100.0**	**100.0**	**100.0**	**100.0**	**100.0**	**100.0**
Basis of eligibility:									
Aged (65 years and over)	27.7	26.4	24.4	23.7	23.1	23.0	21.6	20.7	20.7
Blind and disabled	42.9	43.2	43.3	43.7	43.3	43.4	43.3	43.3	43.6
Adults in families with dependent children[b]	10.3	10.6	11.0	11.5	12.0	11.8	12.3	12.4	12.7
Children under age 21[c]	15.7	15.9	16.8	17.1	17.2	17.1	18.8	19.4	19.3
Other Title XIX[d]	3.4	3.9	4.5	4.0	4.5	4.6	3.9	4.2	3.9
Race and Hispanic origin:[e]									
White	—	—	54.1	53.8	53.4	52.7	52.1	50.7	50.2
Black or African American	—	—	19.6	19.7	19.8	20.0	20.4	20.8	20.8
American Indian or Alaska Native	—	—	1.1	1.2	1.2	1.2	1.2	1.2	1.3
Asian or Pacific Islander	—	—	2.8	2.4	2.5	2.7	2.8	2.8	2.7
Hispanic or Latino	—	—	9.7	10.6	10.7	12.2	12.8	13.1	13.7
Multiple race or unknown	—	—	12.6	12.2	12.3	11.2	10.8	11.4	11.3
Payments per beneficiary[f]					Amount				
All beneficiaries	$3,819	$3,936	$4,328	$4,487	$4,639	$4,764	$4,657	$4,862	$5,051
Basis of eligibility:									
Aged (65 years and over)	11,268	11,929	13,370	13,677	13,687	14,402	13,276	14,141	14,766
Blind and disabled	9,832	10,559	12,470	13,303	13,714	14,536	13,982	14,194	14,839
Adults in families with dependent children[b]	2,104	2,030	2,093	2,292	2,471	2,585	2,622	2,753	2,912
Children under age 21[c]	1,282	1,358	1,545	1,606	1,664	1,729	1,825	1,951	2,036
Other Title XIX[d]	1,532	1,778	2,718	2,474	2,896	2,383	2,255	2,622	2,335
Race and Hispanic origin:[e]									
White	—	—	5,721	5,870	6,026	6,429	6,199	6,390	6,674
Black or African American	—	—	3,733	3,944	4,158	4,398	4,358	4,669	4,929
American Indian or Alaska Native	—	—	3,774	4,001	4,320	4,627	4,489	4,826	5,229
Asian or Pacific Islander	—	—	3,562	3,327	3,513	3,712	3,696	3,863	4,120
Hispanic or Latino	—	—	2,215	2,463	2,563	2,822	2,831	2,960	3,177
Multiple race or unknown	—	—	4,338	4,396	4,493	3,816	3,770	4,106	3,979

—Data not available.

[a]Beneficiaries include Medicaid enrollees who received services and those enrolled in managed care plans.

[b]Includes adults who meet the requirements for the Aid to Families with Dependent Children (AFDC) program that were in effect in their state on July 16, 1996, or, at state option, more liberal criteria (with some exceptions). Includes adults in the Temporary Assistance for Needy Families (TANF) program. Starting with 2001 data, includes women in the Breast and Cervical Cancer Prevention and Treatment Program and unemployed adults.

[c]Includes children (including those in the foster care system) in the TANF program.

[d]Includes some participants in the Supplemental Security Income program and other people deemed medically needy in participating states. Prior to 2001, includes unemployed adults. Excludes foster care children and includes unknown eligibility.

[e]Race and Hispanic origin are as determined on initial Medicaid application. Categories are mutually exclusive. Starting with 2001 data, the Hispanic category included Hispanic persons, regardless of race. Persons indicating more than one race were included in the multiple race category.

[f]Medicaid payments exclude disproportionate share hospital (DSH) payments ($10.7 billion in fiscal year 2008) and DSH mental health facility payments ($1.9 billion in fiscal year 2008).

Notes: Data are for fiscal year ending September 30. Hawaii and Utah had not reported 2008 data as of the date accessed. Some data have been revised and differ from previous editions of *Health, United States*.

SOURCE: "Table 143. Medicaid Beneficiaries and Payments, by Basis of Eligibility, and Race and Hispanic Origin: United States, Selected Fiscal Years 1999–2008," in *Health, United States, 2010: With Special Feature on Death and Dying*, Centers for Disease Control and Prevention, National Center for Health Statistics, 2011, http://www.cdc.gov/nchs/data/hus/hus10.pdf (accessed February 1, 2012)

A, Part B, and possibly other Medicare services, such as prescription drug coverage. A Medigap policy is not needed with a Medicare Advantage Plan. Even though there are generally lower co-payments (the amounts patients pay for each medical service) and extra benefits with Medicare Advantage Plans versus the Original Medicare Plan, patients must typically see physicians who belong to the plan and go to certain hospitals to get services. Medicare Advantage Plans include Medicare Health Maintenance Organizations, Medicare Preferred Provider Organizations, Medicare Special Needs Plans (designed for specific groups of people), and Medicare Private Fee-for-Service Plans.

OTHER MEDICARE HEALTH PLANS. Other types of Medicare Health Plans include Medicare Cost Plans, Demonstrations, and Programs of All-inclusive Care for the Elderly (PACE). Medicare Cost Plans are limited in number and combine features of both Medicare Advantage Plans and the Original Medicare Plan. Demonstrations are special projects that test possible future improvements in Medicare costs, coverage, and quality of care. PACE provides services for frail elderly Americans.

MEDICARE PRESCRIPTION DRUG PLANS (PART D). On January 1, 2006, Medicare began providing insurance coverage for prescription drugs to everyone with Medicare. Its Medicare Prescription Drug Plans typically pay half a person's prescription drug costs. Most people pay a monthly premium for this coverage. Medicare Prescription Drug Plans are available with the Original Medicare Plan, Medicare Advantage Plans, and the other Medicare Health Plans. Table 9.3 shows that in 2008, 32.1 million Americans were enrolled in Part D (prescription drug plans). Of the $468.1 billion in total Medicare expenditures, $49.3 billion (10.5%) was spent on Part D prescription drug expenses.

Medicaid and the State Children's Health Insurance Program

The Medicaid health insurance program, which was enacted under Title XIX of the Social Security Act, provides medical assistance to low-income people, including those with disabilities and members of families with dependent children. The 2010 health care reform legislation expanded the eligibility for Medicaid to everyone under the age of 65 years who has an income (or, if children, whose family has an income) at or below 133% of the federal poverty level. Previously, adults under the age of 65 years who were neither disabled nor pregnant and had no children did not qualify for Medicaid. Children aged one to six years were covered if their family income was below 133% of the federal poverty threshold, but children aged seven to 19 years were covered only if their family income was below 100% of the federal poverty threshold. The coverage for adults with children

varied by state. Jointly financed by federal and state governments, Medicaid coverage includes hospitalization, physicians' services, laboratory fees, diagnostic screenings, and long-term nursing home care.

In 1997 Congress built on Medicaid by enacting the State Children's Health Insurance Program. The intent of the program is to provide medical insurance coverage for children of low-income families who are uninsured but who do not qualify for Medicaid. In February 2009 President Obama signed a bill that reauthorized the program and expanded its coverage so that more children can be covered.

Even though people aged 65 years and older made up only 7.1% of all Medicaid recipients in 2008, they received 20.7% of all Medicaid benefits. (See Table 9.4.) The average payment was $14,766 per older adult, compared with $14,839 for the blind and disabled, $2,912 for adults in families with dependent children, and $2,036 for children under the age of 21 years.

WHO PAYS FOR END-OF-LIFE CARE?

Sherry L. Murphy, Jiaquan Xu, and Kenneth D. Kochanek reveal in "Deaths: Preliminary Data for 2010" (*National Vital Statistics Reports*, vol. 60, no. 4, January 11, 2012) that 72.8% of those who died in 2010 were aged 65 years and older. Medicare covers the medical expenses of these older adults during the terminal stage of their life. Medicaid also covers older adults who have exhausted their Medicare benefits, as well as poor and disabled younger patients. Health programs under the U.S. Department of Veterans Affairs and the U.S. Department of Defense also pay for terminal care.

In "Long-Term Trends in Medicare Payments in the Last Year of Life" (*Health Services Research*, vol. 45, no. 2, April 2010), Gerald F. Riley and James D. Lubitz note that costs in the last year of life for Americans aged 65 years and older decreased from 28.3% in 1978 to 25.1% in 2006. Reasons for this decline may include increased hospice use, which focuses on comfort care at the end of life instead of aggressive medical treatment, and an increase in the proportion of people dying at older ages. Riley and Lubitz note that the costs are lower for people dying at older ages than for those dying at younger ages.

Riley and Lubitz determine that the relative proportions of Medicare services and expenditures during the last year of life changed between 1978 and 2006. In 1978 three-quarters (76.3%) of Medicare expenditures during the last year of life for older Americans were for inpatient hospital care, whereas in 2006 this proportion had declined to half (50.2%). In 2006 dying patients had several other options available to them for end-of-life care than simply remaining in a hospital. As expected, the proportion of expenditures for these other types of services increased from 1978. The proportion of outpatient care expenditures increased from 2.6% in 1978 to 6.8% in 2006. The proportion of hospice expenditures increased because in 1978 Medicare did not pay for hospice. In 2006 hospice care expenditures represented 9.7% of Medicare payments for older Americans who died that year. The proportion of home health care expenditures rose as well, from 1.8% in 1978 to 4.1% in 2006. The proportion of skilled nursing facility expenditures also rose, from 1.9% in 1978 to 10.4% in 2006.

No specific information about the cost of end-of-life care exists for the one-fourth of those who die every year who are under the age of 65 years. Such care is more than likely financed by employer health insurance, personal funds, Medicare, and Medicaid. Nonetheless, aside from funds that are paid out for hospice services, the government has no other information about this group's terminal health care.

Medicare Hospice Benefits

In 1982 Congress created a Medicare hospice benefit program via the Tax Equity and Fiscal Responsibility Act to provide services to terminally ill patients with six months or less to live. In 1989 the U.S. General Accounting Office (GAO; now called the U.S. Government Accountability Office) reported that only 35% of eligible hospices were Medicare certified, in part due to the Health Care Financing Administration's low rates of reimbursement to hospices. That same year Congress gave hospices a 20% increase in reimbursement rates through a provision in the Omnibus Budget Reconciliation Act.

Under the Balanced Budget Act (BBA) of 1997, Medicare hospice benefits are divided into three benefit periods:

- An initial 90-day period

- A subsequent 90-day period

- An unlimited number of subsequent 60-day periods, but only if a patient continues to satisfy the program eligibility requirements

At the start of each period the Medicare patient must be recertified as terminally ill. After the patient's death, the patient's family receives up to 13 months of bereavement counseling.

In 2009 there were 3,407 Medicare-certified hospices, which was a substantial increase from 31 hospices in 1984. (See Table 9.5.) This growth was stimulated in part by increased reimbursement rates that were established by Congress in 1989. Of the 3,407 hospices, 578 were with home health agencies, 531 were affiliated with hospitals, 20 were with skilled nursing facilities, and 2,278 were freestanding hospices. Between 2000 and 2009 the number of Medicare-certified freestanding hospices more than doubled, whereas the other types of hospice facilities decreased in number (home health agencies) or remained

TABLE 9.5

Number of Medicare-certified hospices, by type, 1984–2009

Year	HHA	HOSP	SNF	FSTG	Total
1984	n/a	n/a	n/a	n/a	31
1985	n/a	n/a	n/a	n/a	158
1986	113	54	10	68	245
1987	155	101	11	122	389
1988	213	138	11	191	553
1989	286	182	13	220	701
1990	313	221	12	260	806
1991	325	282	10	394	1,011
1992	334	291	10	404	1,039
1993	438	341	10	499	1,288
1994	583	401	12	608	1,604
1995	699	460	19	679	1,857
1996	815	526	22	791	2,154
1997	823	561	22	868	2,274
1998	763	553	21	878	2,215
1999	762	562	22	928	2,274
2000	739	554	20	960	2,273
2001	690	552	20	1003	2,265
2002	676	557	17	1,072	2,322
2003	653	561	16	1,214	2,444
2004	656	562	14	1,438	2,670
2005	672	551	13	1,648	2,884
2006	650	563	14	1,851	3,078
2007	627	562	18	2,050	3,257
2008	606	552	19	2,169	3,346
2009	578	531	20	2,278	3,407

SNF = Skilled nursing facility-based.
FSTG = Freestanding.
HHA = Home health agency-based.
HOSP = Hospital-based.
Notes: Home health agency-based hospices are owned and operated by freestanding proprietary and nonprofit home-care agencies. Hospital-based hospices are operating units or departments of a hospital.

SOURCE: "Table 1. Number of Medicare-Certified Hospices, by Auspice, 1984–2009," in *Hospice Facts & Statistics*, Hospice Association of America, September 2009, http://www.nahc.org/facts/HospiceStats09.pdf (accessed March 9, 2010). Figure updated by the National Association for Home Care & Hospice, 2010. Reproduced with the express and limited permission from the National Association for Home Care & Hospice. All rights reserved.

relatively static (hospitals and skilled nursing facilities). Medicare pays most of the cost of hospice care.

Terminally ill Medicare patients who stay in a hospice incur less Medicare costs than those who stay in a hospital or skilled nursing facility. In 2009 a one-day stay in a hospice cost Medicare $153, compared with $622 for a skilled nursing facility and $6,200 for a hospital. (See Table 9.6.)

The Hospice Association of America (HAA) contends that terminally ill patients often wait too long to enter hospice care. The HAA believes the difficulty of predicting when death may occur could account for part of the delay, as does the reticence of caregivers, patients, and family to accept a terminal prognosis.

Even though terminal care is often associated with hospice, the hospice Medicare benefit represents a small proportion of the total Medicare dollars that are spent. In fiscal year (FY) 2009, nearly $12 billion (2.8%) of the $434.5 billion in total Medicare benefit payments went to

TABLE 9.6

Comparison of hospital, skilled nursing facility, and hospice Medicare charges, 1999–2009

	1999	2000	2001	2002	2003	2004	2005	2006	2007	2008	2009
Hospital inpatient charges per day	$2,583	$2,762	$3,069	$3,574	$4,117	$4,559	$4,999	$5,475	$5,895	$6,196	$6,200
Skilled nursing facility charges per day	424	413	422	475	487	493	504	519	558	590	622
Hospice charges per covered day of care	113	112	119	125	129	132	138	141	146	150	153

Notes: Hospital data for 2008 & 2009 are updated using the Bureau of Labor Statistics' (BLS) General medical and surgical hospitals Producer Price Index (PPI). SNF data for 2006–2009 are updated using the BLS Nursing care facilities PPI. Hospice data for 2008 & 2009 are updated using the BLS Home health care services PPI. SNF = Skilled nursing facility-based.

SOURCE: "Table 24. Comparison of Hospital, SNF, and Hospice Medicare Charges, 1999–2009," in *Hospice Facts and Statistics*, Hospice Association of America, November 2010, http://www.nahc.org/facts/HospiceStats10.pdf (accessed March 3, 2012). Reproduced with the express and limited permission from the National Association for Home Care & Hospice. All rights reserved.

TABLE 9.7

Medicare benefit payments, fiscal years 2009 and 2010

	2009 (Estimated)		2010 (Projected)	
	Amount ($millions)	% of total	Amount ($millions)	% of total
Total Medicare benefit payments*	434,473	100.0	452,741	100.0
Part A				
Hospital care	132,648	30.5	136,787	30.2
Skilled nursing facility	25,760	5.9	26,268	5.8
Home health	7,152	1.6	7,484	1.7
Hospice	11,953	2.8	12,580	2.8
Managed care	56,789	13.1	60,393	13.3
Total	234,302	53.9	243,512	53.8
Part B				
Physician	62,508	14.4	58,295	12.9
Durable medical equipment	8,265	1.9	8,295	1.8
Carrier lab	4,639	1.1	5,043	1.1
Other carrier	17,168	4.0	17,614	3.9
Hospital	26,546	6.1	34,968	7.7
Home health	11,176	2.6	11,721	2.6
Intermediary lab	3,287	0.8	3,387	0.7
Other intermediary	14,414	3.3	15,023	3.3
Managed care	52,168	12.0	54,885	12.1
Total	200,170	46.1	209,229	46.2

*Figures may not add to totals due to rounding.

SOURCE: "Table 4. Medicare Benefit Payments, FY2009 and FY2010," in *Hospice Facts and Statistics*, Hospice Association of America, November 2010, http://www.nahc.org/facts/HospiceStats10.pdf (accessed March 3, 2012). Reproduced with the express and limited permission from the National Association for Home Care & Hospice. All rights reserved.

TABLE 9.8

Medicaid payments, by type of service, fiscal years 2005 and 2006

	2005 ($millions)	% of total	2006 ($millions)	% of total
Inpatient hospital	35,131.5	12.8	36,268.9	13.5
Nursing home	44,790.3	16.3	45,669.7	17.0
Physician	11,268.9	4.1	10,578.7	3.9
Outpatient hospital	10,011.9	3.6	10,165.7	3.8
Home health[c]	26,019.2	9.5	27,480.4	10.2
Hospice[b]	1,333.2	0.5	1,638.8	0.6
Prescription drugs	42,848.5	15.6	28,128.7	10.5
ICF (MR) services	11,708.7	4.3	11,850.7	4.4
Other	91,739.3	33.4	97,169.8	36.1
Total payments[a]	274,851.4	100.0	268,954.2	100.0

ICF (MR) = Intermediate Care Facilities for the Mentally Retarded.

Notes: Figures may not add to totals due to rounding.
[a]Total outlays include hospice outlays from the Form CMS-64 plus payments for all service types included in the Medicaid Statistical Information Statistics (MSIS), not just the eight service types listed.
[b]Hospice outlays come from Form CMS-64 and do not include Medicaid State Children's Health Insurance Program (SCHIP). All other expenditures come from the MSIS. The federal share of Medicaid's hospice spending in FY 2005, was $779.2 million, or 58.5% of total Medicaid hospice payments. In FY 2006, it was $958.4 million, or 58.5% of total Medicaid hospice payments.
[c]Home health includes both home health and personal support services.

SOURCE: "Table 11. Medicaid Payments, by Type of Service, FY 2005 & FY 2006," in *Hospice Facts and Statistics*, Hospice Association of America, November 2010, http://www.nahc.org/facts/HospiceStats10.pdf (accessed March 4, 2012). Reproduced with the express and limited permission from the National Association for Home Care & Hospice. All rights reserved.

hospice care. (See Table 9.7.) In FY 2010 the projected hospice spending was $12.6 billion (2.8%) of the projected $452.7 billion in total Medicare expenditures.

Medicaid Hospice Benefits

Hospice services also make up a small proportion of Medicaid reimbursements. In FY 2005 Medicaid reimbursements for hospice accounted for $1.3 billion (0.5%) of the $274.9 billion in total expenditures. (See Table 9.8.) In FY 2006 reimbursements for hospice accounted for $1.6 billion (0.6%) of the nearly $269 billion in total expenditures.

Hospice and Diagnoses

Christine Caffrey et al. show in "Home Health Care and Discharged Hospice Care Patients: United States, 2000 and 2007" (April 27, 2011, http://www.cdc.gov/nchs/data/nhsr/nhsr038.pdf) that the primary diagnosis for entering a hospice in 2007 was cancer (43.5%). (See Table 9.9.) Many had diseases of the circulatory system (15.8%) and other ill-defined conditions (12.2%). However, all-listed diagnoses at discharge, which means that the patients were often deceased, were diseases of the circulatory system (50%), cancer (46.4%), and diseases of the respiratory system (21.6%). It should be noted that there are many other diagnoses at discharge on the patient's chart. All-listed diagnoses at discharge do not

TABLE 9.9

Primary and all-listed diagnoses for annual hospice care discharges, 2007

| | Primary diagnoses[a] | | | | All-listed diagnoses[b] | |
| | At admission | | At discharge | | At discharge | |
Diagnosis	Number	Percent distribution	Number	Percent distribution	Number	Percent
Total	**1,045,100**	**100.0**	**1,045,100**	**100.0**	—	—
Infectious and parasitic diseases	6,900†	0.6†	7,100†	0.7†	37,400	3.6
Neoplasms	454,600	43.5	454,200	43.5	491,300	47.0
Malignant neoplasm	447,600	42.8	447,600	42.8	485,300	46.4
Malignant neoplasm of large intestine and rectum	47,000	4.5	46,600	4.5	52,400	5.0
Malignant neoplasm of trachea, bronchus and lung	129,000	12.3	128,700	12.3	161,400	15.4
Malignant neoplasm of bone, connective tissue and skin	15,900	1.5	15,900	1.5	38,200	3.7
Malignant neoplasm of breast	28,700	2.7	28,500	2.7	40,700	3.9
Malignant neoplasm of female genital organs	21,500	2.1	21,400	2.1	25,200	2.4
Malignant neoplasm of prostate	17,100	1.6	16,800	1.6	37,300	3.6
Malignant neoplasm of urinary organs	30,600	2.9	30,600	2.9	35,900	3.4
Malignant neoplasm of hematopoietic tissue	30,600	2.9	31,300	3.0	36,400	3.5
Malignant neoplasm of other and unspecified sites	125,700	12.0	126,000	12.1	193,500	18.5
Endocrine, nutritional, and metabolic diseases and immunity disorders	*	*	*	*	207,900	19.9
Diabetes mellitus	*	*	*	*	127,700	12.2
Diseases of the blood and blood-forming organs	*	*	*	*	70,000	6.7
Anemias	*	*	*	*	64,300	6.2
Mental disorders	69,100	6.6	70,800	6.8	234,300	22.4
Senile dementia or organic brain syndrome	*	*	*	*	14,800*	1.4*
Other mental disorders	61,900	5.9	64,000	6.1	219,400	21.0
Diseases of the nervous system and sense organs	81,400	7.8	80,200	7.7	165,700	15.9
Alzheimer's disease	40,400	3.9	39,400	3.8	64,200	6.1
Parkinson's disease	20,500†	1.9†	21,000†	2.0†	44,900	4.3
All other diseases of the nervous system and sense organs	18,600†	1.8†	18,800†	1.8†	65,100	6.2
Diseases of the circulatory system	165,100	15.8	165,700	15.9	523,000	50.0
Essential hypertension	*	*	*	*	245,500	23.5
Heart disease	115,600	11.1	117,400	11.2	336,300	32.2
Coronary atherosclerosis	*	*	*	*	22,100	2.1
Other chronic ischemic heart disease	7,700*	0.74†	8,200†	0.8†	98,500	9.4
Cardiac dysrhythmias	*	*	*	*	66,000	6.3
Congestive heart failure	66,400	6.4	65,200	6.2	161,200	15.4
Other heart disease	35,300	3.4	37,300	3.6	97,500	9.3
Cerebrovascular disease	46,800	4.5	45,100	4.3	114,000	10.9
Other diseases of the circulatory system	*	*	*	*	67,400	6.4
Diseases of the respiratory system	77,900	7.5	79,900	7.6	225,500	21.6
Pneumonia, all forms	*	*	*	*	38,200	3.7
Chronic obstructive pulmonary disease and allied conditions	49,600	4.7	51,200	4.9	154,800	14.8
Other diseases of the respiratory system	25,800	2.5	25,300	2.4	52,500	5.0
Diseases of the digestive system	18,100	1.7	17,600	1.7	120,300	11.5
Diseases of the genitourinary system	31,700	3.0	32,100	3.1	151,300	14.5
Urinary tract infection	*	*	*	*	30,000	2.9

TABLE 9.9

Primary and all-listed diagnoses for annual hospice care discharges, 2007 [CONTINUED]

| | Primary diagnoses[a] | | | | All-listed diagnoses[b] | |
| | At admission | | At discharge | | At discharge | |
Diagnosis	Number	Percent distribution	Number	Percent distribution	Number	Percent
Diseases of the musculoskeletal system and connective tissue	*	*	*	*	94,300	9.0
Other arthropathies and related disorders	*	*	*	*	26,900	2.6
Osteoporosis	*	*	*	*	25,200	2.4
Other diseases of the musculoskeletal system	*	*	*	*	19,500	1.9
Symptoms, signs, and ill-defined conditions	127,400	12.2	121,700	11.6	216,100	20.7
Injuries and poisonings	*	*	*	*	10,500†	1.0†
Supplementary classification	*	*	*	*	41,300	4.0
Posthospital aftercare	*	*	*	*	22,000	2.1

—Category not applicable.

*Estimate does not meet standards of reliability or precision because the sample size is fewer than 30.

†Estimate does not meet standards of reliability or precision because the sample size is between 30 and 59, or the sample size is greater than 59 but has a relative standard error of 30% or more.

[a]Chiefly responsible for the patient's admission to hospice care.

[b]Up to 16 diagnoses are recorded for each patient at discharge.

Note: Numbers may not add to totals, and percent distributions may not add to 100%, because of rounding and because the denominators for percent distributions may include a category of unknowns not reported in the table.

SOURCE: Christine Caffrey et al., "Table 7. Primary and All-Listed Diagnoses for Annual Hospice Care Discharges: United States, 2007," in *Home Health Care and Discharged Hospice Care Patients: United States, 2000 and 2007*, National Health Statistics Report, no. 38, April 27, 2011, http://www.cdc.gov/nchs/data/nhsr/nhsr038.pdf (accessed March 4, 2012)

add to 100%, because each discharged patient has up to 16 recorded diagnoses.

Home Health Care

The concept of home health care began as postacute care after hospitalization, an alternative to longer, costlier hospital stays. The Centers for Medicare and Medicaid Services explains in *Medicare and Home Health Care* (June 2010, http://www.medicare.gov/Publications/Pubs/pdf/10969.pdf) that in the 21st century Medicare's home health care services provide medical help, prescribed by a doctor, to home-bound people who are covered by Medicare. Having been hospitalized is not a prerequisite. There are no limits to the number of professional visits or to the length of coverage. As long as the patient's condition warrants it, the following services are provided:

- Part-time or intermittent skilled nursing and home health aide services
- Speech-language pathology services
- Physical and occupational therapy
- Medical social services
- Medical supplies
- Durable medical equipment (such as walkers and hospital beds, with a 20% co-pay)

Figure 9.4 divides the Medicare payments made between FYs 2000 and 2009 into the percentage of the total that was paid for each benefit. The percentage of home health care costs of the Medicare budget was 4.3% in FY 2000, but that percentage dropped to 3.5% by FY 2006. It rose to 4.2% by FY 2009. The number of home

FIGURE 9.4

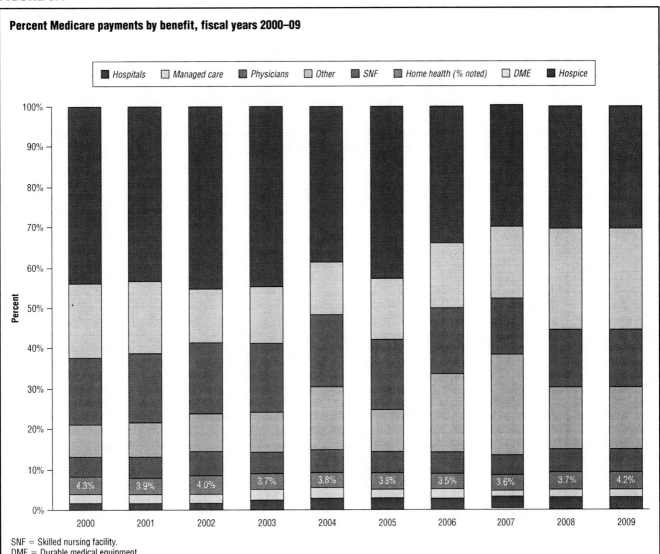

Percent Medicare payments by benefit, fiscal years 2000–09

SNF = Skilled nursing facility.
DME = Durable medical equipment.

SOURCE: "Figure 3. Percent Medicare Payments, by Benefit, Fiscal Years 2000–2009," in *Basic Statistics about Home Care 2010*, National Association for Home Care and Hospice, updated 2010, http://www.nahc.org/facts/10hc_stats.pdf (accessed March 4, 2012). Reproduced with the express and limited permission from the National Association for Home Care & Hospice. All rights reserved.

care agencies that were Medicare certified declined from a high of 10,444 in 1997 to a low of 6,861 in 2001 (excluding 1990 and previous years shown in Table 9.10, when home care was in its infancy). The number then rose to 10,581 in 2009, surpassing the 1997 figure. The National Association for Home Care and Hospice (NAHCH) believes the decline in agencies between 1997 and 2001 is the direct result of changes in Medicare home health reimbursement that were enacted as part of the BBA. The increase since 2001 is likely due to relaxed eligibility criteria for home health care, including the elimination of the requirement of an acute hospitalization before receiving home care in 2003. These relaxed criteria enabled an increased number of beneficiaries to use home health services.

LONG-TERM HEALTH CARE

Longer life spans and life-sustaining technologies have created an increasing need for long-term care. For some older people, relatives provide the long-term care; but those who require labor-intensive, round-the-clock care often stay in nursing homes.

Nursing Home Care

Growth of the home health care industry during the 1980s and early to mid-1990s was only partly responsible for the decline in the numbers of Americans entering nursing homes between 1995 and 2010. (See Table 9.11.) Nursing home declines also occurred in years when the numbers of home health care patients declined after the implementation of the BBA in 1997. Other factors responsible for the decline in the numbers of Americans entering nursing homes are that many elderly people are choosing assisted living and continuing-care retirement communities, which offer alternatives to nursing home care. There is also a trend toward healthy aging—more older adults are living longer with fewer disabilities.

Nonetheless, in 2010 nearly 1.4 million adults were nursing home residents. (See Table 9.11.) The lowest occupancy rates were in Oregon (61.8%), Oklahoma (66.5%), Indiana (67.9%), Missouri (68.3%), and Louisiana (69.8%). The states that had the highest occupancy rates were Alaska (94%), New York (92.4%), Rhode Island (91.4%), Pennsylvania (91.2%), and Minnesota (91%). The District of Columbia (93.5%) also had a high occupancy rate.

TABLE 9.10

Number of Medicare-certified home care agencies, by type, selected years, 1967–2009

Year	Freestanding agencies						Facility-based agencies			Total
	VNA	COMB	PUB	PROP	PNP	OTH	HOSP	REHAB	SNF	
1967	549	93	939	0	0	39	133	0	0	1,753
1980	515	63	1,260	186	484	40	359	8	9	2,924
1990	474	47	985	1,884	710	0	1,486	8	101	5,695
1996	576	34	1,177	4,658	695	58	2,634	4	191	10,027
1997	553	33	1,149	5,024	715	65	2,698	3	204	10,444
1998	460	35	968	3,414	610	69	2,356	2	166	8,080
1999	452	35	918	3,192	621	65	2,300	1	163	7,747
2000	436	31	909	2,863	560	56	2,151	1	150	7,152
2001	425	23	867	2,835	543	68	1,976	1	123	6,861
2002	430	27	850	3,027	563	79	1,907	1	119	7,007
2003	439	27	888	3,402	546	74	1,776	0	113	7,265
2004	446	36	932	3,832	558	69	1,695	1	110	7,679
2005	461	36	1,043	4,321	566	74	1,618	2	103	8,224
2006	459	29	1,132	4,919	562	85	1,547	2	103	8,838
2007	475	31	NA	NA	NA	NA	1,503	2	99	9,284
2008	489	37	1,273	5,849	559	92	1,425	1	99	9,824
2009	516	36	1,392	6,585	598	98	1,311	1	97	10,581

VNA: Visiting Nurse Associations are freestanding, voluntary, nonprofit organizations governed by a board of directors and usually financed by tax-deductible contributions as well as by earnings.
COMB: Combination agencies are combined government and voluntary agencies. These agencies are sometimes included with counts for VNAs.
PUB: Public agencies are government agencies operated by a state, county, city, or other unit of local government having a major responsibility for preventing disease and for community health education.
PROP: Proprietary agencies are freestanding, for-profit home care agencies.
PNP: Private not-for-profit agencies are freestanding and privately developed, governed, and owned nonprofit home care agencies. These agencies were not counted separately prior to 1980.
OTH: Other freestanding agencies that do not fit one of the categories for freestanding agencies listed above.
HOSP: Hospital-based agencies are operating units or departments of a hospital. Agencies that have working arrangements with a hospital, or perhaps are even owned by a hospital but operated as separate entities, are classified as freestanding agencies under one of the categories listed above.
REHAB: Refers to agencies based in rehabilitation facilities.
SNF: Refers to agencies based in skilled nursing facilities.

SOURCE: "Table 1. Number of Medicare-Certified Home Care Agencies, by Auspice, for Selected Years, 1967–2009," in *Basic Statistics about Home Care 2010*, National Association for Home Care and Hospice, updated 2010, http://www.nahc.org/facts/10hc_stats.pdf (accessed March 4, 2012). Data from Centers for Medicare and Medicaid Services, Center for Information Systems, Health Standards and Quality Bureau. Reproduced with the express and limited permission from the National Association for Home Care & Hospice. All rights reserved.

TABLE 9.11

Nursing homes, beds, residents, and occupancy rates, by state, 1995 and 2010

[Data are based on a census of certified nursing facilities]

State	Nursing homes 1995	Nursing homes 2010	Beds 1995	Beds 2010	Residents 1995	Residents 2010	Occupancy rates[a] 1995	Occupancy rates[a] 2010
United States	**16,389**	**15,690**	**1,751,302**	**1,703,398**	**1,479,550**	**1,396,473**	**84.5**	**82.0**
Alabama	221	227	23,353	26,656	21,691	22,968	92.9	86.2
Alaska	15	15	814	682	634	641	77.9	94.0
Arizona	152	139	16,162	16,460	12,382	11,878	76.6	72.2
Arkansas	256	232	29,952	24,548	20,823	17,864	69.5	72.8
California	1,382	1,239	140,203	121,167	109,805	102,591	78.3	84.7
Colorado	219	213	19,912	20,259	17,055	16,302	85.7	80.5
Connecticut	267	239	32,827	29,255	29,948	25,972	91.2	88.8
Delaware	42	47	4,739	4,990	3,819	4,145	80.6	83.1
District of Columbia	19	19	3,206	2,775	2,576	2,595	80.3	93.5
Florida	627	678	72,656	82,226	61,845	71,907	85.1	87.5
Georgia	352	360	38,097	39,960	35,933	34,704	94.3	86.8
Hawaii	34	48	2,513	4,303	2,413	3,880	96.0	90.2
Idaho	76	79	5,747	6,153	4,697	4,388	81.7	71.3
Illinois	827	787	103,230	101,061	83,696	75,224	81.1	74.4
Indiana	556	506	59,538	57,721	44,328	39,167	74.5	67.9
Iowa	419	443	39,959	32,842	27,506	25,463	68.8	77.5
Kansas	429	340	30,016	25,598	25,140	18,985	83.8	74.2
Kentucky	288	285	23,221	26,063	20,696	23,252	89.1	89.2
Louisiana	337	281	37,769	36,098	32,493	25,198	86.0	69.8
Maine	132	109	9,243	7,127	8,587	6,417	92.9	90.0
Maryland	218	231	28,394	29,004	24,716	24,816	87.0	85.6
Massachusetts	550	427	54,532	49,115	49,765	42,880	91.3	87.2
Michigan	432	428	49,473	47,054	43,271	39,894	87.5	84.8
Minnesota	432	385	43,865	32,339	41,163	29,434	93.8	91.0
Mississippi	183	203	16,059	18,589	15,247	16,489	94.9	88.7
Missouri	546	514	52,679	55,393	39,891	37,839	75.7	68.3
Montana	100	88	7,210	6,991	6,415	4,943	89.0	70.7
Nebraska	231	222	18,169	16,065	16,166	12,630	89.0	78.6
Nevada	42	50	3,998	5,856	3,645	4,735	91.2	80.9
New Hampshire	74	79	7,412	7,692	6,877	6,932	92.8	90.1
New Jersey	300	360	43,967	51,101	40,397	45,917	91.9	89.9
New Mexico	83	70	6,969	6,769	6,051	5,555	86.8	82.1
New York	624	635	107,750	117,984	103,409	109,044	96.0	92.4
North Carolina	391	424	38,322	44,392	35,511	37,199	92.7	83.8
North Dakota	87	85	7,125	6,438	6,868	5,629	96.4	87.4
Ohio	943	960	106,884	93,043	79,026	79,234	73.9	85.2
Oklahoma	405	314	33,918	28,932	26,377	19,227	77.8	66.5
Oregon	161	137	13,885	12,218	11,673	7,549	84.1	61.8
Pennsylvania	726	710	92,625	88,829	84,843	81,014	91.6	91.2
Rhode Island	94	86	9,612	8,802	8,823	8,043	91.8	91.4
South Carolina	166	184	16,682	19,474	14,568	17,133	87.3	88.0
South Dakota	114	110	8,296	7,932	7,926	6,497	95.5	81.9
Tennessee	322	318	37,074	37,279	33,929	31,927	91.5	85.6
Texas	1,266	1,173	123,056	130,665	89,354	91,099	72.6	69.7
Utah	91	99	7,101	8,255	5,832	5,361	82.1	64.9
Vermont	23	40	1,862	3,276	1,792	2,931	96.2	89.5
Virginia	271	286	30,070	32,152	28,119	28,314	93.5	88.1
Washington	285	229	28,464	21,837	24,954	18,065	87.7	82.7
West Virginia	129	127	10,903	10,840	10,216	9,557	93.7	88.2
Wisconsin	413	392	48,754	36,113	43,998	30,618	90.2	84.8
Wyoming	37	38	3,035	2,965	2,661	2,427	87.7	81.9

[a]Percentage of beds occupied (number of nursing home residents per 100 nursing home beds).

SOURCE: Adapted from "Table 117. Nursing Homes, Beds, Residents, and Occupancy Rates, by State: United States, Selected Years 1995–2010," in *Health, United States, 2010: With Special Feature on Death and Dying*, Centers for Disease Control and Prevention, National Center for Health Statistics, 2011, http://www.cdc.gov/nchs/data/hus/2010/117.pdf (accessed March 5, 2012). Non-government data from C. M. Cowles, ed., *2010 Nursing Home Statistical Yearbook*, Cowles Research Group, 2011 and previous editions; and Cowles Research Group, unpublished data.

Nursing homes provide terminally ill residents with end-of-life services in a variety of ways:

- Caring for patients in the nursing home

- Transferring patients who request it to hospitals or hospices

- Contracting with hospices to provide palliative care (care that relieves the pain but does not cure the illness) within the nursing home

Medicare does not pay for long-term nursing home services. It pays only for services in a skilled nursing facility for people who are recovering from medical conditions such as a hip fracture, heart attack, or stroke. Medicaid does pay for nursing home care, but only if the individual meets state income and resource requirements for Medicaid assistance. As a result, the costs are paid for by the individuals themselves or by long-term care insurance companies for their policyholders.

The End-Stage Renal Disease Program

Amendments to the Social Security Act in 1972 extended Medicare coverage to include end-stage renal disease (ESRD) patients. ESRD is the final phase of irreversible kidney disease and requires either kidney transplantation or dialysis to maintain life. Dialysis is a medical procedure in which a machine takes over the function of the kidneys by removing waste products from the blood. In 1998 and 2003 more than seven out of 10 (73% in 1998 and 71% in 2003) ESRD patients underwent dialysis and the remaining three out of 10 (27% in 1998 and 29% in 2003) had kidney transplants. (See Table 9.12.) By 2008 the percentage of those who had dialysis dropped to 70%, and the percentage of those who had transplants increased to 30%. The Medicare Payment Advisory Commission notes in *A Data Book: Health Care Spending and the Medicare Program* (June 2011, http://www.medpac.gov/documents/Jun11DataBookEntire Report.pdf) that in 2008 about one-third (34%) of the kidneys used for transplant were from live donors and about two-thirds (66%) were from cadavers.

Medicare beneficiaries with ESRD are high-cost users of Medicare services. According to the Medicare Payment Advisory Commission, patients with ESRD incurred costs that were five times greater than Medicare beneficiaries without ESRD. Between 1998 and 2008 the ESRD population grew by 55.9%. (See Table 9.12.) In 1998 there were 351,400 ESRD patients in the Medicare system, and by 2008 this figure had risen to 548,000 ESRD patients.

PATIENTS WITH TERMINAL DISEASES
Acquired Immunodeficiency Syndrome

The acquired immunodeficiency syndrome (AIDS) is a set of signs, symptoms, and certain diseases that occur together when the immune system of a person who is infected with the human immunodeficiency virus (HIV) becomes extremely weakened. According to the Centers for Disease Control and Prevention (CDC), advances in treatment during the mid- to late 1990s slowed the progression of HIV infection to AIDS, which led to dramatic decreases in AIDS deaths. Lucia Torian et al. of the CDC state in "HIV Surveillance—United States, 1981–2008" (*Morbidity and Mortality Weekly Report*, vol. 60, no. 21, June 3, 2011) that "three decades after the first cases were reported in the United States, HIV infection is no longer inevitably fatal."

Figure 9.5 shows the progression and then the decline of AIDS deaths between 1981 and 2008. AIDS deaths surged between 1981 and 1995, prior to the introduction of highly active antiretroviral therapy (HAART), a powerful medicinal "cocktail" that is effective against the HIV virus and helps keep it from replicating in the human body. After implementation of HAART, AIDS deaths plunged through 1998 and continued a slow decline through 2008. By 2008, 594,496 people had died from AIDS since 1981. Figure 9.5 shows that most of those who are infected with HIV are living with it and being treated with HAART. The figure also shows that the number of people who are living with HIV infection is climbing. In 2008, nearly 1.2 million people were living with HIV infection. Torian et al. report that "nucleic acid testing now can detect HIV as early as 9 days after infection, enhancing the safety of the blood and organ supply and providing opportunities for early detection and disease intervention, including partner notification."

TABLE 9.12

Growth in the number and percentage of Medicare beneficiaries with end stage renal disease, 1998, 2003, and 2008

	1998		2003		2008	
	Patients (thousands)	Percent	Patients (thousands)	Percent	Patients (thousands)	Percent
Total	351.4	100%	449.4	100%	548.0	100%
Dialysis	255.2	73	320.5	71	382.3	70
In-center hemodialysis	225.1	64	291.8	65	350.8	64
Home hemodialysis	2.5	1	1.9	<1	3.8	1
Peritoneal dialysis	26.6	8	25.9	6	26.5	5
Unknown	1.1	<1	0.9	<1	1.2	<1
Functioning graft and kidney transplants	96.2	27	128.9	29	165.6	30

Note: ESRD (end-stage renal disease). Totals may not equal sum of components due to rounding.
Functioning graft patients = patients who have had a successful kidney transplant.

SOURCE: "Chart 11-5. The ESRD Population Is Growing, and Most ESRD Patients Undergo Dialysis," in *A Data Book: Healthcare Spending and the Medicare Program*, Medicare Payment Advisory Commission, June 2011, http://www.medpac.gov/documents/Jun11DataBookEntireReport.pdf (accessed February 5, 2012)

FIGURE 9.5

Estimated numbers of AIDS diagnoses, deaths, persons living with AIDS, and persons living with HIV infection, 1981–2008

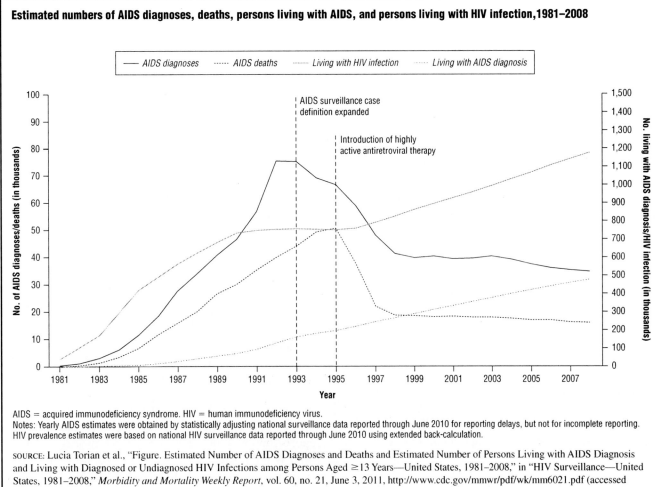

AIDS = acquired immunodeficiency syndrome. HIV = human immunodeficiency virus.
Notes: Yearly AIDS estimates were obtained by statistically adjusting national surveillance data reported through June 2010 for reporting delays, but not for incomplete reporting. HIV prevalence estimates were based on national HIV surveillance data reported through June 2010 using extended back-calculation.

SOURCE: Lucia Torian et al., "Figure. Estimated Number of AIDS Diagnoses and Deaths and Estimated Number of Persons Living with AIDS Diagnosis and Living with Diagnosed or Undiagnosed HIV Infections among Persons Aged ≥13 Years—United States, 1981–2008," in "HIV Surveillance—United States, 1981–2008," *Morbidity and Mortality Weekly Report*, vol. 60, no. 21, June 3, 2011, http://www.cdc.gov/mmwr/pdf/wk/mm6021.pdf (accessed February 5, 2012)

In the fact sheet "U.S. Federal Funding for HIV/AIDS: The President's FY 2012 Budget Request" (October 2011, http://www.kff.org/hivaids/upload/7029-07.pdf), the Henry J. Kaiser Family Foundation (KFF) provides historical federal funding information for HIV/AIDS for FYs 2007 to 2012. The KFF notes that funding began modestly, at less than $100 million. In FY 2007 the federal funding for all aspects of HIV/AIDS had grown to $21.2 billion, and the FY 2012 budget request was for $28.4 billion, including global programs and research.

The KFF shows the categories of funding for HIV/AIDS and compares differences in the categories of funding. The foundation also provides historical category comparisons. Information from these sources reveals that at the beginning of the HIV/AIDS epidemic, 50% of federal funding was spent on research (domestic) because at that time little was known about the disease, how to prevent it, and how to treat people who had contracted it. By FYs 1985 and 1990, as medical researchers learned more about the disease, the proportion that was devoted to research shrank to 36% and 38%, respectively. By FY 2007 about 13% of federal HIV/AIDS funding went to

domestic research. In the FY 2012 budget request, domestic research accounted for 10% of the federal HIV/AIDS funding.

Likewise, the proportion of federal funds targeted for the prevention of HIV/AIDS have decreased over the years. According to the KFF, 25% of federal funding went to prevention in FY 1982, 16% in FY 1985, 13% in FY 1990, 4% in FY 2007, and only 3.5% in the FY 2012 budget request. Conversely, the percentage of federal funds devoted to the care and treatment of people living with HIV/AIDS has increased dramatically as more people acquire the disease and live longer with it. In FY 1982, 25% of federal funding was targeted for care and treatment, whereas in FY 2007, 52% was spent on care and treatment. The FY 2012 budget requested that 52% of funds be targeted for care and treatment.

The KFF also indicates that the federal government spends money on the global fight against this disease. In FY 1990, 3% of the federal annual HIV/AIDS budget was used to help fight this disease globally. By FY 2007 this percentage had grown to nearly 21% of the total federal HIV/AIDS budget, and in FY 2012 the budget request asked that 24% of funds be spent on HIV/AIDS globally.

MEDICAID ASSISTANCE. The financing of health care for AIDS patients has increasingly become the responsibility of Medicaid, the entitlement program that provides medical assistance to low-income Americans. This is due, in large part, to the rising incidence of AIDS among poor people and injection drug users—the groups that are the least likely to have private health insurance. Furthermore, many patients who have private insurance through their employers lose their coverage when they become too ill to work. These individuals eventually turn to Medicaid and other public programs for medical assistance.

Some people, whose employment and economic condition previously afforded the insurance coverage they needed, find that their situation changes once they test positive for HIV. Some may become virtually ineligible for private health insurance coverage. Others require government assistance because insurance companies can declare HIV infection a preexisting condition, making it ineligible for payment of insurance claims. With the implementation of the 2010 health care reform, however, insurance companies will be barred (as of September 23, 2010, for children and January 1, 2014, for adults) from dropping clients due to preexisting conditions or current health status.

THE RYAN WHITE COMPREHENSIVE AIDS RESOURCES EMERGENCY ACT. The Ryan White Comprehensive AIDS Resources Emergency (CARE) Act is a federal program that provides funds for the care, treatment, and support of low-income, uninsured, and underinsured men, women, children, and youth with AIDS. It is the largest federally funded program for helping people with AIDS. The act is named after an Indiana teenager who had AIDS and worked against AIDS-related discrimination. The act was initially passed in 1990 and was reauthorized in 1996, 2000, 2006, and 2009. The 2009 reauthorization (the Ryan White HIV/AIDS Treatment Extension Act) gave the act an additional four years. Before that, however, the Ryan White HIV/AIDS Treatment Modernization Act, which was the 2006 reauthorization, changed somewhat how Ryan White funds could be used and put an emphasis on life-saving and life-extending services for people living with AIDS. The appropriations of CARE funds follow the following formulas:

- Part A (formerly called Title I)—the federal government provides emergency assistance to metropolitan areas that are disproportionately affected by the HIV/AIDS epidemic. To qualify for Part A financing, eligible metropolitan areas must have more than 2,000 cumulative AIDS cases reported during the preceding five years and a population of at least 500,000. The 2006 reauthorization gives priority to urban areas with the highest number of people living with AIDS. In addition, priority is also given to outreach, testing, and helping midsized cities and areas with emerging needs.

- Part B (formerly called Title II)—the federal government provides funds to state governments. Most of the Part B funds are allocated based on AIDS patient counts, and the remaining funds are distributed through competitive grants to public and nonprofit agencies. In addition, states receive funding to support AIDS Drug Assistance Programs, which provide medication to low-income HIV patients who are uninsured or underinsured.

- Part C (formerly called Title III)—federal funds are designated for Early Intervention Services (EIS) and planning. EIS grants support outpatient HIV services for low-income people in existing primary care systems, and planning grants aid those working to develop HIV primary care.

- Part D (formerly called Title IV)—these federal programs focus on the development of assistance for women, infants, and children.

The KFF shows in "Ryan White Funding History by Program, FY91–2010" (2012, http://hab.hrsa.gov/data/reports/funding.html) the annual funding history for the Ryan White CARE Act from its inception in FY 1991 to FY 2010. Between FYs 1991 and 2010 the Ryan White CARE Act experienced more than a 10-fold increase in funding, from $200 million to $2.2 billion. Table 9.13 details the appropriations by program between FYs 2007 and 2010. In FY 2010, $652.6 million (30%) of the Ryan White funding went to Part A (emergency relief) and over $1.2 billion (56%) went to Part B (HIV care).

Cancer

Cancer, in all its forms, is expensive to treat. Compared with other diseases, there are more options for cancer treatment, more adverse side effects that require treatment, and a greater potential for unrelieved pain. According to the American Cancer Society (ACS), in *Cancer Facts and Figures 2012* (2012, http://www.cancer.org/acs/groups/content/@epidemiologysurveilance/documents/document/acspc-031941.pdf), the overall estimated cost of cancer to the nation was $226.8 billion in 2007. Of this amount, $103.8 billion was due to direct medical costs (total of all health expenditures). Of the remainder, $123 billion was the cost of lost productivity due to premature death. It should be noted that the ACS is using a new measure for its medical payments: the Medical Expenditure Panel Survey of the Agency for Healthcare Research and Quality. These nationally representative data give results that will not be projected to the current year.

TABLE 9.13

Funding for the Ryan White Comprehensive AIDS Resources Emergency (CARE) Act, fiscal years 2007–10

[$ = 000's]

Program	Fiscal year 2007	Fiscal year 2008	Fiscal year 2009	Fiscal year 2010
Emergency relief (part A)	$603,993	$627,149	$663,082	$652,551
HIV care (part B)	$1,195,500	$1,195,248	$1,223,791	$1,228,975
(State formula grants)	(405,954)	(386,748)	(408,791)	(3,621,891)
(State AIDS Drug Assistance Program)	(789,546)	(808,500)	(815,000)	(866,786)
Early intervention (part C)	$193,721	$198,754	$201,877	$201,877
Women, infants, children & youth (part D)	$71,794	$73,690	$76,845	$72,583
AIDS ed training centers (part F)	$34,701	$34,094	$34,397	$36,955
Dental reimbursement (part F)	$13,086	$12,857	$13,429	$9,222
SPNS (part F)*				
Total: Ryan White funding	**$2,112,795**	**$2,141,792**	**$2,238,412**	**$2,202,163**

*Special Projects of National Significance: Normally funded with set-asides from parts A, B, C, & D, Appropriation Acts have directed that SPNS shall be funded from Department PHS (Public Health Service Act) evaluation set-asides. The appropriation amounts shown reflect a proportionate redistribution of the $25,000,000 to parts A, B, C, & D.

SOURCE: "Funding: FY07—FY10 Appropriations by Program," in *HRSA HIV/AIDS Programs*, U.S. Department of Health and Human Services, Health Resources and Services Administration, undated, http://hab.hrsa.gov/data/reports/funding.html (accessed February 5, 2012)

MEDICARE, CLINICAL TRIALS, AND CANCER. Some health insurance plans cover all or a portion of the costs that are associated with clinical trials (research studies that offer promising new anticancer drugs and treatment to enrolled patients). Policies vary, and some plans decide whether they will pay for clinical trials on a case-by-case basis. Some health plans limit coverage to patients for whom no standard therapy is available. Others cover clinical trials only if they are not much more expensive than standard treatment, and many choose not to cover any costs that are involved with clinical trials.

On June 7, 2000, President Bill Clinton (1946–) revised Medicare payment policies to enable beneficiaries to participate in clinical trials. Before this policy change, many older adults were prevented from participating in clinical trials because they could not afford the costs that were associated with the trials.

Alzheimer's Disease

The Alzheimer's Association notes in *2012 Alzheimer's Disease Facts and Figures* (2012, http://www.alz.org/downloads/Facts_Figures_2012.pdf) that in 2012 there were 5.4 million people in the United States with Alzheimer's disease (AD). AD is a form of dementia that is characterized by memory loss, behavior and personality changes, and decreasing thinking abilities. In 2012 the cost of medical care for those with AD and other dementias was about $200 billion. As of April 2012, there was no way to prevent AD.

CHAPTER 10
OLDER ADULTS

THE LONGEVITY REVOLUTION

As of the early 21st century, the United States was on the threshold of a longevity revolution. The National Institute on Aging recognizes this revolution when it observes in *Biology of Aging: Research Today for a Healthier Tomorrow* (November 2011, http://www.nia.nih.gov/sites/default/files/biology_on_aging.pdf) that "the facts of aging—what is happening on a biochemical, genetic, and physiological level—remain rich for exploration." What has fueled this new era of long life is a combination of better sanitation (safe drinking water, food, and disposal of waste), improved medical care, and reduced mortality rates for infants, children, and young adults.

The National Center for Health Statistics estimates that in 1900 life expectancy in the United States was 47.3 years at birth; by 1970 it had increased to 70.8 years. (See Table 10.1.) By 2007 it was projected that life expectancy for those born in that year was 77.9 years. Those who were 65 years old in 2007 could expect to live 18.6 more years, with women living an average of 19.9 more years and men 17.2 more years. In 2007 white men and women had longer life expectancies at age 65 than African-American men and women: 18.7 more years versus 17.2 more years.

AGING AMERICANS

According to the U.S. Census Bureau, 35.1 million (12.4%) of the U.S. population were aged 65 years and older in 2000. (See Table 10.2.) Those aged 65 years and older are projected to account for 20.7% of the U.S. population, or 86.7 million people, in 2050. Furthermore, 38.3 million (18.6%) men and 48.4 million (22.7%) women will be over the age of 65 years. Recent statistics show that the "young-old" range is between 65 and 74 years, the "old-old" range is between 75 and 92 years, and the "oldest-old" range is 93 years and older.

Who are the "older" Americans? The White House Council on Women and Girls indicates in *Women in America: Indicators of Social and Economic Well-Being* (March 2011, http://www.whitehouse.gov/sites/default/files/rss_viewer/Women_in_America.pdf) that 95% of people over the age of 65 have been married at least once. At this "older age" in 2009, three times as many women as men had been widowed.

There are also more older women than men. The White House Council on Women and Girls notes that in 2009, 15% of women were over the age of 65 years, whereas only 11% of men were in this age group. Furthermore, both men and women are delaying marriage. During the 1950s both genders married early: women at about age 20 years and men at about age 23 years. However, since then the marriage age has increased tremendously. In 2009 women were married on average at age 25 years and men at age 28 years.

Not only are more older Americans living longer than in previous years but also they are worrying less than younger Americans. Frank Newport and Brett Pelham of the Gallup Organization report in *Don't Worry, Be 80: Worry and Stress Decline with Age* (December 14, 2009, http://www.gallup.com/poll/124655/Dont-Worry-Be-80-Worry-Stress-Decline-Age.aspx) that 26.1% of women and 18.8% of men aged 66 to 70 years responded to pollsters in 2008 and 2009 that they had worried a lot during the previous day. Figure 10.1 shows that this level of worry is much lower than that of younger women and men. Generally, one-third or more of people of both sexes in their 20s, 30s, and 40s responded that they had worried a lot during the previous day. Additionally, as men and women age beyond 70, their level of worry decreases. Only about one out of six men (14.8%) and women (15.6%) who were over the age of 90 responded that they worried a lot during the previous day.

In a more recent survey, Steve Crabtree of the Gallup Organization reports in *U.S. Seniors Maintain Happiness Highs with Less Social Time* (December 12, 2011, http://www.gallup.com/poll/151457/Seniors-Maintain-Happiness-Highs-Less-Social-Time.aspx) that older

TABLE 10.1

Life expectancy at birth, at 65 years of age, and at 75 years of age, by race and sex, selected years 1900–2007

[Data are based on death certificates]

Specified age and year	All races Both sexes	Male	Female	White Both sexes	Male	Female	Black or African American[a] Both sexes	Male	Female
At birth				Remaining life expectancy in years					
1900[b, c]	47.3	46.3	48.3	47.6	46.6	48.7	33.0	32.5	33.5
1950[c]	68.2	65.6	71.1	69.1	66.5	72.2	60.8	59.1	62.9
1960[c]	69.7	66.6	73.1	70.6	67.4	74.1	63.6	61.1	66.3
1970	70.8	67.1	74.7	71.7	68.0	75.6	64.1	60.0	68.3
1980	73.7	70.0	77.4	74.4	70.7	78.1	68.1	63.8	72.5
1990	75.4	71.8	78.8	76.1	72.7	79.4	69.1	64.5	73.6
1995	75.8	72.5	78.9	76.5	73.4	79.6	69.6	65.2	73.9
1999	76.7	73.9	79.4	77.3	74.6	79.9	71.4	67.8	74.7
2000	76.8	74.1	79.3	77.3	74.7	79.9	71.8	68.2	75.1
2001	76.9	74.2	79.4	77.4	74.8	79.9	72.0	68.4	75.2
2002	76.9	74.3	79.5	77.4	74.9	79.9	72.1	68.6	75.4
2003	77.1	74.5	79.6	77.6	75.0	80.0	72.3	68.8	75.6
2004	77.5	74.9	79.9	77.9	75.4	80.4	72.8	69.3	76.0
2005	77.4	74.9	79.9	77.9	75.4	80.4	72.8	69.3	76.1
2006	77.7	75.1	80.2	78.2	75.7	80.6	73.2	69.7	76.5
2007	77.9	75.4	80.4	78.4	75.9	80.8	73.6	70.0	76.8
At 65 years									
1950[c]	13.9	12.8	15.0	—	12.8	15.1	13.9	12.9	14.9
1960[c]	14.3	12.8	15.8	14.4	12.9	15.9	13.9	12.7	15.1
1970	15.2	13.1	17.0	15.2	13.1	17.1	14.2	12.5	15.7
1980	16.4	14.1	18.3	16.5	14.2	18.4	15.1	13.0	16.8
1990	17.2	15.1	18.9	17.3	15.2	19.1	15.4	13.2	17.2
1995	17.4	15.6	18.9	17.6	15.7	19.1	15.6	13.6	17.1
1999	17.7	16.1	19.1	17.8	16.1	19.2	16.0	14.3	17.3
2000	17.6	16.0	19.0	17.7	16.1	19.1	16.1	14.1	17.5
2001	17.7	16.2	19.0	17.8	16.3	19.1	16.2	14.2	17.6
2002	17.8	16.2	19.1	17.9	16.3	19.2	16.3	14.4	17.7
2003	17.9	16.4	19.2	18.0	16.5	19.3	16.4	14.5	17.9
2004	18.2	16.7	19.5	18.3	16.8	19.5	16.7	14.8	18.2
2005	18.2	16.8	19.5	18.3	16.9	19.5	16.8	14.9	18.2
2006	18.5	17.0	19.7	18.6	17.1	19.8	17.1	15.1	18.6
2007	18.6	17.2	19.9	18.7	17.3	19.9	17.2	15.2	18.7
At 75 years									
1980	10.4	8.8	11.5	10.4	8.8	11.5	9.7	8.3	10.7
1990	10.9	9.4	12.0	11.0	9.4	12.0	10.2	8.6	11.2
1995	11.0	9.7	11.9	11.1	9.7	12.0	10.2	8.8	11.1
1999	11.2	10.0	12.1	11.2	10.0	12.1	10.4	9.2	11.1
2000	11.0	9.8	11.8	11.0	9.8	11.9	10.4	9.0	11.3
2001	11.1	9.9	11.9	11.1	9.9	11.9	10.5	9.1	11.4
2002	11.0	9.9	11.9	11.1	9.9	11.9	10.5	9.2	11.4
2003	11.1	10.0	11.9	11.1	10.0	11.9	10.6	9.3	11.5
2004	11.4	10.3	12.2	11.4	10.3	12.2	10.8	9.5	11.7
2005	11.3	10.2	12.1	11.4	10.3	12.1	10.8	9.5	11.7
2006	11.6	10.5	12.3	11.5	10.5	12.3	11.1	9.8	12.0
2007	11.7	10.6	12.5	11.7	10.6	12.4	11.2	9.9	12.1

—Data not available.

[a]Data shown for 1900–1960 are for the nonwhite population.

[b]Death registration area only. The death registration area increased from 10 states and the District of Columbia (D.C.) in 1900 to the coterminous United States in 1933.

[c]Includes deaths of persons who were not residents of the 50 states and D.C.

Notes: Populations for computing life expectancy for 1991–1999 are 1990-based postcensal estimates of U.S. resident population. In 1997, life table methodology was revised to construct complete life tables by single years of age that extend to age 100 (Anderson RN. Method for constructing complete annual U.S. life tables. NCHS. Vital Health Stat 2(129). 1999). Previously, abridged life tables were constructed for 5-year age groups ending with 85 years and over. Life table values for 2000 and later years were computed using a slight modification of the new life table method due to a change in the age detail of populations received from the U.S. Census Bureau. Values for data years 2000–2007 are based on a newly revised methodology that uses vital statistics death rates for ages under 66 and modeled probabilities of death for ages 66 to 100 based on blended vital statistics and Medicare probabilities of dying and may differ from figures previously published. The revised methodology is similar to that developed for the 1999–2001 decennial life tables. Starting with 2003 data, some states allowed the reporting of more than one race on the death certificate. The multiple-race data for these states were bridged to the single-race categories of the 1977 Office of Management and Budget Standards for comparability with other states. Some data have been revised and differ from previous editions of *Health, United States*. Data for additional years are available.

SOURCE: "Table 22. Life Expectancy at Birth, at 65 Years of Age, and at 75 Years of Age, by Race and Sex: United States, Selected Years 1900–2007," in *Health, United States, 2010: With Special Feature on Death and Dying*, Centers for Disease Control and Prevention, National Center for Health Statistics, 2011, http://www.cdc.gov/nchs/data/hus/hus10.pdf (accessed February 1, 2012)

Americans maintain their social "highs" with much less time socializing. Seventy-two percent of seniors reached the highest level of social happiness with six hours of social time during the previous day. In contrast, 51% of 18- to 29 year-olds and 52% of 30- to 39-year-olds required seven to nine or more hours; 60% of 40- to 49-year-olds required

TABLE 10.2

Population and projected population, by age and sex, selected years, 2000–50

[In thousands except as indicated. As of July 1. Resident population.]

Population or percent, sex, and age	2000	2010	2020	2030	2040	2050
Population						
Total						
Total	282,125	308,936	335,805	363,584	391,946	419,854
0–4	19,218	21,426	22,932	24,272	26,299	28,080
5–19	61,331	61,810	65,955	70,832	75,326	81,067
20–44	104,075	104,444	108,632	114,747	121,659	130,897
45–64	62,440	81,012	83,653	82,280	88,611	93,104
65–84	30,794	34,120	47,363	61,850	64,640	65,844
85+	4,267	6,123	7,269	9,603	15,409	20,861
Male						
Total	138,411	151,815	165,093	178,563	192,405	206,477
0–4	9,831	10,947	11,716	12,399	13,437	14,348
5–19	31,454	31,622	33,704	36,199	38,496	41,435
20–44	52,294	52,732	54,966	58,000	61,450	66,152
45–64	30,381	39,502	40,966	40,622	43,961	46,214
65–84	13,212	15,069	21,337	28,003	29,488	30,579
85+	1,240	1,942	2,403	3,340	5,573	7,749
Female						
Total	143,713	157,121	170,711	185,022	199,540	213,377
0–4	9,387	10,479	11,216	11,873	12,863	13,732
5–19	29,877	30,187	32,251	34,633	36,831	39,632
20–44	51,781	51,711	53,666	56,747	60,209	64,745
45–64	32,059	41,510	42,687	41,658	44,650	46,891
65–84	17,582	19,051	26,026	33,848	35,152	35,265
85+	3,028	4,182	4,866	6,263	9,836	13,112
Percent of total						
Total						
Total	100.0	100.0	100.0	100.0	100.0	100.0
0–4	6.8	6.9	6.8	6.7	6.7	6.7
5–19	21.7	20.0	19.6	19.5	19.2	19.3
20–44	36.9	33.8	32.3	31.6	31.0	31.2
45–64	22.1	26.2	24.9	22.6	22.6	22.2
65–84	10.9	11.0	14.1	17.0	16.5	15.7
85+	1.5	2.0	2.2	2.6	3.9	5.0
Male						
Total	100.0	100.0	100.0	100.0	100.0	100.0
0–4	7.1	7.2	7.1	6.9	7.0	6.9
5–19	22.7	20.8	20.4	20.3	20.0	20.1
20–44	37.8	34.7	33.3	32.5	31.9	32.0
45–64	21.9	26.0	24.8	22.7	22.8	22.4
65–84	9.5	9.9	12.9	15.7	15.3	14.8
85+	0.9	1.3	1.5	1.9	2.9	3.8
Female						
Total	100.0	100.0	100.0	100.0	100.0	100.0
0–4	6.5	6.7	6.6	6.4	6.4	6.4
5–19	20.8	19.2	18.9	18.7	18.5	18.6
20–44	36.0	32.9	31.4	30.7	30.2	30.3
45–64	22.3	26.4	25.0	22.5	22.4	22.0
65–84	12.2	12.1	15.2	18.3	17.6	16.5
85+	2.1	2.7	2.9	3.4	4.9	6.1

SOURCE: "Table 2a. Projected Population of the United States, by Age and Sex: 2000 to 2050," in *U.S. Interim Projections by Age, Sex, Race, and Hispanic Origin*, U.S. Census Bureau, March 18, 2004, http://www.census.gov/population/www/projections/usinterimproj/natprojtab02a.pdf (accessed February 5, 2012)

seven hours; and 57% of 50- to 64-year-olds required eight to nine or more hours of social time during the previous day. Crabtree concludes that even though "the relationship is present among all age groups, Americans aged 65 and older are more likely than their younger counterparts to maintain a positive mood with fewer hours of social time."

Baby Boomers

The first children born during the post–World War II baby boom (1946–1964) turned 65 years old in 2011. Baby boomers, the largest single generation in U.S. history, will help swell the 65-and-older population to approximately 54.6 million in 2020. (See Table 10.2.)

The Oldest Demographic

Americans aged 85 years and older account for the most rapidly growing age group in the U.S. population. Predictions vary as to how fast this "oldest old" segment of the population is increasing. The Census Bureau's prediction is that there will be nearly 20.9 million people

FIGURE 10.1

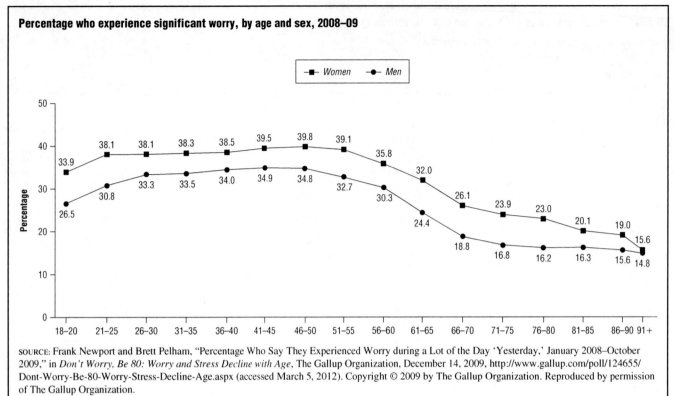

Percentage who experience significant worry, by age and sex, 2008–09

SOURCE: Frank Newport and Brett Pelham, "Percentage Who Say They Experienced Worry during a Lot of the Day 'Yesterday,' January 2008–October 2009," in *Don't Worry, Be 80: Worry and Stress Decline with Age*, The Gallup Organization, December 14, 2009, http://www.gallup.com/poll/124655/ Dont-Worry-Be-80-Worry-Stress-Decline-Age.aspx (accessed March 5, 2012). Copyright © 2009 by The Gallup Organization. Reproduced by permission of The Gallup Organization.

aged 85 years and older by 2050. (See Table 10.2.) However, if life spans continue to increase, the Census Bureau may have to revise its calculation for this portion of the general population.

LEADING CAUSES OF DEATH AMONG THE ELDERLY

Nearly six out of 10 (57%; 1 million out of 1.8 million) people aged 65 years and older who died in 2007 were the victims of diseases of the heart (496,095), malignant neoplasms (cancer; 389,730), or cerebrovascular diseases (stroke; 115,961). (See Table 10.3.)

Coronary Heart Disease

Coronary heart disease (CHD) is the leading cause of death in the United States and remains the leading cause of death among older Americans. Nearly three out of 10 (28.3%; 496,095 out of 1.8 million) people who died of CHD in 2007 were aged 65 years and older. (See Table 10.3.) This figure is down from 1980, when a higher percentage of those aged 65 years and older died of CHD (44.4%; 595,406 out of 1.3 million). This shift is because a greater percentage of people died at a younger age of CHD in 1980 than in 2007. In 1980, 34.9% (148,322 of 425,338) of CHD deaths were in the 45- to 64-year-old age group. In 2007, 32.5% (153,338 of 471,796) of CHD deaths were in this group. In fact, fewer people in the 65-years-and-older age group died of CHD in 2007 than in 1980, even though

the numbers of deaths from all causes in this group rose from 1.3 million in 1980 to nearly 1.8 million in 2007. Nonetheless, CHD is still the leading cause of death among older Americans.

The risk of dying from heart disease increases as a person ages. The death rate from CHD in 2007 for those aged 75 to 84 years was 1,315 deaths per 100,000 population, almost three times the rate for those aged 65 to 74 years (462.9 per 100,000 population). (See Table 10.4.) For those aged 85 years and older, the death rate rose sharply to 4,267.7 deaths per 100,000 population—nine times the rate for those aged 65 to 74 years. In general, females (200.2 deaths per 100,000 population) had a lower incidence of death from heart disease in 2007 than did males (208.4 deaths per 100,000 population). They also had lower death rates at all age levels.

In the 65-years-and-older age group the death rate for males from heart disease has been consistently higher than the death rate for females of the same age group regardless of the race. For example, the death rate from heart disease for African-American males aged 65 to 74 years was 989.4 deaths per 100,000 population in 2007, whereas the death rate from heart disease for African-American females of the same age group was 563.5 deaths per 100,000 population. (See Table 10.4.) In another example, the death rate from heart disease for Hispanic males aged 65 to 74 years was 477 deaths per 100,000 population in 2007, whereas the death rate from heart disease for Hispanic females of the same age group was 249.7 deaths per 100,000 population.

TABLE 10.3

Leading causes of death and numbers of deaths, by age, 1980 and 2007

[Data are based on death certificates]

Age and rank order	1980 Cause of death	Deaths	2007 Cause of death	Deaths
Under 1 year				
Rank	All causes	45,526	All causes	29,138
1	Congenital anomalies	9,220	Congenital malformations, deformations and chromosomal abnormalities	5,785
2	Sudden infant death syndrome	5,510	Disorders related to short gestation and low birth weight, not elsewhere classified	4,857
3	Respiratory distress syndrome	4,989	Sudden infant death syndrome	2,453
4	Disorders relating to short gestation and unspecified low birthweight	3,648	Newborn affected by maternal complications of pregnancy	1,769
5	Newborn affected by maternal complications of pregnancy	1,572	Unintentional injuries	1,285
6	Intrauterine hypoxia and birth asphyxia	1,497	Newborn affected by complications of placenta, cord and membranes	1,135
7	Unintentional injuries	1,166	Bacterial sepsis of newborn	820
8	Birth trauma	1,058	Respiratory distress of newborn	789
9	Pneumonia and influenza	1,012	Diseases of circulatory system	624
10	Newborn affected by complications of placenta, cord, and membranes	985	Neonatal hemorrhage	597
1–4 years				
Rank	All causes	8,187	All causes	4,703
1	Unintentional injuries	3,313	Unintentional injuries	1,588
2	Congenital anomalies	1,026	Congenital malformations, deformations and chromosomal abnormalities	546
3	Malignant neoplasms	573	Homicide	398
4	Diseases of heart	338	Malignant neoplasms	364
5	Homicide	319	Diseases of heart	173
6	Pneumonia and influenza	267	Influenza and pneumonia	109
7	Meningitis	223	Septicemia	78
8	Meningococcal infection	110	Certain conditions originating in the perinatal period	70
9	Certain conditions originating in the perinatal period	84	In situ neoplasms, benign neoplasms and neoplasms of uncertain or unknown behavior	59
10	Septicemia	71	Chronic lower respiratory diseases	57
5–14 years				
Rank	All causes	10,689	All causes	6,147
1	Unintentional injuries	5,224	Unintentional injuries	2,194
2	Malignant neoplasms	1,497	Malignant neoplasms	959
3	Congenital anomalies	561	Congenital malformations, deformations and chromosomal abnormalities	374
4	Homicide	415	Homicide	346
5	Diseases of heart	330	Diseases of heart	241
6	Pneumonia and influenza	194	Suicide	184
7	Suicide	142	Chronic lower respiratory diseases	118
8	Benign neoplasms	104	Influenza and pneumonia	103
9	Cerebrovascular diseases	95	In situ neoplasms, benign neoplasms and neoplasms of uncertain or unknown behavior	84
10	Chronic obstructive pulmonary diseases	85	Cerebrovascular diseases	83
15–24 years				
Rank	All causes	49,027	All causes	33,982
1	Unintentional injuries	26,206	Unintentional injuries	15,897
2	Homicide	6,537	Homicide	5,551
3	Suicide	5,239	Suicide	4,140
4	Malignant neoplasms	2,683	Malignant neoplasms	1,653
5	Diseases of heart	1,223	Diseases of heart	1,084
6	Congenital anomalies	600	Congenital malformations, deformations and chromosomal abnormalities	402
7	Cerebrovascular diseases	418	Cerebrovascular diseases	195
8	Pneumonia and influenza	348	Diabetes mellitus	168
9	Chronic obstructive pulmonary diseases	141	Influenza and pneumonia	163
10	Anemias	133	Septicemia	160

Since the 1950s deaths from heart disease have consistently declined. (See Table 10.4.) Several factors account for this decrease, including better control of hypertension (high blood pressure) and cholesterol levels in the blood. The expanding use of trained mobile emergency personnel (paramedics) in most urban areas has also contributed to the decrease, and the widespread use of cardiopulmonary resuscitation and new pharmaceutical drugs have increased the likelihood of surviving an initial heart attack. Changes in lifestyle, such as the inclusion of physical exercise and a

TABLE 10.3

Leading causes of death and numbers of deaths, by age, 1980 and 2007 [CONTINUED]

[Data are based on death certificates]

Age and rank order	1980		2007	
	Cause of death	Deaths	Cause of death	Deaths
25–44 years				
Rank	All causes	108,658	All causes	122,178
1	Unintentional injuries	26,722	Unintentional injuries	31,908
2	Malignant neoplasms	17,551	Malignant neoplasms	16,751
3	Diseases of heart	14,513	Diseases of heart	15,062
4	Homicide	10,983	Suicide	12,000
5	Suicide	9,855	Homicide	7,810
6	Chronic liver disease and cirrhosis	4,782	Human immunodeficiency virus (HIV) disease	4,663
7	Cerebrovascular diseases	3,154	Chronic liver disease and cirrhosis	2,954
8	Diabetes mellitus	1,472	Cerebrovascular diseases	2,638
9	Pneumonia and influenza	1,467	Diabetes mellitus	2,594
10	Congenital anomalies	817	Septicemia	1,207
45–64 years				
Rank	All causes	425,338	All causes	471,796
1	Diseases of heart	148,322	Malignant neoplasms	153,338
2	Malignant neoplasms	135,675	Diseases of heart	102,961
3	Cerebrovascular diseases	19,909	Unintentional injuries	32,508
4	Unintentional injuries	18,140	Diabetes mellitus	17,057
5	Chronic liver disease and cirrhosis	16,089	Chronic lower respiratory diseases	16,930
6	Chronic obstructive pulmonary diseases	11,514	Cerebrovascular diseases	16,885
7	Diabetes mellitus	7,977	Chronic liver disease and cirrhosis	16,216
8	Suicide	7,079	Suicide	12,847
9	Pneumonia and influenza	5,804	Nephritis, nephrotic syndrome, and nephrosis	6,673
10	Homicide	4,019	Septicemia	6,662
65 years and over				
Rank	All causes	1,341,848	All causes	1,755,567
1	Diseases of heart	595,406	Diseases of heart	496,095
2	Malignant neoplasms	258,389	Malignant neoplasms	389,730
3	Cerebrovascular diseases	146,417	Cerebrovascular diseases	115,961
4	Pneumonia and influenza	45,512	Chronic lower respiratory diseases	109,562
5	Chronic obstructive pulmonary diseases	43,587	Alzheimer's disease	73,797
6	Atherosclerosis	28,081	Diabetes mellitus	51,528
7	Diabetes mellitus	25,216	Influenza and pneumonia	45,941
8	Unintentional injuries	24,844	Nephritis, nephrotic syndrome, and nephrosis	38,484
9	Nephritis, nephrotic syndrome, and nephrosis	12,968	Unintentional injuries	38,292
10	Chronic liver disease and cirrhosis	9,519	Septicemia	26,362

SOURCE: "Table 27. Leading Causes of Death and Numbers of Deaths, by Age: United States, 1980 and 2007," in *Health, United States, 2010: With Special Feature on Death and Dying*, Centers for Disease Control and Prevention, National Center for Health Statistics, 2011, http://www.cdc.gov/nchs/data/hus/hus10.pdf (accessed February 1, 2012)

healthy diet, have also helped decrease the incidence of heart disease.

Until the 1990s almost all research on heart disease focused on white, middle-aged males. Researchers, physicians, and public health officials agree that more research and prevention efforts should be directed toward women, racial and ethnic minorities, and older adults. In "Facts, Bridging the Gap: CVD and Health Equity" (January 2012, http://www.heart.org/idc/groups/heart-public/@wcm/@adv/documents/downloadable/ucm_301731.pdf), both the American Heart Association and the American Stroke Association suggest that affordable and understandable health care should be available for all races and ethnicities, and should be language-appropriate.

The symptoms of a heart attack can be significantly different for women than for men. Heart disease in women is often due to coronary microvascular dysfunction, in which the small blood vessels of the heart do not dilate (widen) properly to supply sufficient blood to the heart muscle. This dysfunction may occur alone, or in addition to, blockages that reduce blood flow in the large coronary arteries as is often the case in men. When the large vessels are blocked, symptoms may include pain, pressure, burning, aching, and tightness in the chest, along with shortness of breath, sweating, weakness, anxiety, and nausea. When small vessels are blocked, symptoms may be more subtle and may include discomfort spread over a wide chest area, exhaustion, depression, and shortness of breath. Nausea, back or jaw pain, shortness of breath, and chest pain may accompany these symptoms.

Cancer

Cancer (malignant neoplasms) is the second-leading cause of death among older adults. In 2007, 389,730 people aged 65 years and older died of cancer. (See Table 10.3.) The risk of developing many types of cancers increases with age, varies by race and ethnicity, and varies with a variety of other factors such as gender. (See Table 10.5 and Table 10.6.)

TABLE 10.4

Death rates for diseases of the heart, by sex, race, Hispanic origin, and age, selected years 1950–2007

[Data are based on death certificates]

Sex, race, Hispanic origin, and age	1950[a]	1960[a]	1970	1980	1990	2000	2006	2007
All persons				Deaths per 100,000 resident population				
All ages, age-adjusted[b]	588.8	559.0	492.7	412.1	321.8	257.6	200.2	190.9
All ages, crude	356.8	369.0	362.0	336.0	289.5	252.6	211.0	204.3
Under 1 year	4.1	6.6	13.1	22.8	20.1	13.0	8.4	10.0
1–4 years	1.6	1.3	1.7	2.6	1.9	1.2	1.0	1.1
5–14 years	3.9	1.3	0.8	0.9	0.9	0.7	0.6	0.6
15–24 years	8.2	4.0	3.0	2.9	2.5	2.6	2.5	2.6
25–34 years	20.9	15.6	11.4	8.3	7.6	7.4	8.2	7.9
35–44 years	88.3	74.6	66.7	44.6	31.4	29.2	28.3	27.4
45–54 years	309.2	271.8	238.4	180.2	120.5	94.2	88.0	85.3
55–64 years	804.3	737.9	652.3	494.1	367.3	261.2	207.3	200.3
65–74 years	1,857.2	1,740.5	1,558.2	1,218.6	894.3	665.6	490.3	462.9
75–84 years	4,311.0	4,089.4	3,683.8	2,993.1	2,295.7	1,780.3	1,383.1	1,315.0
85 years and over	9,152.5	9,317.8	7,891.3	7,777.1	6,739.9	5,926.1	4,480.8	4,267.7
Male								
All ages, age-adjusted[b]	699.0	687.6	634.0	538.9	412.4	320.0	248.5	237.7
All ages, crude	424.7	439.5	422.5	368.6	297.6	249.8	214.0	208.4
Under 1 year	4.7	7.8	15.1	25.5	21.9	13.3	8.8	10.9
1–4 years	1.7	1.4	1.9	2.8	1.9	1.4	1.1	1.0
5–14 years	3.5	1.4	0.9	1.0	0.9	0.8	0.7	0.6
15–24 years	8.3	4.2	3.7	3.7	3.1	3.2	3.3	3.2
25–34 years	24.4	20.1	15.2	11.4	10.3	9.6	11.2	10.5
35–44 years	120.4	112.7	103.2	68.7	48.1	41.4	39.5	38.6
45–54 years	441.2	420.4	376.4	282.6	183.0	140.2	128.9	124.6
55–64 years	1,100.5	1,066.9	987.2	746.8	537.3	371.7	296.8	288.8
65–74 years	2,310.2	2,291.3	2,170.3	1,728.0	1,250.0	898.3	660.5	624.9
75–84 years	4,825.8	4,742.4	4,534.8	3,834.3	2,968.2	2,248.1	1,743.5	1,656.5
85 years and over	9,661.4	9,788.9	8,426.2	8,752.7	7,418.4	6,430.0	4,819.9	4,621.8
Female								
All ages, age-adjusted[b]	486.6	447.0	381.6	320.8	257.0	210.9	162.2	154.0
All ages, crude	289.7	300.6	304.5	305.1	281.8	255.3	208.0	200.2
Under 1 year	3.4	5.4	10.9	20.0	18.3	12.5	7.9	9.0
1–4 years	1.6	1.1	1.6	2.5	1.9	1.0	0.9	1.1
5–14 years	4.3	1.2	0.8	0.9	0.8	0.5	0.6	0.6
15–24 years	8.2	3.7	2.3	2.1	1.8	2.1	1.8	1.9
25–34 years	17.6	11.3	7.7	5.3	5.0	5.2	5.1	5.3
35–44 years	57.0	38.2	32.2	21.4	15.1	17.2	17.0	16.2
45–54 years	177.8	127.5	109.9	84.5	61.0	49.8	48.5	47.2
55–64 years	507.0	429.4	351.6	272.1	215.7	159.3	124.1	117.9
65–74 years	1,434.9	1,261.3	1,082.7	828.6	616.8	474.0	346.3	325.4
75–84 years	3,873.0	3,582.7	3,120.8	2,497.0	1,893.8	1,475.1	1,136.7	1,079.7
85 years and over	8,798.1	9,016.8	7,591.8	7,350.5	6,478.1	5,720.9	4,322.1	4,099.3
White male[c]								
All ages, age-adjusted[b]	701.4	694.5	640.2	539.6	409.2	316.7	245.2	234.8
All ages, crude	434.2	454.6	438.3	384.0	312.7	265.8	226.9	221.1
45–54 years	424.1	413.2	365.7	269.8	170.6	130.7	119.2	116.2
55–64 years	1,082.6	1,056.0	979.3	730.6	516.7	351.8	278.9	271.4
65–74 years	2,309.4	2,297.9	2,177.2	1,729.7	1,230.5	877.8	636.6	603.0
75–84 years	4,908.0	4,839.9	4,617.6	3,883.2	2,983.4	2,247.0	1,743.3	1,659.3
85 years and over	9,952.3	10,135.8	8,818.0	8,958.0	7,558.7	6,560.8	4,947.1	4,756.1
Black or African American male[c]								
All ages, age-adjusted[b]	641.5	615.2	607.3	561.4	485.4	392.5	320.6	305.9
All ages, crude	348.4	330.6	330.3	301.0	256.8	211.1	191.8	186.5
45–54 years	624.1	514.0	512.8	433.4	328.9	247.2	229.8	216.3
55–64 years	1,434.0	1,236.8	1,135.4	987.2	824.0	631.2	526.4	516.3
65–74 years	2,140.1	2,281.4	2,237.8	1,847.2	1,632.9	1,268.8	1,044.6	989.4
75–84 years[d]	4,107.9	3,533.6	3,783.4	3,578.8	3,107.1	2,597.6	2,129.9	1,999.2
85 years and over	—	6,037.9	5,367.6	6,819.5	6,479.6	5,633.5	4,073.1	3,879.6

Between 2006 and 2008 males had the highest incidence of all types of cancer (44.9% of males versus 38.1% of females; see Table 10.5). Regarding age, the older people become, the higher their probability of developing most types of invasive cancer. For example, the older a man gets, the more likely he is to develop prostate cancer. The chance of dying from prostate cancer also rises with age. The American Cancer Society reports in *Cancer Facts and Figures 2012* (2012, http://www.cancer.org/acs/groups/content/@epidemiologysurveilance/documents/document/acspc-031941.pdf) that of all the men who were diagnosed with genital cancers in 2012, about 71% were newly

TABLE 10.4

Death rates for diseases of the heart, by sex, race, Hispanic origin, and age, selected years 1950–2007 [CONTINUED]

[Data are based on death certificates]

Sex, race, Hispanic origin, and age	1950[a]	1960[a]	1970	1980	1990	2000	2006	2007
American Indian or Alaska Native male[c]				Deaths per 100,000 resident population				
All ages, age-adjusted[b]	—	—	—	320.5	264.1	222.2	170.2	159.8
All ages, crude	—	—	—	130.6	108.0	90.1	95.8	94.1
45–54 years	—	—	—	238.1	173.8	108.5	119.5	112.4
55–64 years	—	—	—	496.3	411.0	285.0	256.2	235.8
65–74 years	—	—	—	1,009.4	839.1	748.2	573.6	521.5
75–84 years	—	—	—	2,062.2	1,788.8	1,655.7	1,176.6	1,129.5
85 years and over	—	—	—	4,413.7	3,860.3	3,318.3	2,066.9	1,901.1
Asian or Pacific Islander male[c]								
All ages, age-adjusted[b]	—	—	—	286.9	220.7	185.5	136.3	126.0
All ages, crude	—	—	—	119.8	88.7	90.6	82.4	79.6
45–54 years	—	—	—	112.0	70.4	61.1	55.7	51.5
55–64 years	—	—	—	306.7	226.1	182.6	145.4	131.5
65–74 years	—	—	—	852.4	623.5	482.5	344.3	321.3
75–84 years	—	—	—	2,010.9	1,642.2	1,354.7	963.3	906.3
85 years and over	—	—	—	5,923.0	4,617.8	4,154.2	2,985.9	2,665.8
Hispanic or Latino male[c, e]								
All ages, age-adjusted[b]	—	—	—	—	270.0	238.2	175.2	165.0
All ages, crude	—	—	—	—	91.0	74.7	67.7	66.6
45–54 years	—	—	—	—	116.4	84.3	75.6	73.3
55–64 years	—	—	—	—	363.0	264.8	202.3	201.9
65–74 years	—	—	—	—	829.9	684.8	505.6	477.0
75–84 years	—	—	—	—	1,971.3	1,733.2	1,308.4	1,233.4
85 years and over	—	—	—	—	4,711.9	4,897.5	3,257.9	2,960.8
White, not Hispanic or Latino male[e]								
All ages, age-adjusted[b]	—	—	—	—	413.6	319.9	250.0	239.8
All ages, crude	—	—	—	—	336.5	297.5	260.3	254.3
45–54 years	—	—	—	—	172.8	134.3	124.5	121.6
55–64 years	—	—	—	—	521.3	356.3	284.5	276.6
65–74 years	—	—	—	—	1,243.4	885.1	644.3	610.9
75–84 years	—	—	—	—	3,007.7	2,261.9	1,767.4	1,685.0
85 years and over	—	—	—	—	7,663.4	6,606.6	5,032.8	4,858.5
White female[c]								
All ages, age-adjusted[b]	479.2	441.7	376.7	315.9	250.9	205.6	158.6	150.5
All ages, crude	290.5	306.5	313.8	319.2	298.4	274.5	224.2	215.5
45–54 years	142.4	103.4	91.4	71.2	50.2	40.9	40.7	40.0
55–64 years	460.7	383.0	317.7	248.1	192.4	141.3	111.4	105.3
65–74 years	1,401.6	1,229.8	1,044.0	796.7	583.6	445.2	325.8	304.4
75–84 years	3,926.2	3,629.7	3,143.5	2,493.6	1,874.3	1,452.4	1,123.9	1,068.9
85 years and over	9,086.9	9,280.8	7,839.9	7,501.6	6,563.4	5,801.4	4,402.6	4,169.6
Black or African American female[c]								
All ages, age-adjusted[b]	538.9	488.9	435.6	378.6	327.5	277.6	212.5	204.5
All ages, crude	289.9	268.5	261.0	249.7	237.0	212.6	174.3	170.0
45–54 years	526.8	360.7	290.9	202.4	155.3	125.0	111.0	107.0
55–64 years	1,210.7	952.3	710.5	530.1	442.0	332.8	251.3	242.5
65–74 years	1,659.4	1,680.5	1,553.2	1,210.3	1,017.5	815.2	578.3	563.5
75–84 years[d]	3,499.3	2,926.9	2,964.1	2,707.2	2,250.9	1,913.1	1,461.7	1,384.0
85 years and over	—	5,650.0	5,003.8	5,796.5	5,766.1	5,298.7	4,049.4	3,962.0
American Indian or Alaska Native female[c]								
All ages, age-adjusted[b]	—	—	—	175.4	153.1	143.6	113.2	99.8
All ages, crude	—	—	—	80.3	77.5	71.9	75.1	69.6
45–54 years	—	—	—	65.2	62.0	40.2	41.8	36.7
55–64 years	—	—	—	193.5	197.0	149.4	125.2	108.7
65–74 years	—	—	—	577.2	492.8	391.8	322.3	288.5
75–84 years	—	—	—	1,364.3	1,050.3	1,044.1	937.9	779.2
85 years and over	—	—	—	2,893.3	2,868.7	3,146.3	1,883.1	1,697.9

diagnosed with prostate cancer. The probability of developing prostate cancer is one in 8,499 for men who are younger than 40 years; one in 38 for 40- to 59-year-olds; and one in 15 for men aged 60 to 69 years. (See Table 10.5.) The odds rise to one in eight for men aged 70 years and older.

In spite of their higher odds of developing cancer, older Americans appear to deal better with their cancer diagnosis than do younger Americans. Dan Witters of the Gallup Organization reports in *Cancer History Linked to 58% Increase in Depression* (April 21, 2010, http://

TABLE 10.4

Death rates for diseases of the heart, by sex, race, Hispanic origin, and age, selected years 1950–2007 [CONTINUED]

[Data are based on death certificates]

Sex, race, Hispanic origin, and age	1950[a]	1960[a]	1970	1980	1990	2000	2006	2007
Asian or Pacific Islander female[c]								
All ages, age-adjusted[b]	—	—	—	132.3	149.2	115.7	87.3	82.0
All ages, crude	—	—	—	57.0	62.0	65.0	64.9	63.9
45–54 years	—	—	—	28.6	17.5	15.9	15.9	12.1
55–64 years	—	—	—	92.9	99.0	68.8	48.4	46.8
65–74 years	—	—	—	313.3	323.9	229.6	187.4	168.5
75–84 years	—	—	—	1,053.2	1,130.9	866.2	639.8	611.4
85 years and over	—	—	—	3,211.0	4,161.2	3,367.2	2,492.6	2,345.6
Hispanic or Latina female[c, e]								
All ages, age-adjusted[b]	—	—	—	—	177.2	163.7	118.9	111.8
All ages, crude	—	—	—	—	79.4	71.5	62.6	60.8
45–54 years	—	—	—	—	43.5	28.2	27.3	23.4
55–64 years	—	—	—	—	153.2	111.2	86.9	81.4
65–74 years	—	—	—	—	460.4	366.3	273.0	249.7
75–84 years	—	—	—	—	1,259.7	1,169.4	894.5	856.6
85 years and over	—	—	—	—	4,440.3	4,605.8	3,078.3	2,888.2
White, not Hispanic or Latina female[e]								
All ages, age-adjusted[b]	—	—	—	—	252.6	206.8	160.9	153.0
All ages, crude	—	—	—	—	320.0	304.9	254.7	245.5
45–54 years	—	—	—	—	50.2	41.9	42.2	42.1
55–64 years	—	—	—	—	193.6	142.9	113.2	107.1
65–74 years	—	—	—	—	584.7	448.5	329.1	308.1
75–84 years	—	—	—	—	1,890.2	1,458.9	1,135.8	1,081.0
85 years and over	—	—	—	—	6,615.2	5,822.7	4,460.8	4,230.8

—Data not available.

[a]Includes deaths of persons who were not residents of the 50 states and the District of Columbia (D.C.).

[b]Age-adjusted rates are calculated using the year 2000 standard population. Prior to 2003, age-adjusted rates were calculated using standard million proportions based on rounded population numbers. Starting with 2003 data, unrounded population numbers are used to calculate age-adjusted rates.

[c]The race groups, white, black, Asian or Pacific Islander, and American Indian or Alaska Native, include persons of Hispanic and non-Hispanic origin. Persons of Hispanic origin may be of any race. Death rates for the American Indian or Alaska Native and Asian or Pacific Islander populations are known to be underestimated.

[d]In 1950, rate is for the age group 75 years and over.

[e]Prior to 1997, excludes data from states lacking an Hispanic-origin item on the death certificate.

Notes: Starting with *Health, United States,* 2003, rates for 1991–1999 were revised using intercensal population estimates based on the 2000 census. Rates for 2000 were revised based on 2000 census counts. Rates for 2001 and later years were computed using 2000-based postcensal estimates. Age groups were selected to minimize the presentation of unstable age-specific death rates based on small numbers of deaths and for consistency among comparison groups. Starting with 2003 data, some states allowed the reporting of more than one race on the death certificate. The multiple-race data for these states were bridged to the single-race categories of the 1977 Office of Management and Budget standards for comparability with other states.

SOURCE: "Table 30. Death Rates for Diseases of Heart, by Sex, Race, Hispanic Origin, and Age: United States, Selected Years 1950–2007," in *Health, United States, 2010: With Special Feature on Death and Dying,* Centers for Disease Control and Prevention, National Center for Health Statistics, 2011, http://www.cdc.gov/nchs/data/hus/hus10.pdf (accessed February 1, 2012)

www.gallup.com/poll/127475/Cancer-Diagnosis-Linked-Increase-Depression.aspx) that in 2008 and 2009, 18.5% of those aged 65 years and older who had been diagnosed with cancer said they had also been diagnosed with depression. (See Table 10.7.) By contrast, 48.5% of Americans aged 18 to 29 years who had been diagnosed with cancer said they had also been diagnosed with depression. The proportion of those diagnosed with cancer reporting that they had also been diagnosed with depression decreased with age. Interestingly, the proportion of those never diagnosed with cancer reporting that they had been diagnosed with depression increased with age. Those who had been diagnosed with cancer and reported that they experienced physical pain the day before increased slightly with age, until age 65 years, and then it went down.

Stroke

Stroke (cerebrovascular disease) is the third-leading cause of death and the principal cause of serious disability among older adults. In 2007, 115,961 people aged 65 years and older died from stroke. (See Table 10.3.) The death rate from stroke increases markedly with age. In 2007 the death rate from stroke for those aged 65 to 74 years was 93 deaths per 100,000 population. (See Table 10.8.) This death rate from stroke more than tripled for each successive decade of age after that, to 322.3 deaths per 100,000 population for those aged 75 to 84 years and to 1,015.5 deaths per 100,000 population for those aged 85 years and older.

Men aged 65 to 74 years and 75 to 84 years were more likely to have suffered a stroke in 2007 than females in the same age groups (105.2 versus 82.7 per 100,000 population, and 333.2 versus 314.9 per 100,000 population, respectively). (See Table 10.8.) However, in the 85-years-and-older age group, women were more likely than men to have suffered a stroke (1,072.4 versus 895.7 per 100,000 population). This pattern was consistent overall between 1960 and 2007.

TABLE 10.5

Probability of developing invasive cancers over selected age intervals, by sex, 2006–08[a]

[In percent]

	Birth to 39		40 to 59		60 to 69		70 and older		Birth to death	
All sites[b]										
Male	1.45	(1 in 69)	8.68	(1 in 12)	16.00	(1 in 6)	38.27	(1 in 3)	44.85	(1 in 2)
Female	2.15	(1 in 46)	9.10	(1 in 11)	10.34	(1 in 10)	26.68	(1 in 4)	38.08	(1 in 3)
Urinary bladder[c]										
Male	0.02	(1 in 5,035)	0.38	(1 in 266)	0.92	(1 in 109)	3.71	(1 in 27)	3.84	(1 in 26)
Female	0.01	(1 in 12,682)	0.12	(1 in 851)	0.25	(1 in 400)	0.98	(1 in 102)	1.15	(1 in 87)
Breast										
Female	0.49	(1 in 203)	3.76	(1 in 27)	3.53	(1 in 28)	6.58	(1 in 15)	12.29	(1 in 8)
Colon & rectum										
Male	0.08	(1 in 1,236)	0.92	(1 in 109)	1.44	(1 in 70)	4.32	(1 in 23)	5.27	(1 in 19)
Female	0.08	(1 in 1,258)	0.73	(1 in 137)	1.01	(1 in 99)	3.95	(1 in 25)	4.91	(1 in 20)
Leukemia										
Male	0.16	(1 in 614)	0.22	(1 in 445)	0.34	(1 in 291)	1.24	(1 in 81)	1.57	(1 in 64)
Female	0.14	(1 in 737)	0.15	(1 in 665)	0.21	(1 in 482)	0.81	(1 in 123)	1.14	(1 in 88)
Lung & bronchus										
Male	0.03	(1 in 3,631)	0.91	(1 in 109)	2.26	(1 in 44)	6.69	(1 in 15)	7.66	(1 in 13)
Female	0.03	(1 in 3,285)	0.76	(1 in 132)	1.72	(1 in 58)	4.91	(1 in 20)	6.33	(1 in 16)
Melanoma of the skin[d]										
Male	0.15	(1 in 677)	0.63	(1 in 158)	0.75	(1 in 133)	1.94	(1 in 52)	2.80	(1 in 36)
Female	0.27	(1 in 377)	0.56	(1 in 180)	0.39	(1 in 256)	0.82	(1 in 123)	1.83	(1 in 55)
Non-Hodgkin lymphoma										
Male	0.13	(1 in 775)	0.45	(1 in 223)	0.60	(1 in 167)	1.77	(1 in 57)	2.34	(1 in 43)
Female	0.09	(1 in 1,152)	0.32	(1 in 313)	0.44	(1 in 228)	1.41	(1 in 71)	1.94	(1 in 51)
Prostate										
Male	0.01	(1 in 8,499)	2.63	(1 in 38)	6.84	(1 in 15)	12.54	(1 in 8)	16.48	(1 in 6)
Uterine cervix										
Female	0.15	(1 in 650)	0.27	(1 in 373)	0.13	(1 in 771)	0.18	(1 in 549)	0.68	(1 in 147)
Uterine corpus										
Female	0.07	(1 in 1,373)	0.77	(1 in 130)	0.87	(1 in 114)	1.24	(1 in 81)	2.61	(1 in 38)

[a]For people free of cancer at beginning of age interval.
[b]All sites excludes basal and squamous cell skin cancers and in situ cancers except urinary bladder.
[c]Includes invasive and in situ cancer cases.
[d]Statistic is for whites only.

SOURCE: "Probability of Developing Invasive Cancers over Selected Age Intervals, by Sex, 2006–08," in *Cancer Facts and Figures 2012*, American Cancer Society, 2012, http://www.cancer.org/acs/groups/content/@epidemiologysurveilance/documents/document/acspc-031941.pdf (accessed March 30, 2012). Atlanta: American Cancer Society, Inc. Copyright © 2012 American Cancer Society, Inc. Reprinted with permission. Data from the National Cancer Institute.

Stroke and Alzheimer's disease are the two primary causes of dementia. Death rates from stroke have declined dramatically since the 1950s. (See Table 10.8.) Regardless, stroke leaves approximately one-third of survivors with severe disabilities, and they require continued care.

DEMENTIA

Older people with cognitive (mental) problems were once labeled "senile," which had a derogatory connotation and meant an elderly person who was cognitively impaired. Researchers have found that physical disorders can cause progressive deterioration of cognitive and neurological functions. In the 21st century these disorders produce symptoms that are collectively known as dementia. Symptoms of dementia include loss of language functions, inability to think abstractly, inability to care for oneself, personality change, emotional instability, and loss of a sense of time or place.

Dementia has become a serious health problem in developed countries, including the United States, because older adults are living longer than ever before. One indicator of diminished cognitive functioning in older adults is memory loss. However, Roger E. Kelley and Alireza Minagar note in "Memory Complaints and Dementia" (*Medical Clinics of North America*, vol. 93, no. 2. March 2009) that some memory loss occurs in all people as they age and has been termed "benign forgetfulness of senescence." A physician can test for the presence of dementia and distinguish it from forgetfulness that is benign and not part of a disease process.

TABLE 10.6

Trends in 5-year survival rates[a] by race, 1975–2007

[In percent]

	All races			White			African American		
	1975–77	1987–89	2001–2007	1975–77	1987–89	2001–2007	1975–77	1987–89	2001–2007
All sites	**49**	**56**	**67[b]**	**50**	**57**	**69[b]**	**39**	**43**	**59[b]**
Brain	22	29	35[b]	22	28	34[b]	25	31	40[b]
Breast (female)	75	84	90[b]	76	85	91[b]	62	71	77[b]
Colon	51	60	65[b]	51	61	67[b]	45	53	55[b]
Esophagus	5	10	19[b]	6	11	20[b]	3	7	13[b]
Hodgkin lymphoma	72	79	86[b]	72	80	88[b]	70	72	81[b]
Kidney & renal pelvis	50	57	71[b]	50	57	71[b]	49	55	68[b]
Larynx	66	66	63[b]	67	67	65	59	56	52
Leukemia	34	43	57[b]	35	44	57[b]	33	36	50[b]
Liver & intrahepatic bile duct	3	5	15[b]	3	6	15[b]	2	3	10[b]
Lung & bronchus	12	13	16[b]	12	13	17[b]	11	11	13[b]
Melanoma of the skin	82	88	93[b]	82	88	93[b]	58	79	73
Myeloma	25	28	41[b]	25	27	42[b]	30	30	41[b]
Non-Hodgkin lymphoma	47	51	70[b]	47	52	71[b]	48	46	62[b]
Oral cavity & pharynx	53	54	63[b]	54	56	65[b]	36	34	45[b]
Ovary	36	38	44[b]	35	38	43[b]	42	34	36
Pancreas	2	4	6[b]	3	3	6[b]	2	6	4[b]
Prostate	68	83	100[b]	69	85	100[b]	61	72	98[b]
Rectum	48	58	68[b]	48	59	69[b]	45	52	61[b]
Stomach	15	20	27[b]	14	19	26[b]	16	19	27[b]
Testis	83	95	96[b]	83	95	97[b]	73[c]	88	86
Thyroid	92	95	97[b]	92	94	98[b]	90	92	95
Urinary bladder	73	79	80[b]	74	80	81[b]	50	63	64[b]
Uterine cervix	69	70	69	70	73	70	65	57	61
Uterine corpus	87	83	83[b]	88	84	85[b]	60	57	61

[a]Survival rates are adjusted for normal life expectancy and are based on cases diagnosed in the SEER 9 areas from 1975–77, 1987–89, and 2001 to 2007, and followed through 2008.
[b]The difference in rates between 1975–1977 and 2001–2007 is statistically significant (p <0.05).
[c]Survival rate is for cases diagnosed in 1978–1980.

SOURCE: "Trends in 5-Year Survival Rates (%) by Race, US, 1975–2007," in *Cancer Facts and Figures 2012*, American Cancer Society, 2012, http://www .cancer.org/acs/groups/content/@epidemiologysurveilance/documents/document/acspc-031941.pdf (accessed March 30, 2012). Atlanta: American Cancer Society, Inc. Copyright © 2012 American Cancer Society, Inc. Reprinted with permission. Data from the SEER National Statistics Review.

TABLE 10.7

Cancer diagnosis, depression, and physical pain, by age group, 2008–09

2008–2009 results

	% diagnosed with depression	% that experienced physical pain yesterday
18- to 29-year-olds diagnosed with cancer	48.5	38.3
18- to 29-year-olds not diagnosed with cancer	13.9	16.1
30- to 44-year-olds diagnosed with cancer	37.3	39.2
30- to 44-year-olds not diagnosed with cancer	15.9	19.4
45- to 64-year-olds diagnosed with cancer	31.8	39.7
45- to 64-year-olds not diagnosed with cancer	19.2	26.8
65-year-olds and older diagnosed with cancer	18.5	31.3
65-year-olds and older not diagnosed with cancer	14.8	25.8

SOURCE: Dan Witters, "Cancer Diagnosis Elevates Depression and Physical Pain across All Age Groups, 2008–2009 Results," in *Cancer History Linked to 58% Increase in Depression*, The Gallup Organization, April 21, 2010, http://www.gallup.com/poll/127475/Cancer-Diagnosis-Linked-Increase-Depression.aspx (accessed February 5, 2012). Copyright © 2010 by The Gallup Organization. Reproduced by permission of The Gallup Organization.

Alzheimer's Disease

Alzheimer's disease (AD) is the single most common cause of dementia. It is a progressive, degenerative disease that attacks the brain and results in severely impaired memory, thinking, and behavior. First described in 1906 by the German physician Alois Alzheimer (1864–1915), the disorder may strike people in their 40s and 50s, but most victims are over the age of 65 years.

Alzheimer's autopsy of a severely demented 55-year-old woman revealed deposits of neuritic plaques (clumps of proteins and dying nerve cell fibers that accumulate outside the nerve cells of the brain) and neurofibrillary tangles. The latter characteristic, the presence of twisted and tangled fibers in the brain cells, is the anatomical hallmark of the disease.

SYMPTOMS. The onset of dementia in AD is gradual, and the decline of cognitive function progresses over time. Mild or early AD is not easily distinguishable from the characteristics of normal aging—mild episodes of forgetfulness and disorientation. Gradually, the AD patient may experience confusion; language problems, such as trouble finding words; impaired judgment;

TABLE 10.8

Death rates for cerebrovascular diseases, by sex, race, Hispanic origin, and age, selected years 1950–2007

[Data are based on death certificates]

Sex, race, Hispanic origin, and age	1950[a]	1960[a]	1970	1980	1990	2000	2006	2007
All persons				Deaths per 100,000 resident population				
All ages, age-adjusted[b]	180.7	177.9	147.7	96.2	65.3	60.9	43.6	42.2
All ages, crude	104.0	108.0	101.9	75.0	57.8	59.6	45.8	45.1
Under 1 year	5.1	4.1	5.0	4.4	3.8	3.3	3.4	3.1
1–4 years	0.9	0.8	1.0	0.5	0.3	0.3	0.3	0.3
5–14 years	0.5	0.7	0.7	0.3	0.2	0.2	0.2	0.2
15–24 years	1.6	1.8	1.6	1.0	0.6	0.5	0.5	0.5
25–34 years	4.2	4.7	4.5	2.6	2.2	1.5	1.3	1.2
35–44 years	18.7	14.7	15.6	8.5	6.4	5.8	5.1	4.9
45–54 years	70.4	49.2	41.6	25.2	18.7	16.0	14.7	14.6
55–64 years	194.2	147.3	115.8	65.1	47.9	41.0	33.3	32.1
65–74 years	554.7	469.2	384.1	219.0	144.2	128.6	96.3	93.0
75–84 years	1,499.6	1,491.3	1,254.2	786.9	498.0	461.3	335.1	322.3
85 years and over	2,990.1	3,680.5	3,014.3	2,283.7	1,628.9	1,589.2	1,039.6	1,015.5
Male								
All ages, age-adjusted[b]	186.4	186.1	157.4	102.2	68.5	62.4	43.9	42.5
All ages, crude	102.5	104.5	94.5	63.4	46.7	46.9	37.0	36.4
Under 1 year	6.4	5.0	5.8	5.0	4.4	3.8	3.9	3.5
1–4 years	1.1	0.9	1.2	0.4	0.3	*	0.3	0.2
5–14 years	0.5	0.7	0.8	0.3	0.2	0.2	0.3	0.2
15–24 years	1.8	1.9	1.8	1.1	0.7	0.5	0.5	0.5
25–34 years	4.2	4.5	4.4	2.6	2.1	1.5	1.4	1.2
35–44 years	17.5	14.6	15.7	8.7	6.8	5.8	5.3	5.3
45–54 years	67.9	52.2	44.4	27.2	20.5	17.5	16.4	16.2
55–64 years	205.2	163.8	138.7	74.6	54.3	47.2	38.7	38.0
65–74 years	589.6	530.7	449.5	258.6	166.6	145.0	108.0	105.2
75–84 years	1,543.6	1,555.9	1,361.6	866.3	551.1	490.8	345.5	333.2
85 years and over	3,048.6	3,643.1	2,895.2	2,193.6	1,528.5	1,484.3	932.4	895.7
Female								
All ages, age-adjusted[b]	175.8	170.7	140.0	91.7	62.6	59.1	42.6	41.3
All ages, crude	105.6	111.4	109.0	85.9	68.4	71.8	54.4	53.5
Under 1 year	3.7	3.2	4.0	3.8	3.1	2.7	2.9	2.6
1–4 years	0.7	0.7	0.7	0.5	0.3	0.4	0.4	0.4
5–14 years	0.4	0.6	0.6	0.3	0.2	0.2	0.2	0.2
15–24 years	1.5	1.6	1.4	0.8	0.6	0.5	0.5	0.4
25–34 years	4.3	4.9	4.7	2.6	2.2	1.5	1.2	1.3
35–44 years	19.9	14.8	15.6	8.4	6.1	5.7	4.8	4.6
45–54 years	72.9	46.3	39.0	23.3	17.0	14.5	13.0	12.9
55–64 years	183.1	131.8	95.3	56.8	42.2	35.3	28.2	26.6
65–74 years	522.1	415.7	333.3	188.7	126.7	115.1	86.5	82.7
75–84 years	1,462.2	1,441.1	1,183.1	740.1	466.2	442.1	328.0	314.9
85 years and over	2,949.4	3,704.4	3,081.0	2,323.1	1,667.6	1,632.0	1,089.8	1,072.4
White male[c]								
All ages, age-adjusted[b]	182.1	181.6	153.7	98.7	65.5	59.8	41.7	40.2
All ages, crude	100.5	102.7	93.5	63.1	46.9	48.4	37.7	37.0
45–54 years	53.7	40.9	35.6	21.7	15.4	13.6	12.8	13.0
55–64 years	182.2	139.0	119.9	64.0	45.7	39.7	31.5	31.4
65–74 years	569.7	501.0	420.0	239.8	152.9	133.8	97.1	94.3
75–84 years	1,556.3	1,564.8	1,361.6	852.7	539.2	480.0	338.5	323.1
85 years and over	3,127.1	3,734.8	3,018.1	2,230.8	1,545.4	1,490.7	941.3	905.0
Black or African American male[c]								
All ages, age-adjusted[b]	228.8	238.5	206.4	142.0	102.2	89.6	67.1	67.1
All ages, crude	122.0	122.9	108.8	73.0	53.0	46.1	39.3	39.5
45–54 years	211.9	166.1	136.1	82.1	68.4	49.5	43.5	41.0
55–64 years	522.8	439.9	343.4	189.7	141.7	115.4	105.9	99.8
65–74 years	783.6	899.2	780.1	472.3	326.9	268.5	218.7	223.3
75–84 years[d]	1,504.9	1,475.2	1,445.7	1,066.3	721.5	659.2	471.1	491.9
85 years and over	—	2,700.0	1,963.1	1,873.2	1,421.5	1,458.8	882.0	866.9

disorientation in place and time; and changes in mood, behavior, and personality. The speed with which these changes occur varies, but eventually the disease leaves patients unable to care for themselves.

In the terminal stages of AD, patients require care 24 hours per day. They no longer recognize family members and need help with simple daily activities, such as eating, dressing, bathing, and using the toilet. Eventually, they may

142 Older Adults

Death and Dying

TABLE 10.8

Death rates for cerebrovascular diseases, by sex, race, Hispanic origin, and age, selected years 1950–2007 [CONTINUED]

[Data are based on death certificates]

Sex, race, Hispanic origin, and age	1950[a]	1960[a]	1970	1980	1990	2000	2006	2007
American Indian or Alaska Native male[c]				Deaths per 100,000 resident population				
All ages, age-adjusted[b]	—	—	—	66.4	44.3	46.1	25.8	31.1
All ages, crude	—	—	—	23.1	16.0	16.8	14.4	16.5
45–54 years	—	—	—	*	*	13.3	16.3	13.9
55–64 years	—	—	—	72.0	39.8	48.6	35.0	37.0
65–74 years	—	—	—	170.5	120.3	144.7	82.9	83.3
75–84 years	—	—	—	523.9	325.9	373.3	174.3	266.0
85 years and over	—	—	—	1,384.7	949.8	834.9	344.5	481.0
Asian or Pacific Islander male[c]								
All ages, age-adjusted[b]	—	—	—	71.4	59.1	58.0	39.8	35.5
All ages, crude	—	—	—	28.7	23.3	27.2	23.6	22.0
45–54 years	—	—	—	17.0	15.6	15.0	13.4	14.7
55–64 years	—	—	—	59.9	51.8	49.3	36.3	31.5
65–74 years	—	—	—	197.9	167.9	135.6	108.9	90.7
75–84 years	—	—	—	619.5	483.9	438.7	294.9	274.2
85 years and over	—	—	—	1,399.0	1,196.6	1,415.6	865.9	748.7
Hispanic or Latino male[c, e]								
All ages, age-adjusted[b]	—	—	—	—	46.5	50.5	35.9	34.4
All ages, crude	—	—	—	—	15.6	15.8	14.3	14.1
45–54 years	—	—	—	—	20.0	18.1	17.0	16.5
55–64 years	—	—	—	—	49.2	48.8	41.1	42.9
65–74 years	—	—	—	—	126.4	136.1	100.1	94.6
75–84 years	—	—	—	—	356.6	392.9	292.8	263.6
85 years and over	—	—	—	—	866.3	1,029.9	581.9	594.6
White, not Hispanic or Latino male[e]								
All ages, age-adjusted[b]	—	—	—	—	66.3	59.9	41.7	40.3
All ages, crude	—	—	—	—	50.6	53.9	42.6	41.9
45–54 years	—	—	—	—	14.9	13.0	12.1	12.3
55–64 years	—	—	—	—	45.1	38.7	30.3	30.0
65–74 years	—	—	—	—	154.5	133.1	96.5	93.8
75–84 years	—	—	—	—	547.3	482.3	340.5	326.3
85 years and over	—	—	—	—	1,578.7	1,505.9	960.2	922.4
White female[c]								
All ages, age-adjusted[b]	169.7	165.0	135.5	89.0	60.3	57.3	41.1	39.9
All ages, crude	103.3	110.1	109.8	88.6	71.6	76.9	57.9	57.0
45–54 years	55.0	33.8	30.5	18.6	13.5	11.2	10.4	10.0
55–64 years	156.9	103.0	78.1	48.6	35.8	30.2	24.1	22.5
65–74 years	498.1	383.3	303.2	172.5	116.1	107.3	79.3	75.8
75–84 years	1,471.3	1,444.7	1,176.8	728.8	456.5	434.2	321.5	310.5
85 years and over	3,017.9	3,795.7	3,167.6	2,362.7	1,685.9	1,646.7	1,102.2	1,083.8
Black or African American female[c]								
All ages, age-adjusted[b]	238.4	232.5	189.3	119.6	84.0	76.2	57.0	55.0
All ages, crude	128.3	127.7	112.2	77.8	60.7	58.3	46.5	45.6
45–54 years	248.9	166.2	119.4	61.8	44.1	38.1	31.3	33.0
55–64 years	567.7	452.0	272.4	138.4	96.9	76.4	61.1	58.4
65–74 years	754.4	830.5	673.5	361.7	236.7	190.9	148.9	143.8
75–84 years[d]	1,496.7	1,413.1	1,338.3	917.5	595.0	549.2	415.6	387.9
85 years and over	—	2,578.9	2,210.5	1,891.6	1,495.2	1,556.5	1,060.5	1,050.6
American Indian or Alaska Native female[c]								
All ages, age-adjusted[b]	—	—	—	51.2	38.4	43.7	30.9	28.4
All ages, crude	—	—	—	22.0	19.3	21.5	19.8	19.7
45–54 years	—	—	—	*	*	14.4	*	10.0
55–64 years	—	—	—	*	40.7	37.9	16.2	23.7
65–74 years	—	—	—	128.3	100.5	79.5	78.8	83.4
75–84 years	—	—	—	404.2	282.0	391.1	267.6	198.7
85 years and over	—	—	—	1,095.5	776.2	931.5	648.1	599.9

become incontinent, blind, and unable to communicate. The course of the disease varies widely, but Orazio Zanetti, Sebastiano Bruno Solerte, and F. Cantoni suggest in "Life Expectancy in Alzheimer's Disease (AD)" (*Archives of Gerontology and Geriatrics*, vol. 49, suppl. 1, 2009) that people who are diagnosed with AD when in their 60s and early 70s might expect to live seven to 10 years after diagnosis, with life expectancy decreasing as the age of diagnosis increases. People who are diagnosed when in their 90s might expect to live three years or less after diagnosis.

TABLE 10.8

Death rates for cerebrovascular diseases, by sex, race, Hispanic origin, and age, selected years 1950–2007 [CONTINUED]

[Data are based on death certificates]

Sex, race, Hispanic origin, and age	1950[a]	1960[a]	1970	1980	1990	2000	2006	2007
Asian or Pacific Islander female[c]								
All ages, age-adjusted[b]	—	—	—	60.8	54.9	49.1	34.9	33.2
All ages, crude	—	—	—	26.4	24.3	28.7	26.7	26.4
45–54 years	—	—	—	20.3	19.7	13.3	10.4	9.9
55–64 years	—	—	—	43.7	42.1	33.3	28.8	25.2
65–74 years	—	—	—	136.1	124.0	102.8	80.8	72.6
75–84 years	—	—	—	446.6	396.6	386.0	284.2	259.7
85 years and over	—	—	—	1,545.2	1,395.0	1,246.6	777.0	802.4
Hispanic or Latina female[c, e]								
All ages, age-adjusted[b]	—	—	—	—	43.7	43.0	32.3	30.8
All ages, crude	—	—	—	—	20.1	19.4	17.5	17.1
45–54 years	—	—	—	—	15.2	12.4	11.8	11.0
55–64 years	—	—	—	—	38.5	31.9	27.8	25.4
65–74 years	—	—	—	—	102.6	95.2	76.9	71.6
75–84 years	—	—	—	—	308.5	311.3	240.6	244.2
85 years and over	—	—	—	—	1,055.3	1,108.9	742.9	684.5
White, not Hispanic or Latina female[e]								
All ages, age-adjusted[b]	—	—	—	—	61.0	57.6	41.5	40.3
All ages, crude	—	—	—	—	77.2	85.5	65.5	64.7
45–54 years	—	—	—	—	13.2	10.9	10.1	9.8
55–64 years	—	—	—	—	35.7	29.9	23.5	22.1
65–74 years	—	—	—	—	116.9	107.6	79.0	75.9
75–84 years	—	—	—	—	461.9	438.3	325.9	314.4
85 years and over	—	—	—	—	1,714.7	1,661.6	1,118.7	1,103.7

*Rates based on fewer than 20 deaths are considered unreliable and are not shown.
—Data not available.
[a]Includes deaths of persons who were not residents of the 50 states and the District of Columbia (D.C.).
[b]Age-adjusted rates are calculated using the year 2000 standard population. Prior to 2003, age-adjusted rates were calculated using standard million proportions based on rounded population numbers. Starting with 2003 data, unrounded population numbers are used to calculate age-adjusted rates.
[c]The race groups, white, black, Asian or Pacific Islander, and American Indian or Alaska Native, include persons of Hispanic and non-Hispanic origin. Persons of Hispanic origin may be of any race. Death rates for the American Indian or Alaska Native and Asian or Pacific Islander populations are known to be underestimated.
[d]In 1950, rate is for the age group 75 years and over.
[e]Prior to 1997, excludes data from states lacking an Hispanic-origin item on the death certificate.
Notes: Starting with *Health, United States, 2003*, rates for 1991–1999 were revised using intercensal population estimates based on the 2000 census. Rates for 2000 were revised based on 2000 census counts. Rates for 2001 and later years were computed using 2000-based postcensal estimates. Age groups were selected to minimize the presentation of unstable age-specific death rates based on small numbers of deaths and for consistency among comparison groups. Starting with 2003 data, some states allowed the reporting of more than one race on the death certificate. The multiple-race data for these states were bridged to the single-race categories of the 1977 Office of Management and Budget standards for comparability with other states.

SOURCE: "Table 31. Death Rates for Cerebrovascular Diseases, by Sex, Race, Hispanic Origin, and Age: United States, Selected Years 1950–2007," in *Health, United States, 2010: With Special Feature on Death and Dying*, Centers for Disease Control and Prevention, National Center for Health Statistics, 2011, http://www.cdc.gov/nchs/data/hus/hus10.pdf (accessed February 1, 2012).

PREVALENCE. In 2007, 73,797 deaths from AD were reported for those aged 65 years and older. (See Table 10.3.) In that year AD was the fifth-leading cause of death in the 65-years-and-older age group, whereas in 1980 AD was not even in the top 10 leading causes of death for this age group. According the Alzheimer's Association, in *2011 Alzheimer's Disease Facts and Figures* (2011, http://www.alz.org/downloads/Facts_Figures_2011.pdf), the number of deaths from AD increased by 66% between 2000 and 2008, whereas the percentage change in the numbers of deaths from stroke, prostate cancer, breast cancer, heart disease, and the human immunodeficiency virus had all decreased.

The Alzheimer's Association notes the estimated lifetime risk for developing AD by age and sex. At the age of 65 years the estimated lifetime risk for women developing AD is 17.2%, and that risk rises to 20.3% at the age of 85 years. Men aged 65 to 85 years have about a one in 11 to a one in eight chance of developing dementia. At the age of 65 years the estimated lifetime risk for men developing AD is 9.1%, and that risk rises to 12.1% at the age of 85 years. (Even though lifetime risk usually means risk from birth to death, dementia [including AD] only infrequently occurs before the age of 65 years.)

DEPRESSION

The National Institute of Mental Health notes in the fact sheet "Older Adults: Depression and Suicide Facts" (September 27, 2010, http://www.nimh.nih.gov/health/publications/older-adults-depression-and-suicide-facts.shtml) that depression is estimated to occur in less than 1% to about 5% of older people in the general population, but the estimate rises to 11.5% in elderly hospital patients and to 13.5% in elderly home health care patients. Family members and health care professionals often fail to recognize depression among the elderly. Older people usually suffer from comorbidity (the presence of more than one chronic illness at one time), so depression may be masked by the symptoms of other disorders. In addition, older adults suffering from depression may mistakenly think that their depression is simply a reaction to an illness or loss, or is a consequence of aging. Also, many sufferers fail to divulge their depression because of the stigma that is associated with mental illness.

Suicide

According to the National Institute of Mental Health, in "Older Adults," depression is commonly associated with suicide in older people. Most suicidal older adults, up to 75%, visit their primary care physician during the month before ending their life. However, their depression apparently is not accurately diagnosed or effectively treated.

Depression is especially common in nursing homes and in other types of aged-care facilities and residences. Tanya E. Davison, Marita P. McCabe, and David Mellor determine in "An Examination of the 'Gold Standard' Diagnosis of Major Depression in Aged-Care Settings" (*American Journal of Geriatric Psychiatry*, vol. 17, no. 5, May 2009) that the usual screening methods used to detect depression among residents in aged-care settings underreport the condition. The researchers note that including additional informant interviews with the usual individual patient clinical interviews revealed that 22% of a large sample of aged-care setting residents with an average age of approximately 85 years and with normal cognitive functioning suffered from clinical depression, whereas the usual screening method alone revealed a rate of only 16%. (An informant interview is conducted with a nursing home staff member who knows the patient well.) Not only is depression in long-term and aged-care settings underreported or unrecognized but also when recognized it may be undertreated, treated inadequately, or treated inappropriately.

Feeling lonely or abandoned or suffering financial woes, many depressed nursing home and other aged-care setting residents end their life by nonviolent means such as by starving themselves, failing to take prescribed medications, or ingesting large amounts of prescribed medications. This type of suicide, as a result of depression, is different from that committed by the terminally ill who, not wishing to prolong the dying process, refuse life-sustaining medical treatment.

In the United States the suicide rate generally increases with age. In 2007 those aged 75 to 84 years and 85 years and older had a rate of 16.3 and 15.6 suicides, respectively, per 100,000 population. (See Table 6.1 in Chapter 6.) However, those aged 45 to 54 years had a higher rate, at 17.7 suicides per 100,000 population.

Men have a higher suicide rate than women. Men aged 85 years and older had the highest suicide rate of 41.8 suicides per 100,000 population in 2007, whereas the rate among women of that age was 3.1 suicides per 100,000 population. (See Table 6.1.)

Of men aged 65 years and older by race, non-Hispanic white men had the highest suicide rate in 2007 at 32.2 suicides per 100,000 population. (See Table 6.1.) In contrast, African-American men of this age had the lowest suicide rate of 8.7. One generally held theory about the high rates of suicide among aged white men is that they have traditionally been in positions of power and thus have great difficulty adjusting to a life that they may consider useless or diminished.

OLDER WOMEN
Women Live Longer Than Men

In the United States the life expectancy in 2007 for females born in that year was five years more than for males—80.4 years and 75.4 years, respectively. (See Table 10.1.) As the population ages, these differences in life expectancies show up in the sex ratios of older people. A sex ratio is the number of men per 100 women. Sex ratios under 100 mean that there are more women than men, and sex ratios over 100 mean that there are more men than women.

In *An Aging World: 2008* (June 2009, http://www .census.gov/prod/2009pubs/p95-09-1.pdf), Kevin Kinsella and Wan He of the Census Bureau show the sex ratios for those aged 65 to 79 years and for those aged 80 years and older for both developed and developing countries. In 2008 in developed countries (which includes the United States) there were 76 men for every 100 women aged 65 to 79 years. For those aged 80 years and older there were 48 men for every 100 women. By 2040 the sex ratios in developed countries are expected to rise, indicating that the life expectancy of men will rise in relation to women. By 2040 the sex ratio in the 65-to-79-year-old age group will rise to 84, and in the 80-plus age group the sex ratio will rise to 56. The story in developing countries is different. Sex ratios in the 65-to-79-year-old age group are expected to remain stable between 2008 and 2040 and to decline in the 80-plus age group.

Elderly Women Have More Chronic Diseases Than Do Elderly Men

Older women are more likely than men of the same age to suffer from chronic conditions, such as arthritis, osteoporosis and related bone fractures, AD, and incontinence. Women are also more likely to have more than one chronic disorder at a time (comorbidity). At any given age, women are frailer than men, even though they have a lower mortality rate.

GERIATRICS

Geriatrics is the medical subspecialty that is concerned with the prevention and treatment of diseases in the elderly. In 1909 the American physician Ignatz L. Nascher (1863–1944) coined the term *geriatrics* from the Greek *geras* (old age) and *iatrikos* (physician). Geriatricians are physicians trained in internal medicine or family practice who obtain additional training and certification in the diagnosis and treatment of older adults. Geriatricians rely on the findings of researchers and gerontologists (nonphysician professionals who conduct scientific studies of aging and older adults) to help older adults maintain function and independence.

Gerontology was unheard of before the 19th century, when most people died at an early age. Those who reached old age accepted their deteriorating health as a part of aging. Gerontology was born during the early 20th century, when scientists began investigating the pathological changes that accompany the aging process. Even though many developed countries have recognized the need for increased geriatrics education, the United States' medical education continues to lag in this regard. According to the Institute of Medicine, in *Retooling for an Aging America: Building the Healthcare Workforce* (April 2008, http://www .iom.edu/Reports/2008/Retooling-for-an-Aging-America-Building-the-Health-Care-Workforce.aspx), the number of people aged 65 years and older will nearly double between 2005 and 2030, from 37 million to 70 million, and will account for almost 20% of the U.S. population.

The Association of American Medical Colleges responded to this need by developing minimum geriatrics-specific competencies that can be used in U.S. medical schools to guide geriatrics training. The competencies establish performance benchmarks for medical school graduates who will care for geriatric patients when they are first-year residents. The competencies are organized under eight general areas: medication management; cognitive and behavioral disorders; self-care capacity; falls, balance, and gait disorders; health care planning and promotion; atypical presentation of disease; palliative care (care that relieves the pain but does not cure the illness); and hospital care for elders.

Decline in Numbers of Geriatricians in the United States

The American Geriatrics Society (AGS) reports in "The Demand for Geriatric Care and the Evident Shortage of Geriatrics Healthcare Providers" (July 2011, http://www .americangeriatrics.org/files/documents/Adv_Resources/Pay Reform_fact5.pdf) that there is a tremendous deficit in the number of physicians who are specializing in geriatrics and geriatric psychiatry. According to the AGS, as of March 2011 there were only 7,162 active certified geriatricians practicing in the United States (one for every 2,620 people aged 75 years and older) and 1,751 certified geriatric psychiatrists (one for every 10,865 people aged 75 years and older). By 2030 the ratio of geriatricians to Americans 75 years and older is projected to decline to one in 3,798 and the ratio of geriatric psychiatrists to one in 12,557.

The AGS suggests that low Medicare reimbursement rates leave geriatricians with much lower salaries than physicians in other fields, a situation that has become a primary factor in the declining numbers of geriatricians and geriatric psychiatrists that graduate from U.S. medical schools. According to the U.S. Senate Democratic Policy Committee, in "Summary of Health Care and Revenue Provisions" (September 17, 2010, http://dpc.senate.gov/ healthreformbill/healthbill62.pdf), the 2010 health care reform legislation attempted to address this problem. The committee explains that the reform legislation "improves Medicare payments for primary care which will protect access to these vital services."

CHAPTER 11
PUBLIC OPINION ABOUT LIFE AND DEATH

LIFE AFTER DEATH

Since the dawn of history, many people have believed that human beings do not simply cease to exist once they die. Many religions and cultures teach that the physical body may die and decompose but that some element of the person goes on to what many call the afterlife.

Between 1972 and 1982, when the Roper Center for Public Opinion Research (http://www.ropercenter.uconn .edu/) asked the American public, "Do you believe there is life after death?," 70% said they believed in an afterlife. In 1996, when the Roper Center asked the same question, 73% of respondents said "yes." The National Opinion Research Center at the University of Chicago reveals similar results in its General Social Survey 2002 (http://www.cpanda.org/cpanda/getDDI.xq?studyID=a00079). Seventy-two percent of those polled said they believe there is life after death. Likewise, the Harris Poll notes in "What People Do and Do Not Believe In" (December 15, 2009, http://www.harrisinteractive.com/vault/Harris_Poll _2009_12_15.pdf) that in 2009, 71% of Americans said they believe there is life after death.

Frank Newport of the Gallup Organization notes in *Americans More Likely to Believe in God Than the Devil, Heaven More Than Hell* (June 13, 2007, http://www.gallup .com/poll/27877/Americans-More-Likely-Believe-God-Than -Devil-Heaven-More-Than-Hell.aspx) that when asked in polls about an afterlife and what that "eternal destination" might be, many Americans expressed a belief in heaven, where people who led a good life are eternally rewarded after death, and in hell, where unrepentant people who led a bad life are eternally punished. Newport indicates that belief in the existence of heaven and hell increased over time. Between 1997 and 2007 a majority of respondents (72% in 1997 and 81% in 2007) acknowledged a belief in heaven. In addition, a majority of respondents (56% in 1997 and 69% in 2007) acknowledged a belief that hell exists in the afterlife.

The percentages of people believing in the existence of heaven and hell from the Harris poll results differ slightly from the Gallup poll results. In 2007, 75% of Harris poll respondents said they believed in the existence of heaven, whereas 81% of Gallup poll respondents expressed this belief. In 2009 the Harris poll figure remained steady at 75%. In 2007, 62% of Harris poll respondents said that they believed in the existence of hell, whereas 69% of Gallup poll respondents expressed this belief. In 2009 the Harris poll figure remained somewhat steady at 61%. Harris researchers also determine that in 2009, 82% of respondents believed in God, 72% in angels, 60% in the devil, and 20% in reincarnation.

FEAR AND ANXIETY ABOUT DEATH

R. J. Russac et al. of the University of North Florida conducted studies not only to examine the consistent assertion in the medical literature that young adults typically report higher levels of concern about death than do older adults but also to examine the assertion that women typically report higher levels of concern about death than do men. The researchers report in "Death Anxiety across the Adult Years: An Examination of Age and Gender Effects" (*Death Studies*, vol. 31, no. 6, July 2007) that the results of their studies support these findings and that anxiety about death peaks at about the age of 20. Their results also support previous findings that women report higher levels of concern about death than do men. However, the results also show that the decline in death anxiety after the age of 20 differed between men and women. Concern about death declined after the age of 20 in both sexes, but in women a secondary peak in anxiety about death occurred during their early 50s.

Fearful Aspects of Dying

Russac et al. wonder why younger people would be more anxious and fearful of dying than older people. Other researchers, they note, suggest that older Americans come to terms with death as they age. Other hypotheses include that death is more appealing to older people (especially to older people with chronic conditions and illnesses) than to younger people, that older people are more religious and this affects their views, and that older people have more experience with death over their lifetime so they are less anxious about it. Russac et al. suggest that it might have to do with the concurrent peak in younger people's reproductive years. Their concerns might actually be about their children and wondering what would happen to their children if they were to die. Likewise, some researchers suggest that women report more anxiety about death than men because they are the primary caretakers, not only of children but also of the elderly and those who might be dying. One hypothesis for women's secondary peak of anxiety about death in their 50s is that women reach menopause during those years and this change of life may remind them that they are getting older and closer to death.

Ann Bowling et al. reveal in "Fear of Dying in an Ethnically Diverse Society: Cross-Sectional Studies of People Aged 65+ in Britain" (*Postgraduate Medical Journal*, vol. 86, no. 1014, April 2010) that fears about dying differ among social and ethnic groups. The researchers determine that in an ethnically diverse sample of study participants aged 65 years and older, the Pakistani participants expressed the greatest fear of dying, whereas the Chinese participants expressed the least fear. Bowling et al. conclude that when the combined ethnically diverse group of older participants was compared with an ethnically homogeneous group of older British participants, the "older people from ethnic minorities had more anxieties about dying than others, and were more likely to express fears the more extensive their family support."

The Seriously Ill Have Different Concerns

In "What Matters Most in End-of-Life Care: Perceptions of Seriously Ill Patients and Their Family Members" (*Canadian Medical Association Journal*, vol. 174, no. 5, February 28, 2006), Daren K. Heyland et al. find that when patients with advanced chronic illnesses and advanced cancer were asked whether they agreed or strongly agreed about the importance of a variety of end-of-life issues, their concerns were quite different from those of the general population. Even though dying at home appears to be a priority for many Americans, dying in the location of choice (home or hospital) was 24th on the patients' ranked list of concerns. Their top priorities (very or extremely important) were trusting their physician (ranked first), not being kept on life support when there is little hope (ranked second), having their physician communicate with them honestly (ranked third), and completing things and preparing for death (resolving conflicts and saying good-bye) (ranked fourth). Seriously ill patients also revealed they did not want to be a physical or emotional burden on their families (ranked fifth), wanted to

have an adequate plan of home care and health services when discharged from the hospital (ranked sixth), and wanted to have relief from their symptoms (ranked seventh).

GETTING OLDER

Living to Age 100

The ABC News/*USA Today* poll "Most Wish for a Long Life—Despite Broad Aging Concerns" (October 24, 2005, http://abcnews.go.com/images/Politics/995a1Longevity.pdf) reveals that in 2005 only one-quarter of a random national sample of 1,000 adults wanted to live to be 100 years and older. Twenty-three percent stated they would like to live into their 90s and 29% into their 80s.

Those surveyed by the ABC News/*USA Today* poll were asked how likely they thought it was that they would live to be 100 years old and still have a good quality of life. Thirty-five percent thought it was very or somewhat likely, whereas 64% thought it was somewhat or very unlikely.

Concerns about Aging

The aging of the baby boomers (people born between 1946 and 1964) and the growing number of people living longer have focused much attention on concerns that come with aging. The ABC News/*USA Today* poll finds that even though respondents wanted to live longer, most were concerned about losing their health (73%). Seven out of 10 worried about losing their mental abilities (69%) and losing their ability to care for themselves (70%). The respondents were also worried about being a burden to their families (54%) and living in a nursing home (52%).

Opinions on Nursing Homes

The Henry J. Kaiser Family Foundation conducted a national survey that included questions about nursing homes and reported its findings in *Toplines: Update on the Public's Views of Nursing Homes and Long-Term Care Services* (December 2007, http://www.kff.org/kaiserpolls/upload/7719.pdf). When asked if they thought that during the past five years "the quality of nursing homes in this country has gotten better, gotten worse, or stayed about the same," only 14% of respondents thought nursing homes have gotten better. Thirty-one percent thought nursing homes have gotten worse, whereas 32% felt that they have stayed about the same.

More than half (53%) of respondents felt nursing homes are understaffed, and only 19% believed nursing homes "have staff who are concerned about the well-being of their patients." Forty-three percent thought there is not enough government regulation of these facilities.

Only 12% believed nursing homes provide high-quality services.

Since that time, Data.Medicare.gov (2012, https://data .medicare.gov/browse?tags=nursing+home) has developed a complete website that compares nursing home surveys from across the country. Many nursing homes in various areas had surveys on health, fire safety, number of beds, occupancy rate, and installation of sprinklers (for fire suppression). There is a portion of the website that describes complaints, enforcements, staff information, provider information, and survey deficiencies.

SUICIDE

The General Social Survey 2002, 2004, and 2010 were all conducted by the National Opinion Research Center (http://www3.norc.org/GSS+Website/). The center indicates that 58% of respondents in the 2002 and 2004 surveys and 55% in the 2010 survey approved of suicide if a person had an incurable disease, but only a small minority approved of it if the person had gone bankrupt (8% in 2002, 11% in 2004, and 8% in 2010), had dishonored his or her family (9% in 2002, 11% in 2004, and 8% in 2010), or was simply tired of living (15% in 2002, 16% in 2004, and 15% in 2010). In 2010, when asked another question about suicide and an incurable illness, 68% found it acceptable.

According to the Centers for Disease Control and Prevention (April 2012, http://www.cdc.gov/injury/wisqars/ index.html), in 2009 suicide was the 10th-leading cause of death in the United States for everyone aged from birth to 85 years and older. It was also the second-leading cause of death among young people aged 25 to 34 years, and the third-leading cause of death among young people aged 15 to 24 years.

In *In More Religious Countries, Lower Suicide Rates* (July 3, 2008, http://www.gallup.com/poll/108625/ More-Religious-Countries-Lower-Suicide-Rates.aspx), Brett Pelham and Zsolt Nyiri of the Gallup Organization indicate that in 2008 the United States' suicide rate of 11.05 deaths per 100,000 population was near the median (middle) suicide rate when compared with other countries of the world. The United States also fell near the median level of scores on the Gallup Religiosity Index, which is a measure of the importance of religion in people's lives. Pelham and Nyiri determine that the suicide rates of countries worldwide rise and fall with their level of religiosity: those having a higher level of religiosity (a higher score) have a lower suicide rate. Conversely, those having a lower level of religiosity (a lower score) have a higher suicide rate. The religiosity score for the United States on the Gallup Religiosity Index was 61 and the suicide rate was 11.05 deaths per 100,000 population in 2008. In comparison, the religiosity score for Kuwait was 83 and the suicide rate was 1.95 deaths per 100,000 population. The

religiosity score for Russia was 28 and the suicide rate was 36.15 deaths per 100,000 population.

In *Knocking on Heaven's Door? Protestantism and Suicide* (June 10, 2011, http://www2.warwick.ac.uk/fac/ soc/economics/research/workingpapers/2011/twerp_966 .pdf), Sascha O. Becker and Ludger Woessmann show that suicides are higher in countries that are mainly Protestant than in countries that are mainly Catholic. The researchers compare data from the Prussian countries during the 19th century and more recent data from the Organization for Economic Co-operation and Development. The data clearly show that in all circumstances, more people committed suicide in Protestant countries than in Catholic countries. Becker and Woessmann suggest that "sociological and theological differences between Protestants and Catholics make suicide more likely among the former group." However, when the hypothesis was tested, the researchers determined that this was true: "Still, our results hold conditional on proxies for economic development, suggesting that religious denomination in the form of Protestantism is a main independent driver of regional differences in suicide rates."

BELIEF IN GOD/UNIVERSAL SPIRIT

Newport explains in *More Than 9 in 10 Americans Continue to Believe in God* (June 3, 2011, http://www .gallup.com/poll/147887/Americans-Continue-Believe-God .aspx) that in May 2010 Gallup pollsters asked people whether they believed in God or in a universal spirit. Eighty percent said they believe in God, while an additional 12% said that they believe in a universal spirit. (See Table 11.1.) Six percent said that they believe in neither. One year later the Gallup Organization conducted another poll, and this time it combined the sample for two questions: "Do you believe in God?" and "Do you believe in God or a universal spirit?" Table 11.2 shows the results by demographics. Ninety-two percent of respondents said they believe in God. Of this sample, 90% were men and 94% were women. Age ranges were quite close to being equal, except for the 18- to 29-year-old age group. Educationally, 94% were college grads, but 87% had a postgraduate education. The greatest proportion came from the South (96%) and the lowest proportion from the East (86%). The conservatives were well represented (98%), as were the moderates (91%) and liberals (85%). Concerning political party affiliation, Republicans (98%) had the highest representation, whereas Independents (89%) and Democrats (90%) were somewhat lower.

PHYSICIAN-ASSISTED SUICIDE AND EUTHANASIA

Many advocates of physician-assisted suicide believe that people who have an incurable disease and are dying should be allowed to end their life with a lethal dose of

TABLE 11.1

Belief in God or universal spirit, 2010

WHICH OF THE FOLLOWING STATEMENTS COMES CLOSEST TO YOUR BELIEF ABOUT GOD—YOU BELIEVE IN GOD, YOU DON'T BELIEVE IN GOD, BUT YOU DO BELIEVE IN A UNIVERSAL SPIRIT OR HIGHER POWER, OR YOU DON'T BELIEVE IN EITHER?

	Believe in God	Believe in universal spirit	Don't believe in either	Other (vol.)	No opinion
2010 May 3–6	80%	12	6	1	1

(vol.) = Volunteered response.

SOURCE: Frank Newport, "Which of the following statements comes closest to your belief about God—you believe in God, you don't believe in God, but you do believe in a universal spirit or higher power, or you don't believe in either?" in *More Than 9 in 10 Americans Continue to Believe in God*, The Gallup Organization, June 3, 2011, http://www.gallup.com/poll/147887/Americans-Continue-Believe-God.aspx (accessed February 7, 2012). Copyright © 2011 by The Gallup Organization. Reproduced by permission of The Gallup Organization.

TABLE 11.2

Belief in God by demographic characteristics, 2011

COMBINED SAMPLE FOR TWO QUESTIONS: "DO YOU BELIEVE IN GOD?" AND "DO YOU BELIEVE IN GOD OR A UNIVERSAL SPIRIT?"

	Belief in God %
National adults	92
Men	90
Women	94
18 to 29	84
30 to 49	94
59 to 64	94
65+	94
High school or less	92
Some college	93
College grad	94
Postgraduate education	87
East	86
South	96
Midwest	91
West	92
Conservatives	98
Moderates	91
Liberals	85
Republicans	98
Independents	89
Democrats	90

SOURCE: Frank Newport, "Belief in God, by Demographic Categories," in *More than 9 in 10 Americans Continue to Believe in God*, The Gallup Organization, June 3, 2011, http://www.gallup.com/poll/147887/Americans-Continue-Believe-God.aspx (accessed February 7, 2012). Copyright © 2011 by The Gallup Organization. Reproduced by permission of The Gallup Organization.

medication that is prescribed by their physician. Joseph Carroll of the Gallup Organization notes in *Public Divided over Moral Acceptability of Doctor-Assisted Suicide* (May 31, 2007, http://www.gallup.com/poll/27727/Public-Divided-Over-Moral-Acceptability-DoctorAssisted-Suicide.aspx) that U.S. public opinion rose slowly between 1996 and 2001 in favor of physician-assisted suicide, from 52% in 1996 to 68% in 2001. After 2001 a slow decline occurred, with 56% in favor of physician-assisted suicide in 2007.

According to Carroll, in 2007 more Democrats than Republicans supported euthanasia (77% versus 64%, respectively) and physician-assisted suicide (62% versus 49%, respectively). Support of both euthanasia and physician-assisted suicide also varied by the frequency of attendance of religious services. Those who seldom or never attended services were the most supportive of both euthanasia (84%) and physician-assisted suicide (73%). Those who attended almost weekly or attended monthly were the next most supportive: 70% supported euthanasia and 52% supported physician-assisted suicide. The least supportive were those who attended religious services each week: 47% supported euthanasia and 35% supported physician-assisted suicide.

Table 11.3 shows the division in 2011 among Americans regarding the perceived moral acceptability of certain behaviors and social policies. The percentage of those who think that physician-assisted suicide is morally acceptable goes down as people age. For those aged 18 to 34 years, 46% thought it is acceptable; for those aged 35 to 54 years, 45% thought it is acceptable; and for those aged 55 years and older, 43% thought it is acceptable. There was a difference of three percentage points between the youngest group and the oldest group.

Oregon Physician-Assisted Suicide Law

In 1994 Oregon became the first jurisdiction in the world to legalize physician-assisted suicide when its voters passed the Death with Dignity Act. Under the act, Oregon law permits physician-assisted suicide for patients with less than six months to live. Patients must request physician assistance three times, receive a second opinion from another doctor, and wait 15 days to allow time to reconsider.

Before the Death with Dignity Act could take effect, opponents of the law succeeded in obtaining an injunction against it. Three years later, in November 1997, Oregon's legislature let the voters decide whether to

TABLE 11.3

Public opinion on the moral acceptability of doctor-assisted suicide, by age, 2011

% Morally acceptable, ranked by "difference"

	18 to 34 years	35 to 54 years	55 and older	Difference, 18 to 34 minus 55 and older
	%	%	%	pct. pts.
Pornography	42	29	19	+23
Gay/lesbian relations	66	56	47	+19
Premarital sex	71	58	53	+18
Out-of-wedlock births	62	56	46	+16
Gambling	71	65	59	+12
Polygamy	19	8	8	+11
Abortion	44	42	34	+10
Cloning humans	18	10	9	+9
Cloning animals	36	32	28	+8
Embryonic stem cell research	66	59	62	+4
Doctor-assisted suicide	46	45	43	+3
Divorce	72	66	70	+2
Extramarital affairs	8	7	7	+1
Use of animal fur for clothing	55	57	56	−1
Suicide	14	13	19	−5
Death penalty	56	67	70	−14
Medical testing on animals	47	57	61	−14

SOURCE: Lydia Saad, "U.S. Perceived Moral Acceptability of Behaviors and Social Policies—by Age" in *Doctor-Assisted Suicide Is Moral Issue Dividing Americans Most*, The Gallup Organization, May 31, 2011, http://www.gallup.com/poll/147842/Doctor-Assisted-Suicide-Moral-Issue-Dividing-Americans.aspx (accessed February 7, 2012). Copyright © 2011 by The Gallup Organization. Reproduced by permission of The Gallup Organization.

repeal or retain the law. Voters reaffirmed the Death with Dignity Act. Harris Interactive indicates in "Majorities of U.S. Adults Favor Euthanasia and Physician-Assisted Suicide by More Than Two-to-One" (April 27, 2005, http://community.compassionandchoices.org/document.doc?id=486) that in 1997, before the law was reaffirmed in Oregon, 68% of those surveyed said

they would approve of a similar law allowing physician-assisted suicide in their state. Asked again in 2001 whether they would favor or oppose such a law in their own state, 61% of respondents indicated they favored such legislation.

The National Foundation and the Regence Foundation conducted a poll in 2010 and 2011 to ask Oregonians, Washingtonians, and Americans in general many questions regarding death and dying and reported their findings in "Living Well at the End of Life Poll: Topline Results" (July 2011, http://syndication.nationaljournal.com/communications/NationalJournalRegenceSeattle Toplines.pdf). Overall, Oregonians and Washingtonians seem to know a lot more about palliative care and end-of-life options than Americans nationally. For example, when asked if they were familiar with "some different terms related to health care," 32% of Oregonians, 26% of Washingtonians, and 24% of Americans said they were familiar with the term *palliative care*; 78% of Oregonians, 77% of Washingtonians, and 65% of Americans were familiar with the term *end-of-life care*; and 94% of Oregonians, 87% of Washingtonians, and 86% of Americans were familiar with the term *hospice care*. Oregonians and Washingtonians were asked how confident they were that if they needed such end-of-life care it would be available to them or their family; 76% of Oregonians and 72% of Washingtonians were totally confident. When asked about their support of the program Physicians Orders for Life-Sustaining Treatment, in which physicians can sign a medical order that compels other physicians to follow the order, whether it be to shorten the patient's life or prolong it, 91% of Oregonians said they approved of it as did 85% of Washingtonians. Likewise, there was strong support for the Death with Dignity Act, which 77% of Oregonians and 70% of Washingtonians said they supported.

IMPORTANT NAMES
AND ADDRESSES

AARP
601 E St. NW
Washington, DC 20049
1-888-687-2277
E-mail: member@aarp.org
URL: http://www.aarp.org/

Aging with Dignity
PO Box 1661
Tallahassee, FL 32302-1661
(850) 681-2010
1-888-594-7437
FAX: (850) 681-2481
E-mail: fivewishes@agingwithdignity.org
URL: http://www.agingwithdignity.org/

Alzheimer's Association
225 N. Michigan Ave., 17th Floor
Chicago, IL 60601-7633
(312) 335-8700
1-800-272-3900
FAX: 1-866-699-1246
E-mail: info@alz.org
URL: http://www.alz.org/

American Association of Suicidology
5221 Wisconsin Ave. NW
Washington, DC 20015
(202) 237-2280
FAX: (202) 237-2282
URL: http://www.suicidology.org/

American Cancer Society
250 Williams St. NW
Atlanta, GA 30303
1-800-227-2345
URL: http://www.cancer.org/

American Foundation for Suicide Prevention
120 Wall St., 29th Floor
New York, NY 10005
(212) 363-3500
1-888-333-2377
FAX: (212) 363-6237

E-mail: inquiry@afsp.org
URL: http://www.afsp.org/

Centers for Disease Control and Prevention
1600 Clifton Rd.
Atlanta, GA 30333
1-800-232-4636
E-mail: cdcinfo@cdc.gov
URL: http://www.cdc.gov/

Children's Hospice International
1101 King St., Ste. 360
Alexandria, VA 22314
(703) 684-0330
1-800-242-4453
URL: http://www.chionline.org/

Compassion & Choices
PO Box 101810
Denver, CO 80250
1-800-247-7421
FAX: 1-866-312-2690
E-mail: info@compassionandchoices.org
URL: http://www.compassionandchoices.org/

Hastings Center
21 Malcolm Gordon Rd.
Garrison, NY 10524
(845) 424-4040
E-mail: mail@thehastingscenter.org
URL: http://www.thehastingscenter.org/

Health Resources and Services Administration Information Center
5600 Fishers Lane
Rockville, MD 20857
1-888-275-4772
E-mail: ask@hrsa.gov
URL: http://www.hrsa.gov/

March of Dimes
1275 Mamaroneck Ave.
White Plains, NY 10605
(914) 997-4488
URL: http://www.marchofdimes.com/

National Association for Home Care and Hospice
228 Seventh St. SE
Washington, DC 20003
(202) 547-7424
FAX: (202) 547-3540
URL: http://www.nahc.org/

National Council on Aging
1901 L St. NW, Fourth Floor
Washington, DC 20036
(202) 479-1200
URL: http://www.ncoa.org/

National Hospice and Palliative Care Organization
1731 King St., Ste. 100
Alexandria, VA 22314
(703) 837-1500
FAX: (703) 837-1233
E-mail: nhpco_info@nhpco.org
URL: http://www.nhpco.org/

National Institute on Aging
Bldg. 31, Rm. 5C27
31 Center Dr., MSC 2292
Bethesda, MD 20892
(301) 496-1752
1-800-222-2225
FAX: (301) 496-1072
E-mail: niaic@nia.nih.gov
URL: http://www.nia.nih.gov/

National Right to Life Committee
512 10th St. NW
Washington, DC 20004
(202) 626-8800
E-mail: NRLC@nrlc.org
URL: http://www.nrlc.org/

Older Women's League
1625 K St. NW, Ste. 1275
Washington, DC 20006
(202) 567-2606

1-877-653-7966
FAX: (202) 332-2949
E-mail: info@owl-national.org
URL: http://www.owl-national.org/

Patients Rights Council
PO Box 760
Steubenville, OH 43952
(740) 282-3810

1-800-958-5678
URL: http://www.internationaltaskforce.org/

United Network for Organ Sharing
700 N. Fourth St.
Richmond, VA 23219
(804) 782-4800
1-888-894-6361
FAX: (804) 782-4817
URL: http://www.unos.org/

Visiting Nurse Associations of America
900 19th St. NW, Ste. 200
Washington, DC 20006
(202) 384-1420
FAX: (202) 384-1444
E-mail: vnaa@vnaa.org
URL: http://vnaa.org/vnaa/
siteshelltemplates/homepage_navigate.htm

RESOURCES

The National Center for Health Statistics (NCHS) provides in its annual publication *Health, United States* a statistical overview of the nation's health. The NCHS periodical *National Vital Statistics Reports* supplies detailed U.S. birth and death data. The Centers for Disease Control and Prevention (CDC) reports on nationwide health trends in its *Advance Data* reports, *HIV Surveillance Report*, *Longitudinal Studies of Aging*, *Morbidity and Mortality Weekly Report*, and *Trends in Health and Aging*. The Centers for Medicare and Medicaid Services reports on the nation's spending for health care.

The U.S. Census Bureau publishes a wide variety of demographic information on American life. *U.S. Interim Projections by Age, Sex, Race, and Hispanic Origin* (March 2004) incorporates the results of the 2000 census and makes projections to 2050.

The Alliance for Aging Research promotes scientific research on human aging and conducts educational programs to increase communication and understanding among professionals who serve the elderly.

The mission of the National Hospice and Palliative Care Organization (NHPCO) is "improving end of life care and expanding access to hospice care with the goal of profoundly enhancing quality of life for people dying in America and their loved ones." The Hospice Association of America represents hospices, caregivers, and volunteers who serve terminally ill patients and their families. The NHPCO and the Hospice Association of America both collect data about hospice care.

The United Network for Organ Sharing manages the national transplant waiting list, maintains data on organ transplants, and distributes organ donor cards. The primary goals of the U.S. Organ Procurement and Transplantation Network (OPTN) are to "increase and ensure the effectiveness, efficiency and equity of organ sharing in the national system of organ allocation" and to "increase the supply of donated organs available for transplantation." The Scientific Registry of Transplant Recipients (SRTR) evaluates the scientific and clinical status of organ transplantation in the United States. Valuable information on these topics is available in the OPTN/SRTR annual reports.

The National Right to Life Committee provides the "Will to Live," an alternative living will, whereas Compassion & Choices provides news and bulletins on Oregon's Death with Dignity Act and other end-of-life legislation. The American Bar Association Commission on Law and Aging publishes information that is related to advance directives.

For cancer statistics, a premier source is the American Cancer Society's annual *Cancer Facts & Figures*.

Journals that frequently publish studies dealing with life-sustaining treatment, medical ethics, and medical costs include *American Family Physician*, *American Journal of Hospice and Palliative Medicine*, *American Journal of Nursing*, *American Journal of Transplantation*, *Annals of Internal Medicine*, *Archives of Disease in Childhood*, *Archives of Internal Medicine*, *Archives of Physical Medicine and Rehabilitation*, *BMC Medicine*, *Current Opinion in Critical Care*, *Harvard Women's Health Watch*, *Health Services Research*, *Journal of the American Medical Association*, *Journal of Clinical Nursing*, *Journal of General Internal Medicine*, *Journal of Medical Education*, *Journal of Medical Ethics*, *Journal of Neurology*, *Journal of Palliative Medicine*, *Mayo Clinic Proceedings*, *Neurology*, *New England Journal of Medicine*, *Nursing Ethics*, *Pediatrics*, *Physical Therapy*, *Psychological Science*, and *Trends in Cognitive Sciences*.

The Gallup Organization, Harris Interactive, and the Roper Center for Public Opinion Research have all conducted opinion polls on topics that are related to death and dying.

The Henry J. Kaiser Family Foundation provides a wealth of information on Medicare, Medicaid, health insurance, prescription drugs, HIV/AIDS, and nursing homes.

INDEX

Page references in italics refer to photographs. References with the letter t following them indicate the presence of a table. The letter f indicates a figure. If more than one table or figure appears on a particular page, the exact item number for the table or figure being referenced is provided.

A

AAN. *See* American Academy of Neurology

ABC News, 148

Abe Perlmutter, Michael J. Satz, State Attorney for Broward County, Florida v., 97–98

Abe Perlmutter, Michael J. Satz etc. v., 98

Academy of Nutrition and Dietetics, 30

Accidents, 23

ACP (advanced care planning), 32

Acquired immunodeficiency syndrome (AIDS). *See* HIV/AIDS

Active euthanasia, 56

AD. *See* Alzheimer's disease

Adkins, Janet, 70

Adolescents

end-of-life decisions for, 53

fear of death among, 147

high school students who attempted suicide, whose suicide attempt required medical attention, by sex, race/ethnicity, grade, 63(*t*6.4)

high school students who attempted suicide, whose suicide attempt required medical attention, by sex/selected U.S. sites, 64*t*–65*t*

high school students who felt sad or hopeless, by sex, race/ethnicity, grade, 65(*t*6.6)

high school students who felt sad or hopeless, by sex, selected U.S. sites, 67*t*

high school students who seriously considered attempting suicide, who

made suicide plan, by sex, race/ethnicity, grade, 66*t*

suicidal ideation, suicide attempts, injuries among students in grades 9–12, by sex, grade level, race, Hispanic origin, 62*t*–63*t*

suicide among LGBT adolescents, 61–65

suicide among young people, 57–58, 60–61

"Adolescents with Life-Threatening Illnesses" (Knapp), 53

Adults

fear of death among, 147

older, end-of-life costs, 118–119

See also Older adults

Advance directives

advance health-care directive, sample of, 89*t*–91*t*

artificial nutrition and hydration, 88–91

combined advance directive laws, 92

communication for end-of-life care, 93

cost for end-of-life care and, 93

cultural differences in, 21

DNR order in, 28

durable power of attorney for health care, 88

"Five Wishes," states in which it is legally valid, 92*f*

health care power of attorney and combined advance directive legislation, 78*t*–87*t*

history of, 77

living wills, 77, 88

on mechanical ventilation, 30

need to create, 32

Patient Self-Determination Act, 93

relief from pain, 91–92

Advanced care planning (ACP), 32

Advantage Plans, Medicare, 116, 118

African-Americans

coronary heart disease and, 134

infant death among, 39

life expectancy of, 131

patient autonomy, cultural differences in, 20, 21

suicide among young people, 60

suicide death rate for, 57

suicide rate for elderly, 145

Age

Alzheimer's disease and, 141–144

cancer among elderly and, 136–139

cancer diagnosis, depression, physical pain, by age group, 141(*t*10.7)

cancers, probability of developing invasive, over selected age intervals, by sex, 140*t*

coronary heart disease, among elderly, 134–136

death rates, by age, for 15 leading causes of death, 25*t*–28*t*

death rates for cerebrovascular diseases, by sex, race, Hispanic origin, and age, 142*t*–144*t*

death rates for diseases of the heart, by sex, race, Hispanic origin, and age, 137*t*–139*t*

death rates for suicide, by sex, race, Hispanic origin, age, 58*t*–60*t*

of hospice care discharges, 4

leading causes of death and, 23–24

leading causes of death/numbers of deaths, by age, 135*t*–136*t*

life expectancy and, 131

life expectancy at birth, at 65 years of age, at 75 years of age, by race, sex, 132*t*

of patients requesting assisted suicide/euthanasia, 66

population/projected population, by age and sex, 133*t*

stroke among elderly and, 139–140

suicide among young people by, 57–58, 60–61

suicide death rate by, 57

worry, percentage who experience significant, by age/sex, 134f

Stem, brain, 10

Stevens, John Paul, 104, 107

Stolzle, Hayley, 46

Storar, Dorothy, 97

Storar, John, 97

Stroke

death rates for cerebrovascular diseases, by sex, race, Hispanic origin, and age, 142t–144t

as leading cause of death among elderly, 139–140

Students. *See* High school students

Subjective test, 98–99

Substituted judgment

court cases on, 96–97

Cruzan, Nancy Beth, case, 103–104

Suffocation, 61

Suicide

average annual number/percentage of adults aged 18 years+ who had suicidal thoughts, made a plan, or attempted suicide during previous year, 61t

cultural/religious views on, 56–57

death rates for suicide, by sex, race, Hispanic origin, age, 58t–60t

high school students who attempted suicide, whose suicide attempt required medical attention, by sex, race/ethnicity, grade, 63(t6.4)

high school students who attempted suicide, whose suicide attempt required medical attention, by sex/selected U.S. sites, 64t–65t

high school students who felt sad or hopeless, by sex, race/ethnicity, grade, 65(t6.6)

high school students who felt sad or hopeless, by sex and selected U.S. sites, 67t

high school students who seriously considered attempting suicide, and who made a suicide plan, by sex, race/ethnicity, and grade, 66t

among LGBT adolescents, 61–65

in older adults, 145

Oregon physician-assisted suicide law, 150–151

physician-assisted, 149–150

public opinion on life/death, 149–151

Roman Catholicism on, 13

suicidal ideation, suicide attempts, injuries among students in grades 9–12, by sex, grade level, race, Hispanic origin, 62t–63t

suicide deaths, death rates, age-adjusted death rates, by mechanism of suicide, 68(t6.10)

suicide-related behaviors, trends in, 68(t6.9)

in U.S., 57

among young people, 57–58, 60–61

See also Physician-assisted suicide

"Suicide and Suicide Risk in Lesbian, Gay, Bisexual, and Transgender Populations: Review and Recommendations" (Haas et al.), 62–65

Suicide Prevention Resource Center, 62–65

"Suicides in Japan Spiked after Earthquake" (Agence France-Presse), 56–57

"Summary of Health Care and Revenue Provisions" (U.S. Senate Democratic Policy Committee), 109, 146

Superintendent of Belchertown State School et al. v. Joseph Saikewicz, 96–97

Superior Court of the State of California, Barber v., 99

Supreme Court of Florida, 98

Surrogate

in absence of durable power of attorney for health care, 88

designation of, 21

feeding tube, court case, 98–99

liability of doctors, court case on, 99

See also Proxy

Suttee, 56

Sutton, Paul D., 47

Swetz, Keith M., 21

Switzerland

assisted suicide in, 75–76

right-to-die ruling, 75

Symptoms

of Alzheimer's disease, 141–143

of heart attack, 136

T

Talmud, 15

Tax Equity and Fiscal Responsibility Act, 119

Tay-Sachs disease, 41

"Teaching End-of-Life Issues in US Medical Schools: 1975 to 2005" (Dickinson), 19

Teenagers. *See* Adolescents

Tennessee, 85t

Tenzin Gyatso, 16

Teradyon, Hanina ben, 15

Terminal illness

DNR order and, 28

euthanasia/assisted suicide, ethics of, 21–22

euthanasia/physician-assisted suicide worldwide, 75–76

passive euthanasia and, 56

patient autonomy and, 20

See also Diseases

Terminally ill patients

artificial nutrition and hydration for, 30–31

hospice care costs for, 119

See also Patients

Termination of Life on Request and Assisted Suicide (Review Procedures) Act, 75

Terri's Law (House Bill 35-E), 105

Tests, 98–99

Texas, 85t

Thomas, Ken, 72

Thomas Aquinas, Saint

on end of life, 13

views on suicide, 56

The Tibetan Book of Living and Dying (Rinpoche), 16

Tissue transplantation

organ/tissue donor card, 35f

transplantable tissues, 32, 33f

Toplines: Update on the Public's Views of Nursing Homes and Long-Term Care Services (KFF), 148

Torah, 15

Torian, Lucia, 126

Transmission, of HIV/AIDS, 24

Transplants. *See* Organ transplants

Treatments. *See* Life-sustaining treatments; Medical treatments

Trends in Spina Bifida and Anencephalus in the United States, 1991–2006 (Mathews), 42, 44

"Trials for Parents Who Chose Faith over Medicine" (Johnson), 52

Tuberculosis, 3

Tushkowski, Joseph, 71

Twentieth century, death in, 3–4

"Twenty Years since Cruzan and the Patient Self-Determination Act: Opportunities for Improving Care at the End of Life in Critical Care Settings" (Rushton, Kaylor, & Christopher), 31–32

2010 Death with Dignity Act Report (Washington State Department of Health), 74

2011 Alzheimer's Disease Facts and Figures (Alzheimer's Association), 144

2012 Alzheimer's Disease Facts and Figures (Alzheimer's Association), 129

U

Undertakers, 3

Uniform Anatomical Gift Act of 1968, 37

Uniform Determination of Death Act

guidelines of, 8

states adoption of, 9

Uniform Health-Care Decisions Act (UHCDA)

living will in, 88

overview of, 92

Unitarian Universalist Association, 15

United Network for Organ Sharing (UNOS)

management of national transplant waiting list, 32, 34–35